ENT Emergencies

Disclaimer

This publication has been provided as a service to the medical community, in good faith, and every effort has been made to ensure the accuracy of the material. However, in view of the possibility of human error or changes in "ever-evolving" medical science, neither the authors/editors nor the publishers, nor any other party involved in preparation/publication of this work warrants (guarantees) that the information contained herein is in every respect accurate or complete, and they are not responsible for any error or omissions or the results obtained from the use of such information. Esteemed readers are, therefore, requested to confirm the information contained herein with other available sources, to keep in touch with the latest available literature, to check the product information sheet included in the package of each drug (regarding indication, dosage, contraindications, and date of manufacture/expiry) and follow or alter their management protocols, accordingly.

ENT Emergencies

Editors

Parmod Kalsotra
MBBS MS DNB
Professor and Head
Department of ENT—Head and Neck Surgery
Sri Maharaja Gulab Singh Hospital
Government Medical College
Jammu, Jammu & Kashmir, India
drpkalsotra@yahoo.co.in

Subirendra Kumar
MBBS MS DNB
Former Associate Professor
All India Institute of Medical Sciences
New Delhi, India
Senior Consultant
Program Director—Otology Fellowship
Oman Medical Specialty Board
Department of ENT
Al-Nahdha Hospital, MOH, Oman
subir555@gmail.com

Alok Thakar
MBBS MS DNB DLO FRCS Ed
Professor and Head
Department of ENT—Head and Neck Surgery
All India Institute of Medical Sciences
New Delhi, India
drathakar@gmail.com

Forewords

Santosh Kumar Kacker
K Vijay Kumar

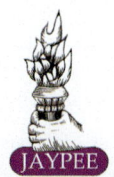

JAYPEE BROTHERS MEDICAL PUBLISHERS
The Health Sciences Publisher
New Delhi | London

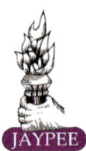 **Jaypee Brothers Medical Publishers (P) Ltd.**

Headquarters
Jaypee Brothers Medical Publishers (P) Ltd
EMCA House, 23/23-B
Ansari Road, Daryaganj
New Delhi 110 002, India
Landline: +91-11-23272143, +91-11-23272703
+91-11-23282021, +91-11-23245672
Email: jaypee@jaypeebrothers.com

Corporate Office
Jaypee Brothers Medical Publishers (P) Ltd
4838/24, Ansari Road, Daryaganj
New Delhi 110 002, India
Phone: +91-11-43574357
Fax: +91-11-43574314
Email: jaypee@jaypeebrothers.com

Overseas Office
JP Medical Ltd.
83, Victoria Street, London
SW1H 0HW (UK)
Phone: +44 20 3170 8910
Fax: +44 (0)20 3008 6180
Email: info@jpmedpub.com

Website: www.jaypeebrothers.com
Website: www.jaypeedigital.com

© 2024, Jaypee Brothers Medical Publishers

The views and opinions expressed in this book are solely those of the original contributor(s)/author(s) and do not necessarily represent those of editor(s) or publisher of the book.

All rights reserved. No part of this publication may be reproduced, stored or transmitted in any form or by any means, electronic, mechanical, photo copying, recording or otherwise, without the prior permission in writing of the publishers.

All brand names and product names used in this book are trade names, service marks, trademarks or registered trademarks of their respective owners. The publisher is not associated with any product or vendor mentioned in this book.

Medical knowledge and practice change constantly. This book is designed to provide accurate, authoritative information about the subject matter in question. However, readers are advised to check the most current information available on procedures included and check information from the manufacturer of each product to be administered, to verify the recommended dose, formula, method and duration of administration, adverse effects and contra indications. It is the responsibility of the practitioner to take all appropriate safety precautions. Neither the publisher nor the author(s)/editor(s) assume any liability for any injury and/or damage to persons or property arising from or related to use of material in this book.

This book is sold on the understanding that the publisher is not engaged in providing professional medical services. If such advice or services are required, the services of a competent medical professional should be sought.

Every effort has been made where necessary to contact holders of copyright to obtain permission to reproduce copyright material. If any have been inadvertently overlooked, the publisher will be pleased to make the necessary arrangements at the first opportunity.

Inquiries for bulk sales may be solicited at: jaypee@jaypeebrothers.com

ENT Emergencies

First Edition: **2024**

ISBN: 978-93-5696-212-5

Printed: at Replika Press Pvt. Ltd.

Dedicated to

Our teachers for being the guiding light and anchor in our academic and professional journey.

Our students for giving inspiration to write this book.

Our family for their constant support.

Parmod Kalsotra
Subirendra Kumar
Alok Thakar

Contributors

Ajit Man Singh
MBBS MS DNB DLO FRCS Ed
Principal Consultant
Department of ENT—Head and
Neck Surgery
Max Super Speciality Hospital
New Delhi, India

Alok Thakar
MBBS MS DNB DLO FRCS Ed
Professor and Head
Department of ENT—Head and
Neck Surgery
All India Institute of Medical Sciences
New Delhi, India

Amit Manhas MBBS PGDMLS MD
Associate Professor
Department of Anesthesia
Super Speciality Hospital
Government Medical College
Jammu, Jammu & Kashmir, India

Arvind Kairo MBBS MS
Additional Professor
Department of ENT
All India Institute of Medical Sciences
New Delhi, India

C Preetam Chappity
MS DNB MNAMS FACS MBA
Additional Professor
Department of ENT—Head and
Neck Surgery
All India Institute of Medical Sciences
Bhubaneswar, Odisha, India

Ghanshyam Saini
MBBS MD (Pediatrics)
Professor and Head
Department of Pediatrics
Sri Maharaja Gulab Singh Hospital
Government Medical College
Jammu, Jammu & Kashmir, India

Gopika Kalsotra
MBBS MS (PGIMER)
Associate Professor
Department of ENT
Sri Maharaja Gulab Singh Hospital
Government Medical College
Jammu, Jammu & Kashmir, India

Jemy Jose MBBS MS FRCS (ORL-HNS)
Consultant
Department of ENT—Head and
Neck Surgery
Hull University Teaching Hospitals
Hull, UK

Kapil Sikka MBBS MS DNB FACS
Professor
Department of ENT—Head and
Neck Surgery
All India Institute of Medical Sciences
New Delhi, India

Monica Manhas MBBS PGDMLS MD
Associate Professor
Department of Physiology
Government Medical College
Jammu, Jammu & Kashmir, India

Parmod Kalsotra MBBS MS DNB
Professor and Head
Department of ENT—Head and
Neck Surgery
Sri Maharaja Gulab Singh Hospital
Government Medical College
Jammu, Jammu & Kashmir, India

Parveen Akhter Lone
BDS MDS (OMFS) FICD
Professor and Head
Postgraduate Department of Oral
and Maxillofacial Surgery
Indira Gandhi Government
Dental College
Jammu, Jammu & Kashmir, India

Contributors

P Ghosh MBBS MS (ENT) DLO
Former Professor and Head
Department of ENT—Head and
Neck Surgery
All India Institute of Medical Sciences
New Delhi, India

Rakesh Kumar MBBS MS
Commonwealth Fellow (Facial Plastic Surgery)
Professor
Department of ENT—Head and
Neck Surgery
All India Institute of Medical Sciences
New Delhi, India

Sachin Gupta MBBS MS (ENT)
Lecturer
Department of ENT
Sri Maharaja Gulab Singh Hospital
Government Medical College
Jammu, Jammu & Kashmir, India

Sahil Kalsotra MBBS
Resident Medical Officer
(Casuality/Emergency)
SDDM Hospital
Jammu, Jammu & Kashmir, India

Shallu Jamwal MBBS MS (Gyne & Obs)
Assistant Professor
Department of Gynecology and
Obstetrics
Government Medical College
Kathua, Jammu & Kashmir, India

Shyam Gupta
MBBS MS MRCS FRCS (Glasgow) MNAMS
Assistant Professor
Department of Surgery
Government Medical College
Jammu, Jammu & Kashmir, India

Subirendra Kumar
MBBS MS DNB
Former Associate Professor
All India Institute of Medical Sciences
New Delhi, India
Senior Consultant
Program Director—Otology Fellowship
Oman Medical Specialty Board
Department of ENT
Al-Nahdha Hospital, MOH, Oman

**Venkata Surya Phani Bhushan
Durvasula** MBBS MS FRCS (ENT) Ed
Staff Physician El Dorado Arkansas and
Adjunct Faculty Instructor
Department of Otolaryngology, Head
and Neck Surgery
University of Arkansas for
Medical Sciences
Little Rock, Arkansas, USA

Vikas Gupta MBBS MS
Additional Professor and Head
Department of ENT—Head and
Neck Surgery
All India Institute of Medical Sciences
Bhopal, Madhya Pradesh, India

Foreword

Dealing with medical emergencies is the most important aspect in clinical practice, especially in ENT. *ENT Emergencies* covers 14 chapters which have been updated according to recent trends in medical literature. This book provides a clear emphasis on important aspects like acute vertigo, neck and faciomaxillary trauma, acute facial nerve palsy in addition to other important chapters.

Well-directed algorithms of management of acute facial nerve paralysis, acute vertigo, neck trauma, epistaxis, caustic ingestion, are quite elucidative and will definitely stimulate young ENT specialists to frame certain guidelines in their mind, to manage emergent patients.

For proper diagnosis and management of patients, it is important to attain sound and core knowledge and guidance about the subject. By providing a step-by-step approach to ENT emergencies, this book will act as a bridge between resident doctors and patients.

It will motivate young budding ENT surgeons to refer their standard textbooks for clearing their doubts and misconceptions and will definitely boost the confidence of resident doctors while dealing the ENT emergencies. The aim of this book is to establish minimum standard protocol for management of patients reporting to the emergency ward.

This book will be a significant addition to the library of medical professionals as well.

My best wishes to authors and readers.

Santosh Kumar Kacker
MBBS MS FRCS (London) FAMS
Former Director and Professor
Department of ENT—Head and Neck Surgery
All India Institute of Medical Sciences
New Delhi, India

Esteemed readers are requested to consult following textbooks for further reading:

1. Watkinson JC, Clarke RW. Scott-Brown's Otorhinolaryngology and Head and Neck Surgery, 8th edition (Volume 1, 2, and 3). Florida: CRC Press; 2018.
2. Flint P, Haughey B, Lund V, Robbins K, Thomas JR, Lesperance M, et al. Cummings Otolaryngology Head and Neck Surgery, 7th edition. New York: Elsevier; 2020.
3. Paparella MM, da Costa SS, Fagan JJ. Paparella's Otolaryngology: Head and Neck Surgery, Volume 1. New Delhi: Jaypee Brothers Medical Publishers; 2019.
4. Malik NA. Textbook of Oral and Maxillofacial Surgery, 2nd edition. New Delhi: Jaypee Brothers Medical Publishers; 2008.

Foreword

Otorhinolaryngology as a subspecialty has made great advances in recent years. The advances in endoscopic sinus surgery, skull base surgery, cosmetic surgeries such as rhinoplasty, head and neck surgeries and neuro-otological surgeries has increased the scope and garnered interest of the clinicians from all around the world. With increase in the dimensions of the specialty, the clinicians need to be conversant with the advancements along with a sound knowledge of the core subject. Emergencies in ENT is one such aspect which require thorough knowledge, alert mind and diligent skills on the part of caregiver to provide adequate care to the patients. This, however, makes the young surgeons and residents go search for books which precisely deal with the emergencies in ENT to manage them properly.

ENT Emergencies is a precise and compact source to guide the young budding ENT surgeons to deal with ENT emergencies. It is written in a very lucid language so that resident doctors can grasp it in less time. This book will definitely help the ENT surgeons who deal with emergencies for proper management of the patients. The Authors have put their best in making this book coherent and comprehensible.

My best wishes to authors and readers.

K Vijay Kumar (IPS)
Former Advisor to the Hon'ble Governor
Jammu and Kashmir, India

Preface

The purpose of this book remains as a quick and concise guide for the residents to see and treat emergency problems in the field of otolaryngology—head and neck surgery. The book has been published in good faith and every attempt has been made to ensure accuracy of the material.

But medical science being ever changing, it is worthwhile to request all the readers to keep in touch with the latest available literature and alter their management protocol as per the circumstances, available infrastructure, and latest acquired knowledge. Also, any latest additional information may kindly be sent to the authors to keep this book up to the mark.

Though, the text has been updated, it is bound to inherit some lacunae and drawbacks. In case of any inadvertent error(s), mistake or omission, it is our sincere request to forgive us and inform us so that in the next edition we can rectify the problem.

Parmod Kalsotra
Subirendra Kumar
Alok Thakar

Acknowledgments

We acknowledge with gratitude the help and assistance that we received from our respected teachers and colleagues in the preparation of this manuscript.

We are grateful to (*Late*) *Mr Navin Bhasin* for his excellent typesetting and helpful criticism during the manuscript writing.

We are thankful to Mr Rohan and his team (Global Village, Kachi Chawni, Jammu) for helping us preparing the handbook.

We are thankful to Drs Vipin Magotra (Professor, Radiology), Rajeev Gupta (Professor and Head, Preventive and Social Medicine), Sunil Dutt (Professor, Pediatrics), Vivek Mahajan (Lecturer, Pharmacology), Naveed Gul, Aditiya Saraf, Neharika Pathak, Arun Manhas, Sandeep Singh, Aadil Bashir, Shivane Thakur, Youshita Mahajan, Danish Fayaz, Inna Fayaz, for their help in preparation of the present handbook. Special thanks to Dr Samiksha Bhagat for her sincerity and hard work and keeping up with pace under undue pressure of time limit.

We also express our thanks to M/s Jaypee Brothers Medical Publishers (P) Ltd, New Delhi, India, for publishing this book so well. We also thank Shri Jitendar P Vij (Group Chairman), Mr Ankit Vij (Managing Director), Mr MS Mani (Group President), Ms Chetna Malhotra (Senior Director-Professional Publishing, Marketing and Business Development), Ms Pooja Bhandari (Director-Production), and Mr Ashwani Kumar Singh (Manager) for their help, guidance and timely active intervention in publishing of the book.

Contents

1. **Wound Management** 1
   Sahil Kalsotra, Shallu Jamwal, Shyam Gupta

2. **Acute Vertigo** 11
   *Monica Manhas, Ajit Man Singh, Rakesh Kumar,
   Subirendra Kumar, P Ghosh*

3. **Acute Facial Palsy** 48
   Subirendra Kumar, Ajit Man Singh, Monica Manhas

4. **Epistaxis** 61
   C Preetam Chappity, Vikas Gupta, Parmod Kalsotra

5. **Foreign Bodies** 75
   Arvind Kairo, Amit Manhas, Kapil Sikka

6. **Acute Upper Airway Obstruction** 86
   Amit Manhas, C Preetam Chappity, Rakesh Kumar

7. **Faciomaxillary Trauma** 99
   Gopika Kalsotra, Parveen Akhter Lone, Subirendra Kumar

8. **Neck Trauma** 131
   *Venkata Surya Phani Bhushan Durvasula,
   Jemy Jose, Parmod Kalsotra*

9. **Deep Neck Space Infections** 147
   *Parmod Kalsotra, Venkata Surya Phani Bhushan Durvasula,
   Jemy Jose*

10. **Pediatric Stridor** 171
    Sahil Kalsotra, Gopika Kalsotra, Ghanshyam Saini

11. **Sudden Sensorineural Hearing Loss** 187
    *Sachin Gupta, Venkata Surya Phani Bhushan Durvasula,
    Arvind Kairo*

12. **Caustic Ingestion** 192
    Shallu Jamwal, Shyam Gupta, Parmod Kalsotra

13. **Complicated Otitis Media** 200
    Parmod Kalsotra, Sachin Gupta, Kapil Sikka

14. **Complicated Rhinosinusitis** 224
    *Venkata Surya Phani Bhushan Durvasula,
    Vikas Gupta, Parmod Kalsotra*

Index 243

CHAPTER 1

Wound Management

Sahil Kalsotra, Shallu Jamwal, Shyam Gupta

■ INTRODUCTION

Trauma is one of the most common causes of morbidity and mortality. An ENT surgeon, being an integral part of the "trauma care team", should be well versed in basics of airway management, trauma care and wound management.

Most important aspect prior to medicosurgical management of wound is taking a proper and relevant "history" of:
- Etiology of wound (self-induced trauma, human or animal bite, road traffic accident, exogenously inflicted trauma)
- Patient's existing medical conditions
- Any medications that the patient is receiving (anticoagulants)
- Drug allergy (to local anesthesia, antibiotics, analgesics)
- Tetanus immunization status

During *examination*, look for the following:
- Age and medical fitness of the patient
- Potential degree of contamination of wound
- Any potential for bone, cartilage, muscle or nerve injury

■ STEPS OF WOUND MANAGEMENT

The steps of *wound management* will include:
- Analgesia
- Assessment of wound
- Irrigation of wound (wound cleansing) and removal of foreign bodies
- Debridement
- Closure
- Antitetanus/antirabies management
- Regular follow-up

Analgesia

This may be either local, local block, oral or parenteral.

Local: Local anesthetic agent (2% xylocaine—plain or with adrenaline) can be safely injected into the wound edges after sensitivity test.

Local block: This is indicated in those areas where local injection into the wound will cause tissue distortion, e.g., lips and ears.

Parenteral: It is indicated in complicated wounds that require extensive cleansing and debridement and cannot be treated with only local anesthesia.

Assessment of Wound

Assessment of wound and irrigation go hand-in-hand. Traumatic wounds are usually irregular in outline, single or multiple, symmetrical or irregular in shape and usually painful. The tissue injury may be "partial thickness", i.e., limited to the epidermis and superficial dermis with no damage to the dermal blood vessels. Healing can take place by regeneration of epithelial tissue. The "full thickness injury" involves loss of the dermis and extends to deeper tissue layers and disrupts dermal blood vessels. Wound, if left untreated, will involve the formation of several types of tissue and scar formation.

During assessment, look for location (indicates which wound needs special attention), size and depth of wound and examine the "wound bed" (clean or needs removal of necrotic/devitalized tissue).

Also, during examination, one must look for underlying loss of muscle or bone, damage to big parts or organs, nerves, and blood vessels. Occasionally, avulsive trauma may involve tearing away of tissue from the body, e.g., explosions, gun-shots, animal and human bites. The avulsed tissue can be usually saved by wrapping it in a sterile dressing and placing it in a cool container. It must be ensured that the tissue is not inadvertently frozen and not dipped in water or saline.

Radiology/imaging is indicated in certain situations:
- *Plain X-ray:* Glass foreign bodies are easily picked up.
- *CT scan:* It is indicated in deep-seated foreign bodies and for assessment of underlying bony trauma. Limitation is in case of wood, plastic, and vegetative foreign bodies.
- *MRI:* It can pick up wooden foreign bodies.
- *Ultrasound:* This can detect radiolucent foreign bodies.

Irrigation (Wound Cleansing)

The commonly used agents are:
- Antimicrobial cleansers such as chlorhexidine:
- Warm saline
- Warm saline with dilute hydrogen peroxide
- Warm saline with dilute povidone iodine

Irrigation entails removal of any foreign bodies, debris, dust, soil, necrotic tissue from the wound and any bacteria (this procedure also abolishes anaerobic conditions which favor germination of tetanus spores) and involves flushing the wound with "normal saline" with a disposable syringe. Wound edges are injected with local anesthetic to provide analgesia. Surrounding skin is cleaned by scrubbing with a sponge and antiseptic solution. Normal saline solution effectively removes contaminants and being isotonic, does not damage the cells.

Debridement

It involves the removal of dead tissue and can be accomplished by:
- *Sharp surgical debridement:* It is the fastest and most preferred method using a 15 number scalpel blade and tissue forceps. The devitalized tissue and jagged wound edges are debrided.
- *Laser debridement:* This is again a fast method of debridement but this facility is not available everywhere.
- *Mechanical debridement:* This is accomplished by allowing a moist coarse-mesh gauze placed on the wound to dry. This allows the necrotic tissue to adhere to these dressings which is then removed. It is useful on wounds that present with moderate necrotic debris.

Closure

The decision to whether or not the wound should be closed and the type of closure depends on the age, location, depth or extent and degree of contamination of the wound. Ideally, a wound that is >12 hours old should not be closed primarily. But in highly vascular area such as head and neck, this "golden period of 12 hours" is not valid and wound can be closed with minimal risk of infection up to *24 hours*. Otherwise, highly contaminated wounds (e.g., animal bites, human bites) are often irrigated and left open and may be considered for delayed closure.

Prerequisites for closure/repair:
- Informed written consent prior to repair
- Photograph of wound is desirable
- Shift the patient to well illuminated minor/major OT
- Fine instruments such as fine-toothed forceps, small needle holder, skin hooks, suture scissors, fine scissors, 11 and 15 number blades
- Loupe magnification as desirable

Suturing: Eversion is an important aspect of suturing to counter the scar contracture. If wound edges are flat after reapproximation, scar will invert after healing because of contracture. For closure, drape the area with sterile sheet after proper cleaning of the wound and provide adequate analgesia. The wound may be closed by any of the following techniques:

Interrupted suture: Insert the needle at about 2–3 mm from the edge of the wound, at a 90° angle to the skin and drive the needle through the epidermis,

dermis and subcutaneous tissue, in a curve that conforms to the curvature of the needle. Drive the needle through the wound until it exits approximately 2–3 mm from the opposing side of the wound. Equal bites of tissue should be taken from each side of the wound and edges should be slightly everted when the sutures have been tied. In case of "beveled edged" wound, a bite close to the skin edge should incorporate a large chunk of subcutaneous tissue and is taken on the larger edge and then a needle along with suture is passed to other side, taking a bite farther from the skin edge as it would be incorporating less subcutaneous tissue in its bite and then the knot is applied. Interrupted sutures are most commonly used technique because of its simplicity and even if one suture breaks, the remaining sutures will continue to hold the wound in approximation.

Horizontal mattress suture: It everts the wound edges and spreads tension along the wound edge **(Fig. 1)**. This makes it ideal for holding fragile skin as well as skin under high tension such as distant edges of a large laceration. This can be helpful to prevent wound bleeding but it can also cause strangulation and skin necrosis if tied too tightly. The needle is inserted at 90° angle to the skin, approximately 4–8 mm from one of the wound edges and run through the subcutaneous tissue until it exits approximately 4–8 mm from the opposite wound edge. The needle is then reinserted about 1–2 mm

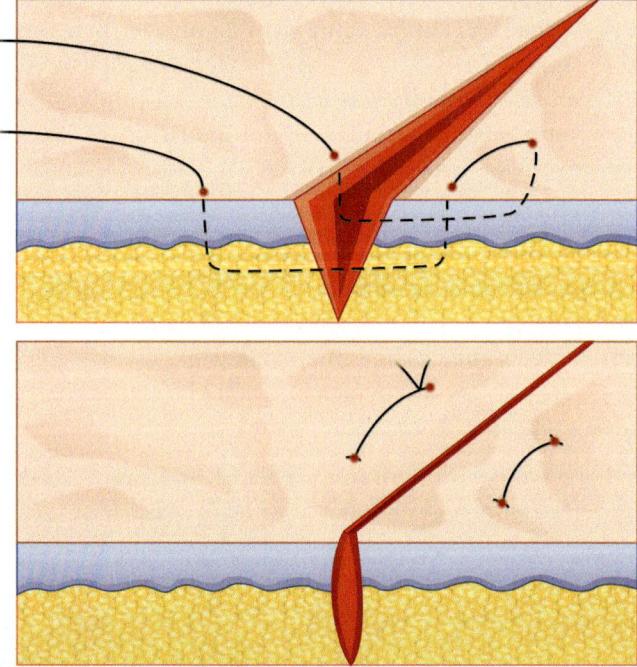

Fig. 1: Horizontal mattress suture.

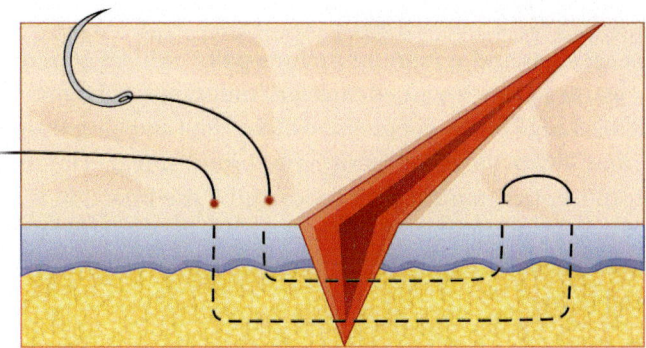

Fig. 2: Vertical mattress suture.

away at the same level from the opposite wound edge and driven in an arc until it exits 4–8 mm from the first wound edge. Both ends of the sutures are then tied gently at their exit from the first wound edge. The width of the suture is to be increased depending upon the tension on the wound edge, higher the tension wider the stitch.

Vertical mattress suture: It is indicated for lacerations that are under a significant amount of tension, e.g., wound over joints or gaping wounds, scalp wounds. The needle is inserted at 90° angle to the skin, approximately 4–8 mm from one of the wound edges **(Fig. 2)** and runs deep into the dermis until it exits approximately 4–8 mm from the opposite wound edge. The needle is then reinserted approximately 1–2 mm from the opposite wound edge and runs superficially at 1 mm depth driven in an arc until it exits 1–2 mm from the first wound edge.

Continuous suture: It is generally recommended for clean wounds which are not under lot of tension. To apply continuous suture, begin approximately 2 mm from the wound edge, insert the needle through the tissue at 90° angle to the skin and drive the needle through tissue following the curvature of the needle and make it come out at approximately 2 mm back from the opposite side of the wound. Reinsert the needle at 90° angle from the wound edge and begin the next stitch. This procedure is continued until the wound is closed and ties placed at both ends of the suture line. Although, the continuous suture is cosmetically superior to other techniques, the main drawback is, if the suture breaks or gets infected, full length of wound gets affected.

Skin stapling: It is mainly indicated in scalp and neck wounds. But due to high costs, it is not routinely used in emergencies. Evert the wound edges with tissue forceps or pinch the wound together with nondominant hand, align the skin stapler along the wound edge and squeeze the trigger to apply staples.

Management of Infected Wound

The classical signs and symptoms include pain, redness of periwound skin which is warm to touch and edematous/indurated or boggy, presence of purulent discharge (yellow or green) which is foul smelling along with fever, malaise and leukocytosis on peripheral blood smear. The management includes antiseptics, topical antibiotics and if the infection is severe then oral or systemic antibiotics must be used. An incision and drainage may be needed to evacuate the pus from the abscess cavity or to remove the devitalized tissue.

Special Consideration:
- *Lip:* Wounds involving lip require proper and meticulous reapproximation of mucosal, muscular and cutaneous layers individually. Special precautions must be taken for vermilion border by placing a prime suture to accurately align vermilion-cutaneous junction. Avulsion injury of the lip (<1/3 of lip) should be managed with local flap reconstruction. While large avulsion will require microvascular surgeon role for reimplantation.
- *Pinna:* Full thickness laceration requires accurate reapproximation of the cartilage (only suturing of skin and perichondrium without cartilage suturing is sufficient). Avulsed auricle will require replantation. De-epithelize full cartilage and bury it in postauricular subcutaneous pocket.
  Some advocate de-epithelization of only the posterior aspect of the avulsed cartilage and suturing the anterior skin margin to postauricular scalp flap. Some advocate microvascular reimplantation.
- *External nose:* It needs special consideration from esthetic point of view. Mucosa is closed first of all without achieving a watertight closure. Skin is approximated in meticulous way. Deep suture may be required through perichondrium or cartilage to establish proper shape and maintain integrity of cartilaginous framework. Avulsed small segment can be replanted back. Local or regional flaps can be utilized to repair the defect. Large segment avulsion or amputation requires microvascular anastomosis. If microvascular surgeon is not available, simple reimplantation and proper wound care with intravenous antibiotics helps to preserve at least some of the original structure.

Wound Cleansers:
Antiseptics: These include povidone iodine, hydrogen peroxide or silver compounds. While "chlorhexidine" is limited largely to surgical scrub and irrigation of wound, hydrogen peroxide (H_2O_2) has a weak antibacterial and antiviral (including HIV) action. The mechanical effect of effervescence, because of ready release of oxygen is probably more useful in wound cleansing, especially infective slough. "Povidone iodine" significantly reduces bacterial

load 10 minutes after the application but the effect does not persist for long. It is still most widely accepted and used as local antiseptic, even though a few studies have reported a retardation of the wound healing process. Topical formulation of povidone iodine is available in concentration of 4–10% and on application, release free iodine from a complex and this free iodine has a broad-spectrum activity against bacteria, fungi, viruses, protozoa, cysts, spores, etc. "Silver compound" (silver sulfadiazine) is mostly indicated in burn wounds and has broad-spectrum (bactericidal) activity against gram-positive, gram-negative bacteria including *Pseudomonas aeruginosa*, and is also active against some fungi including yeast.

Topical antibiotics:
- *Neomycin:* Neomycin A, B and C is obtained from *Streptomyces fradiae*. "Neomycin B" is available alone for topical use as "framycetin" and is effective against *Staphylococcus aureus* infection but can induce rapid resistance and contact allergy.
- *Polymyxin B sulfate:* This is obtained from *Bacillus polymyxa* and used topically in combination with neomycin sulfate, bacitracin zinc to treat skin infections and infected wounds. It has excellent bactericidal action and stimulating role in healing process.
- *Bacitracin zinc:* This is obtained from *Bacillus licheniformis* or *Bacillus subtilis* and is effective against gram-positive (including *Staphylococci, Streptococci* and *Clostridia*) and gram-negative (*Neisseria* and *Haemophilus influenzae*) organisms.
- *Fusidic acid:* This is very effective but can increase resistance among community methicillin susceptible *Staphylococcus aureus* (MSSA).
- Feracrylum gel is a biodegradable and biocompatible polymer. It has hygroscopic property which maintains a moist environment around its application on the wound site thus promoting wound healing and painless removal of dressing. Additionally, it has hemostatic activity suitable for oozing wounds. It is antimicrobial against a wide range of gram-positive, gram-negative, aerobic and anaerobic bacteria apart from various pathogenic fungi.
- *Colloidal silver solution:* It has a broad-spectrum antimicrobial action owing to its ability to disrupt the bacterial cell wall and inhibit the bacterial cell respiration. It also prevents the bacterial cell multiplication by attacking the bacterial DNA and hence facilitates to cleanse the wound, reduces bioburden, and accomplishes the goals of wound bed preparation in a biocompatible, safe, and effective way.

Systemic antibiotics: Broad-spectrum antibiotics are given empirically. Good quality swab sample from the infected wound is sent for "culture and sensitivity" and the systemic antibiotics (oral or intravenous) can be tailored as per the report.

Wound is managed by changing the dressing daily. The process of dressing includes—cleaning the wound with antiseptic, applying antimicrobial ointment, placing a sterile gauze piece on the wound, which is fixed with sticking plaster or a dressing. This process is repeated every day when the wound is fresh. As the wound heals, alternate day dressing may be used.

Antitetanus and Antirabies Management

"Antitetanus prevention" in a particular wound depends upon the immune status of the patient.
- If the patient had completed the course of tetanus toxoid or a booster dose within the past 5 years, nothing more is required.
- If the patient had completed the course of tetanus toxoid a booster dose >5 years ago but within last 10 years, tetanus toxoid single dose (0.5 mL) is given.
- In patients who completed the course of tetanus toxoid or a booster dose >10 years back, tetanus toxoid single dose (0.5 mL) and human tetanus immunoglobulin (250–500 IU) is given.
- In cases where the course of toxoid is not completed, or the immune status is unknown, 1,500 units of antitetanus serum (ATS) or 250–500 units of human immunoglobulin is administered in one arm and 0.5 mL of tetanus toxoid is administered into the other arm or given into the gluteal region. These patients should then be followed up with another dose of 0.5 mL of tetanus toxoid at 6 weeks and a third dose after 1 year. The antitoxin provides immediate temporary protection, and the toxoid is for long lasting protection.

Antirabies management: Local management of wound is of utmost importance and should be done at the earliest to prevent the virus absorption at the local nerve endings. The local area of the wound of the animal bite should be immediately flushed and washed thoroughly with plenty of soap and running water for at least 15 minutes thus help removal of virus, as much as possible from the wound site. Punctured wound can be irrigated with catheter. "Virucidal" agents such as alcohol tincture (400–700 mL/liter) or 0.01% aqueous solution of iodine or povidone iodine can be used for cleaning the wound to inactivate the virus. Attempts at closing the bite wound immediately should be avoided as this might help in spreading the virus into deeper tissues. Suturing of the wound, if necessary, can be performed 24–48 hours later, and this should be accomplished using minimum possible stitches after antirabies serum has been applied locally or infiltrated around the wound.

Antirabies treatment depends upon state of wound **(Table 1)**. If there are only minor scratches, abrasions without bleeding, licks on broken skin or nibbling of uncovered skin, administer antirabies vaccine immediately. In cases of single or multiple transdermal bites or scratches, contamination of mucus membrane with saliva; administer rabies immunoglobulin and

TABLE 1: Categories of contact with suspected rabid animal.

Category	Postexposure prophylaxis
First: Touching/feeding animal, lick on intact skin	Nil
Second: • Nibbling of uncovered skin • Minor scratch/abrasion but no bleeding	• Immediate rabies vaccination • Local wound treatment
Third: • Single/multiple transdermal scratch/bite • Lick on broken skin • Mucus membrane contamination with saliva from licking • Contact with bats	• Immediate rabies vaccination and administration • Rabies immunoglobulin • Local wound treatment

vaccine immediately. Stop treatment in both above-mentioned cases if animal remains healthy throughout the observation period of 10 days or if animal is killed humanely and found to be negative for rabies by appropriate laboratory technique.

It is very important to seek timely consultation from the Department of PSM/Community Medicine and/or Medicine Department for Anti-Rabies Management.

Follow-up

All patients should be kept under regular follow-up to look for any wound infection and dehiscence which will require further management. Dressing should be removed on 3rd day while in wounds which are more prone for infection (i.e., bites, heavily contaminated wounds), dressing may be removed after 24 hours to reassess the wounds. Sutures in the head and neck region are generally removed after 5 days and Steri-strips™ (Ethistrips) should be placed over the wound.

Standard precautions are to be followed while managing all types of emergencies. It is extremely important to handle and dispose off contaminated items and equipment in the patient's environment in an appropriate manner thus preventing the transmission of infectious agents. These standard precautions include:

Hand Hygiene

- Avoid unnecessary touching of surfaces in the vicinity of the patient.
- Always wash hands thoroughly with a soap and water or alcohol-based hand rub as a part of hand hygiene. This is necessary:
  - Before touching patients.
  - In case of inadvertent contact with body fluids, mucous membranes, non-intact skin or blood.

- After touching a patient to feel a pulse or palpation or lifting a patient.
- If hands are moved from a contaminated area to a clean area during patient care.
- After using the medical equipment near a patient.
■ Not to wear artificial fingernails or extenders.

Personal protective equipment (PPE): Always wear PPE, when dealing with an ENT emergency because it is associated with a high risk of contact with blood or body fluid of the patient and prevents contamination of one's clothing and skin.

■ *Gloves:* "Wear" disposable gloves while handling the emergency because of reasonably high risk of contact with blood and other potentially infectious materials, mucus membranes, nonintact skin, or potentially contaminated intact skin.
  - Remove gloves and dispose them appropriately using proper techniques to prevent hand contamination.
  - Change the gloves in between patients, for the care of more than one patient.
  - Never reuse gloves.
  - "Change" the gloves during patient care if the gloved hands needed to change from a contaminated body site to a noncontaminated area.
■ *Gowns:* A gown must be worn to prevent contamination of clothing while managing an emergency. Before leaving the patient's environment all the gowns and gloves must be removed and disposed off and should never be reworn.
■ *Mouth, nose, and eye protection:* Wear a face shield covering the front and sides of the face, a mask with attached shield, or a mask and goggles (in addition to gloves and gown).

■ FURTHER READING

1. Baranork S, Ayello EA. Wound Care Essentials: Practices Principles, 2nd edition, Ambler, PA: Lippincott/Williams and Wilkins; 2016.
2. Carville K. Wound Care Manual, 5th edition. Perth: Silver Chain; 2005.
3. Stone S, Carter WA. Wound Preparation. In: Tintinalli JE, Kelen GD, Stapczyniki JS, Ma OJ, Clin DM (Eds). Tintinalli's Emergency Medicine, 6th edition. New York: The McGraw-Hill Companies Inc.; 2004. pp. 284-7.

CHAPTER 2

Acute Vertigo

*Monica Manhas, Ajit Man Singh, Rakesh Kumar,
Subirendra Kumar, P Ghosh*

■ INTRODUCTION

Subjective feeling of vertigo encompasses variable expressions:
- Definite sense of rotation
- About to faint
- Feeling of loss of balance without any special sensation in head
- Feeling of light headedness
- Oscillopsia.

Vertigo, by definition, is an illusion of motion with a distinct rotational component.

"Acute vertigo attack" (AVA) is a well-defined isolated attack of vertigo with a distinct onset (usually within 3 days) and offset which may be appearing for the first time in a particular patient or the presentation may be recurrent attacks of vertigo. *Acute vestibular syndrome (AVS)* is characterized by an acute onset (over seconds to hours) of objective rotatory vertigo, nausea/vomiting, and gait unsteadiness along with head motion intolerance and nystagmus that could last for days to weeks.

To treat a vertigo attack, one must have working knowledge of neuro-otology involved in Body Balance System (BBS). The proper body balance and posture stabilization utilizes the vestibular, visual, and proprioceptive sensations that are then, centrally integrated and its effective and finely tuned motor control.

■ THE VESTIBULAR END ORGANS

These are of two types, (1) semicircular canals (SCCs) and (2) otolith organs (utricle and saccule). The SCCs act as velocity transducers during high velocity (angular acceleration) impulsive head movements to stabilize vision, involving vestibulo-ocular reflex (VOR). These "three SCCs" are oriented roughly at 90° to one another in all three planes of space, the lateral canals of each side are coplanar, as are the anterior canal (AC) on one side and the posterior canal on the other. When the head turns rapidly to one side, ipsilateral input increases dramatically and contralateral input decreases to a lesser degree making the eye deviate equal and opposite to the head movement via 3rd, 4th, and 6th cranial nerve nuclei.

The *"utricle and saccule"*, on the other hand, provide information to the brain regarding gravitational orientation and linear acceleration input (utricle—horizontal and saccule—vertical orientation), which help in maintaining head and trunk posture via medial and lateral vestibulospinal tracts (VSTs) [vestibulospinal reflex (VSR)].

The midline cerebellum modulates the finer motor activity triggered by VOR and VSR. Vestibular input provides an inhibitory influence in the cerebellum and fine tunes ocular and postural movements thus plays a pivotal role in appropriate interaction among vestibular, visual, and proprioceptive inputs. Other regulatory mechanisms are in the mesencephalon and cerebral cortex, involved via vestibulocortical pathways, are thalamus, superior Sylvian gyrus and inferior intraparietal sulcus, which integrate the three main (vestibular, proprioceptive, and visual) signals to provide a conscious awareness of body orientation.

In case of *"unilateral SCC"* dysfunction, brainstem senses only the input from contralateral side, due to the absent dysfunctional side and interprets it as circular motion in the direction of normal ear/side. This defective VOR causes eyes to slowly drift to the impaired side (due to contralateral vestibular apparatus) which then snap back to the normal side (due to stimulation from ipsilateral cerebral cortex), resulting in spontaneous nystagmus (SPN) opposite to the side of the dysfunction. Also, with head turning rapidly toward impaired side, the normal side alone cannot stabilize gaze leading to vertigo due to inadequate VOR.

In cases of *"bilateral SCC"* dysfunction, the vertigo is absent or minimal because the brainstem does not perceive any asymmetry. However, head movement in any direction leads to blurring of vision because of slippage of images across the retina (oscillopsia).

On the other hand, *unilateral loss of "otolith"* input causes postural instability with a deviation in upright stance due to impaired VSR. The head tilts and body leans toward the suppressed side because there is loss in extensor tone on the affected side. With *bilateral loss of otolith* inputs, there is loss of sense of gravity that causes the patient to become more dependent on proprioceptive and visual input. These patients present with a difficulty in walking in the dark or on walking on uneven surfaces.

■ VISUAL SYSTEM

Following ocular functions are involved for visual cues for orientation:
- *VOR:* It minimizes slipping of image on retina in motion (retinal slip) and thus maximizing visual acuity during high velocity head movements and rotations.
- *Smooth pursuit system (SPS):* It is closely related to optokinetic reflex (OKR) and helps in tracking of slow-moving objects using foveal stimulation. The smooth pursuit function has its most efficient range for frequencies <1 Hz.

- *Saccadic system:* It helps in refixation on a new target. Saccade movements are conjugate, high velocity (200–600°/s), accurate (do not overshoot or undershoot), and of short latency (<250 ms). The brainstem reticular formation and frontal lobe control velocity, latency, and conjugate movement, while midline cerebellum and fastigial nuclei control the accuracy.
- *Optokinetic Reflex (OKR):* It corrects the visual information when the peripheral retina is stimulated thus stabilizing the image during motion. It is a combination of smooth pursuit and saccade mechanism.
- *Binocular vision, depth perception, and convergence movements* are other important ocular functions.

■ PROPRIOCEPTIVE INPUT

Pressure receptors in the soles of the feet and joint stretch receptor in the feet, legs, trunk, and neck all combine a rich network of multilevel subcortical and cortical reflex pathways designed to maintain the body's center of gravity. Mainly three tracts: vestibulospinal (medial and lateral) and the reticulospinal tract are involved in this function. Additionally, projections from medial vestibular nucleus (VN) to the ascending and descending portions of the medial longitudinal fasciculus (MLF) plays a major role in the cervical VORs, coordinating the eye-head movements. Diseases such as peripheral neuropathies (diabetes) and corticospinal degeneration interrupt these pathways and create difficulties with posture control.

■ EVALUATION

Posterior circulation infarctions involving the lateral medulla, lateral pontine and inferior cerebellar areas represent 5% of AVS cases in the emergency. Taking a proper, informative, and well-defined history from the patient and/or the attendants is a clinical art which cannot be overemphasized, especially in acute vertigo. Approximately 75% of vertigo patients can be diagnosed just by an appropriate history itself. *It is also important to differentiate between patient suffering from vertigo (a well-defined spinning movement or motion) and dysequilibrium (a result of various sensations).*

The *self-description by the patient* can be categorized in one of the following medical terms:
- Sensation of spatial disorientation—dizziness
- Sensation of movement or motion—vertigo
- Imbalance and problem in walking on uneven surfaces—dysequilibrium
- Difficulty in walking or reading and unable to focus on objects with movement—oscillopsia (that occurs only with eyes open. Vertigo, on the other hand, occurs with eyes open or closed)
- Motion sickness and height vertigo—physiologic dizziness

- Light headedness and impending fainting—presyncope
- Panic attacks and hyperventilation—psychological
- Spinning of head (subjective vertigo)—central dizziness
- Focusing problem—ocular dizziness
- Children may explain their symptoms using their own vocabulary such as being on a merry-go-round

After the patient has described the sensation in his or her own explanatory language, the *"characteristics of the sensation"* are asked which include:

- Frequency—one, multiple, or synchronous.
- Initial spell—when, how long it lasted, and nature of spell.
- Last spell—when, how long it lasted, its nature, and whether different from initial spell.
- Frequency of spells—times per day, week, or month.
- Duration of spell—seconds, second to a few minutes, hours, and days.
- Precipitating factors (provoking events)—position change, exertion, cough, allergic attack, trauma to ear, road traffic accident, viral, bacterial infection, flight, scuba diving, or barotrauma.
- *Presence of nausea and vomiting (N&V):* Nausea and vomiting are because of stimulation of the nucleus tractus solitarius and vagus nuclei located in the medulla. Vertigo associated with nausea or vomiting is seen in acute vestibular neuronitis, severe episodes of Meniere's disease or benign paroxysmal positional vertigo (BPPV). Usually, nausea and vomiting are mild and in proportion to the degree of vertigo in peripheral vestibular lesions and the cases of pontine strokes [e.g., anterior inferior cerebellar artery (AICA) syndrome]. Dorsal medullary stroke [posterior inferior cerebellar artery (PICA) syndrome] on the other hand, produces nausea and vomiting that are violent and out of proportion to the degree of vertigo. Other central vestibular lesions (cerebellum, thalamus, and 4th ventricle floor) produce very mild or may present clinically without nausea and vomiting.

"Past medical history" should be asked to know any predisposing factor and relevant questions are asked regarding any history of allergies (medication, food, and inhalant), illness (endocrine, cardiac, renal, pulmonic, neurologic, psychiatric, etc.), medication (antihypertensive, ototoxic drugs, endocrine, etc.), or any surgical intervention.

Other important aspects to be considered are:
- *Incoordination:* Associated with onset of vertigo, which may be associated with impaired "fine" movements (cerebellar and posterior fossa) or "coarse" movements (extrapyramidal).
  - Voluntary or repeated movements (chorea and epilepsy)
  - Tremors (central lesion)

- *Motor weakness:* Its onset, course, duration, and pattern. Hemiparesis, numbness, or weakness.
- *Paresthesia,* incontinence of bowel and bladder activity.
- *Hearing loss:*
  - Either unilateral (labyrinthine pathology and posterior fossa pathology), or bilateral (ototoxicity)
  - Sudden in onset (infective, viral, traumatic, and idiopathic)
  - Progressive in course (degenerative changes, posterior fossa tumors, and ototoxicity)
  - Duration
  - Fluctuating hearing loss

(*Note*: Peripheral vertigo is generally associated with hearing loss while in central vertigo, the hearing is normal except in cases of cerebrovascular events involving internal auditory artery or AICA)

- *Tinnitus:*
  - Pulsatile or nonpulsatile
  - Unilateral or bilateral
  - High pitch (aminoglycosides) or low pitch (otosclerosis and Meniere's disease)
  - Whether maskable or not (central and psychological)
- *Aural fullness:* Pressure and popping sensation
- *Visual dysfunction:* Presence of visual field defects, diplopia, and abducens paralysis are consistent with diagnosis of benign intracranial hypertension (pseudotumor cerebri). Diplopia may be a cardinal feature of central lesions and Gradenigo's syndrome. Vertical diplopia may be seen because of skew deviation resulting from peripheral or central otolith dysfunction.
- *Ear discharge:* Its onset, unilateral or bilateral, mucoid/mucopurulent or purulent, odor, blood stained, etc.
- *Earache:* Its onset, unilateral/bilateral, its severity, radiation, character, aggravating, and relieving factors. *Ear or mastoid pain, facial weakness, and hearing loss* are generally seen in acute middle ear disease, e.g., otitis media and herpes zoster oticus. Pain accompanying vertigo may also be seen in cases of invasive diseases of temporal bone or meningeal irritation.
- *Palpitation:* In panic disorders and arrhythmias
- *Altered sensorium:* In stroke, drugs, seizure, and Wernicke syndrome
- *Seizures:* Associated aura, duration, type and frequency of attacks, taste, smell, visual distortions, and hallucinations.
- *Loss of consciousness:* Ask for any tongue bite and/or frothing. When loss of consciousness occurs, a central nervous system (CNS) or cardiac abnormality (an arrhythmia resulting in a Stokes–Adams attack) must be ruled out. Also seen in vasovagal syncope, seizures, subarachnoid hemorrhage (SAH).

- *Headache (migraines):* Exact side, location, radiation, severity, aggravating, and relieving factors.
  - Ask for associated photophobia and phonophobia.
  - Occipital headache and speech difficulty are common features of acute cerebellar disease.
- *Deadly Ds:* Dysphagia, dysphonia, dysarthria, diplopia, dysesthesia, drop attacks, and down-up distortion (room tilt illusion)—central lesion.
- *Memory or concentration problems*
- *Facial palsy*
- *Presence of any psychiatric symptoms:* Anxiety, pallor, sweating, diarrhea, depression, restlessness, and irritability.
- *Alcohol abuse*, drug addictions, history of sexually transmitted disease (STD) (e.g., syphilis), and smoking.
- *Cervical rotation*, extension, and postural changes
  - Cervical pain with vertigo suggests cervical vertigo.
  - Neck pain is also associated with vascular dissection.
- *Light-headedness and syncope/near syncope:* Cardiac activity-ask about palpitation, shortness of breath, rhythm disturbances, fainting/passing out attacks. Dyspnea is seen in anemia.
- *Stroke risk factors:* Smoking, hypertension, diabetes, hyperlipidemia, atrial fibrillation, eclampsia, hypercoagulable state, or prior stroke or myocardial infarction.
- *Fever*

■ EXAMINATION

It includes general physical examination and neuro-otologic examination.

General physical examination includes:
- Recording the height, weight, general body built, and five vitals (pulse, blood pressure (BP), respiratory rate, level of consciousness, and body temperature).
- BP is recorded both in lying down as well as in standing position to rule out postural or *orthostatic hypotension* (drop in systolic BP by at least 20 mm Hg or diastolic BP by 10 mm Hg within 3 minutes of standing from supine position), BP is also recorded in both arms (to rule out *subclavian steal syndrome*).
- Cardiac auscultation—for any added sound and look for cervical bruits.
- Complete lymph node examination for any metastatic deposits.
- Thyroid examination, any organomegaly and cervical spine examination.

Otolaryngological examination includes general ear, nose, and throat (ENT) examination, otoscopy (status of tympanic membrane, any perforation or cholesteatoma), tubal patency, mastoid tenderness, fistula sign, Siegel

examination and in any doubt, do the examination under microscope (EUM)/otoendoscopy.
Central nervous system examination includes:
- Any skull abnormalities
- Meningeal irritation signs
- Basic mental status (orientation to time, person, and space)
- Hyperventilation
- Motor system muscle strength and tone of abductors, adductors, flexors and extensors, and any muscle wasting
- *Sensory system:* Pain, temperature, fine and crude touch, and vibration sensation
- *Cerebellar function:* Finger nose test, heel-knee-shin for "dysmetria", dysdiadochokinesia (rapid alternating movements), hypotonia, and decreased tendon reflexes
- Deep tendon reflexes and plantar responses
- Proprioception

Eye Examination

It includes visual acuity, confrontational visual fields, lid examination for ptosis, pupillary size and reactivity, ocular fixation, extraocular movement range, ocular alignment (cover or uncover, crossover test, and Maddox rod), convergence and nystagmus (various characters of nystagmus are described later).

- *Conjugate deviation of eye:* Instruct the patient to look at the examiner who remains directly in front of him. Grasp the patient's head and move it right and left, up and down noting the position of the eyes at each new head position. Failure of conjugate deviation in a lateral direction indicates a gaze deficit (cerebral or brainstem lesion). Acute cerebral dysfunction causes paralysis to contralateral side and brainstem dysfunction to ipsilateral side of lesion, while vertical failure indicates bilateral brainstem lesion.
- *Ophthalmoscopy* will include examination of optic nerve head and retina, any flakes, floaters, or hemorrhage (seek an ophthalmologist opinion).

Cranial Nerve Examination

Examine for all cranial nerves including:
- Eye movements, fields of vision, and pupil size and reflex (III, IV, and VI)
- Corneal reflex (V)
- Test for sensation of face to light touch and pain (V)
- Touch sensation in the skin of the external auditory canal or/and adjacent concha (VII nerve or CPA lesion lesion pressing on the trigeminal tract in brainstem—Hitzelberger sign) (VII)
- Strength of facial muscles on both sides (VII)
- Inspect for elevation of soft palate elevation or gag reflex (IX and X)

- Examine for strength of contraction of sternocleidomastoid and trapezius (XI)
- Protrusion and movements of tongue and inspect for wasting of tongue (XII)

Audiological Tests

These include examination of hearing status by *"whispering and conversation test"*, as a measure of the distance from the speaker. Perception of whispering sound is severely affected in sensory, especially retrocochlear pathologies. *"Tuning fork test"* include Rinne's test, Weber's test, and absolute bone conduction (ABC) test. Preferably 512 Hz tuning fork is used, which can be repeated with 128, 256, 1,024, and 2,048 Hz tuning forks. Hearing loss with positive Rinne's test indicates neurosensory loss in which, Weber's test is lateralized to the better ear and ABC is decreased.

Vestibular Examination

The bedside vestibular examination includes evaluation of:
- Spontaneous nystagmus (SPN)
- Skew deviation
- Vestibulo-ocular reflex
- Maneuver-induced vertigo
- Visual component testing
- Body balance and gait

Spontaneous Nystagmus

This "jerk nystagmus" or vestibular nystagmus is characterized by a slow drift of the eyes (known as slow component) in one direction followed by a compensatory fast jerk (known as fast component) of the eyes in the opposite direction and results from lesions mainly in peripheral vestibular pathways or sometimes from brainstem or cerebellar lesion due to unopposed, relatively high spontaneous neural activity of the intact labyrinth (static imbalance). In contrast, the pendular nystagmus has two opposite slow phases without a jerk component and is usually because of an abnormality in the visual fixation system in the brain.

The slow component is resulted by vestibular stimulation and is mediated through the three-neuron arc from the SCCs to the extraocular muscles. The fast component is mediated by functioning cerebral cortex.

The patient is made to sit or lie comfortably with the head and neck in a straightforward position and gaze directed straight forward. The eyes are then observed with visual fixation for approximately 30 seconds and then without visual fixation for approximately 1 minute. The patient is asked initially to hold his or her eyes in the neutral midline (if present, the nystagmus is named spontaneous) and then to gaze not >30° to the right and 30° to the left, down, and up, for approximately 10 seconds in each direction, named gaze-evoked nystagmus (caution: allowing the patient to gaze for >30° to the either side will evoke physiological end-point nystagmus). Since vestibular nystagmus is suppressed by visual fixation; to avoid the fixation suppression, various techniques are applied, i.e., Frenzel goggle (+20 diopters lenses) or ophthalmoscopic examination with occlusion of the opposite eye or by simply asking the patient to stare at the blank wall. SPN of 5-10°/s is considered within normal limits by some authors while others are of opinion that any observable spontaneous nystagmus in a patient complaining of dizziness is considered a pathologic sign. The suppression by visual fixation is because of intact smooth pursuit and fixation system.

Spontaneous nystagmus is named by the direction of the fast phase as well as by the axis of rotation. "Peripheral nystagmus" (because of inner ear or 8th cranial nerve lesion) is a jerk nystagmus with unidirectional constant-velocity slow phase, which may vary with gaze direction. According to *"Alexander's law"*, the velocity is greatest when looking in the direction of the quick phase.

The *"axis" of rotation of slow phase of nystagmus* is also important because a unilateral vestibular lesion results in slow phase with a primarily horizontal component directed toward the lesioned side and a torsional component to a small degree, with the upper pole of the eyes rotating towards the lesioned side (mixed plane).

Nystagmus may appear with eccentric eye positions, i.e., when eyes gaze beyond 30° to either side, the cause may be physiologic (end-point nystagmus) or pathologic. Physiological end-point nystagmus cannot sustain while pathologic one persists as long as the position is held. Symmetric gaze evoked nystagmus (i.e., equal amplitude on looking to both left and right) results from drug intoxications (phenytoin, alcohol, diazepam, and phenobarbital) or CNS pathologies. Whereas asymmetrical gaze evoked nystagmus results from brainstem or cerebellar pathologies.

"Central SPN" (because of lesion in central vestibular pathway): It is differentiated from peripheral SPN in that it usually has a prominent axis of rotation of slow phase of nystagmus which may be horizontal, torsional, or vertical and is often not suppressed by visual fixation; and ocular smooth pursuit is often lost. Also, the central nystagmus may not change or "reverse" the direction, when gaze is directed towards the direction of the fast component (the later is due to disruption of both, the vestibular pathways and gaze-holding pathways). Moreover, the peripheral nystagmus is accompanied by significant vertigo as compared to central SPN.

Commonly seen, *"centrally-mediated SPN"* are:
- *Downbeat spontaneous nystagmus (DBN):* It is defined as nystagmus with the fast phase beating in downward direction. It is of maximal intensity when the eyes are directed laterally and downward and with the eyes in this position, the nystagmus is directed obliquely, i.e., horizontal, downward

since DBN often goes together with horizontal gaze evoked nystagmus. DBN is because of disorders of vestibulocerebellum (cerebellar floccular lesion) or floor of 4th ventricle lesion, probably because of decreased tonic neural activity to interstitial nucleus of Cajal (INC) from both sides of posterior SCCs. Also, it is seen in Arnold–Chiari malformation, vascular insufficiency, multiple sclerosis (MS), CNS trauma, posterior cranial tumors, and phenytoin or lithium toxicity.

- *Upbeat spontaneous nystagmus (UBN):* It is characterized by upward ocular oscillations when the patient's eyes are in primary neutral gaze. It is mostly from lesion in "brachium conjunctivum" or dorsal upper medullary lesions and not in the cerebellum and probably because of decreased tonic neural activity to INC from both sides anterior SCC. The downward drift in UBN is because of either the lesion is in excitatory pathways (pons) to the elevating extraocular muscle or lesion of inhibitory feedback pathway (medulla) to the flocculus, which in turn leads to decreased excitation of elevating extraocular muscles.
- *Torsional nystagmus*: It is because of decreased tonic neural activity to the INC from anterior and posterior SCC on one side. Its intensity may change with head rotation and may be suppressed completely by visual convergence. It is seen in patients with syringobulbia, syringomyelia, and dorsolateral medullary lesions.
- *Periodic alternating nystagmus (PAN):* It is a type of horizontal nystagmus with eyes in primary gaze with the fast phase changing direction, or alternating, approximately every 2 minutes. It may cease for 5–20 seconds between episodes of direction change. It is seen in degenerative cerebellar disease, multiple sclerosis, anticonvulsant toxicity, neurosyphilis and is probably because of unstable (high gain) neural activity in medial vestibular nucleus.
- *Sea-saw nystagmus:* It is because of unilateral lesion of INC and nucleus of Darkschewitsch, and characterized by the elevation and intorsion of one eye while the other eye depresses and extorts. It is seen in midline compressive lesions in the suprasellar area, brainstem strokes, pituitary tumors, and albinism (congenital type).
- *Ocular palatal myoclonus (OPM):* It is a vertical pendular SPN with synchronous palatal myoclonus. Spasms of facial muscles, vocal cord, and diaphragm may also be seen. It is seen with lesions involving the Guillain-Mollaret triangle (dentate nucleus, the red nucleus, and the inferior olivary nucleus).

Skew Deviation

It is vertical misalignment of the eyes resulting from an imbalance of vestibular tone between right and left sides (i.e., neural firing), particularly the input from the otoliths to the oculomotor system. Each utricle projects to lateral and medial VN and then to medial and lateral VSTs. From medial VN, it also projects to III and IV cranial nerve nuclei via MLF and supplies four extraocular muscles that act vertically. In presence of any lesion in otolith (utricular) pathway, the contralateral excitation of superior rectus and oblique muscle causes elevation and intorsion of the eye on normal side and excitation of ipsilateral inferior rectus and oblique muscle cause depression and extorsion of the eye on involved side, the combination causes skew deviation. Excitation of neck muscles from intact VST causes "head tilt" to ipsilateral side. Also, body leans toward the side of lesion because of loss of extensor tone. Ocular counter roll, head tilt and skew deviation, combined reaction is known as "ocular tilt response" and is caused by ipsilateral lesion in utricle (labyrinthitis), vestibular nerve (vestibular neuritis), and VN (Wallenberg's syndrome) contralateral lesion in MLF and INC. Skew is generally detected by *alternate cover testing* with or without a quantifiable prismatic correction. Ask the patient to look directly at your/examiner's nose. Cover the right and then the left eye alternatively and continue alternating back and forth, every 2 seconds. Slight vertical correction (one side corrects upward and the other corrects downward) is seen in presence of skew deviation. Always focus on one eye (either of the two) since amplitude of correction is small (1-2 mm). Skew has primarily been identified as a sign in the patients with posterior fossa pathology. It is most seen with brainstem lesions (with 98% specificity) and has been observed to be a herald manifestation in cases with basilar occlusion. Differential diagnosis of skew is superior oblique palsy. Skew is comitant in all directions of gaze whereas vertical strabismus decreases significantly when an individual changes position from sitting to supine position.

Vestibulo-ocular Reflex

Vestibulo-ocular reflex dysfunction is because of loss of "dynamic sensitivity" in the VN in the involved side, resulting in decreased gain (eye velocity/head velocity) of the VOR for head movements toward involved side. The bedside tests are:

- *Head impulse test (HIT) (Halmagyi test):* The patient is asked to relax and maintain gaze at the examiner nose or a distant target. Face the patient while holding the patient's head and then briskly turn the head to the right and to the left. Normally, the patient's gaze remains locked to the target or examiner's nose. The test is abnormal if patient's gaze is jerked away from the target. A series of refixation saccades (Halmagyi's sign) bring back gaze to the fixation target. Positive HIT indicates a peripheral lesion. If the test results are abnormal with a right head turn, the lesion is on the right side. This test is called *"Doll's eye test"* if done in comatose patients. (*Note*: Normal VOR and HIT in an acute vertiginous patient indicates strong possibility of a central lesion.)

Posterior circulation pathology can have false negative (abnormal) HIT, especially in AICA or labyrinthine artery stroke wherein infarct involves the area of entry of vestibular nerve into the brainstem. AICA and labyrinthine artery stroke, in addition to abnormal HIT, can present with acute hearing loss that can be picked up by bedside hearing test (especially bone conduction).

- *Head shaking nystagmus (HSN) (Kopfschuttel test):* With "eyes closed", pitching the head down 30°, oscillates the patient's head horizontally two cycles/second, 20 times. Appearance of jerk nystagmus (i.e., horizontal post head-shake nystagmus) indicates a vestibular imbalance (peripheral or central lesion). The presence of HSN typically parallels increasing right/left excitability differences noted on electronystagmography (ENG). The presence of atypical nystagmus (either vertical or rotatory) known as "cross coupling" on HSN requires exclusion of a CNS disorder (cerebellar lesion).
- *Vestibular dynamic visual acuity test (oscillopsia test):* Ask the patient to read a fixed (Snellen's) eye chart with the head still and again with head moving. A loss of more than three lines is considered a positive sign of decreased VOR and subsequent retinal slip. This test assesses whether the VOR is intact bilaterally, e.g., ototoxicity and bilateral Meniere's disease, wherein one often complains of oscillopsia.

Maneuver-induced Vertigo

Certain maneuvers should be performed that may evoke nystagmus.

- *Dix–Hallpike (Nylén–Bárány) test (positioning nystagmus):* It is diagnostic for BPPV. Patient is made to sit on the examination table and head is turned 45° horizontally. The head and trunk are brought straight back "en bloc" so that head is hanging over the edge of the examination table by 20°. Presence of nystagmus is looked for and vertigo feeling is asked for. Patient is brought up slowly to a sitting position with head still turned 45° and nystagmus is looked for again. This test is repeated with the head turned 45° to the other direction.

  In *BPPV*, the nystagmus should begin within 30 seconds, and lasts fewer than 30 seconds, is fatigable, and beats toward the undermost (geotropic), offending ear upon assumption of the provocative position. The nystagmus is repeatable and reverses direction when the patient moves back to the sitting position.

  Positional nystagmus: It is any persistent or long lasting nystagmus which appears after the assumption of different head positions, while positioning nystagmus is believed to be initiated by the semi-circular canals and probably also by the otolith organs and it manifests in cases of both central and peripheral vestibular lesions.

  Ask the patient to assume the head position in which the vertiginous sensation occurs and then one by one, 11 specific positions are tested (five in sitting position—head upright, right side down, left side down, head extended, and head flexed and "six" in supine position, i.e., head straight, right side down, left side down, head hanging, head hanging-turned to right, and head hanging turned to left). Each position should be changed reasonably slowly and head should be maintained in each position for at least 30 seconds. Look for nystagmus thus induced and its characters, i.e., latency, intensity, direction and fatiguability, and accompanying dizziness. Changes in head position in relation to the vector that represents the direction of gravity of the earth may result in provocation of a hitherto unidentified nystagmus or change in existing SPN at rest position and may represent central causes like lesions involving cerebellum or MS or vertebrobasilar insufficiency (VBI). It may also represent peripheral vestibular lesions or BPPV and peripheral nystagmus follows Ewald's laws. *However, this test is rarely performed these days.*

- *Pressure testing (Siegel's speculum):* By applying positive and negative pressure to the external ear canal, nystagmus can be elicited (Hennebert's sign). Same nystagmus may be elicited with tragal compression or loud noise (Tullio's sign) in cases of perilymph fistula (PLF), superior SCC dehiscence, occasionally Meniere's disease, and hypermobile stapes. Valsalva-induced nystagmus is seen in craniocervical junction anomalies, superior canal dehiscence, perilymphatic fistula, and ossicular chain abnormalities. Vibration of mastoid process induces nystagmus in unilateral vestibular loss and fistulas.
- *Hyperventilation:* Ask the patient to breathe deeply for approximately 30–60 seconds and then observe for presence of any nystagmus. Hyperventilation (by alkalosis and changes in ionized calcium) provokes nystagmus either by altering conduction in peripheral (vestibular schwannoma) or central vestibular pathways (MS). It may also reproduce anxiety-related vestibular symptoms and may produce or enhance downbeat nystagmus in patients with cerebellar diseases.

Visual Component Testing

If impaired, indicates brainstem pathology.

Smooth pursuit eye movements: These are slow eye movements with head kept still that assist in maintenance of images of small moving targets on the fovea. With the head still, ask the patient to track a small target moving horizontally and vertically but slowly (10–20°/second). Corrective (catch-up or back-up) saccades are looked for which are because of decreased pursuit gain (gain = eye movement velocity/target velocity) also known as "saccadic pursuit". The involvement of several anatomical structures in integration of smooth pursuit eye movements makes it hard to pinpoint a lesion in case of observed abnormality. Peripheral unilateral vestibule lesion does not impair smooth pursuit movement. Marked asymmetries of smooth pursuit, however, indicate a structural lesion.

Saccadic eye movements (saccades are fast changes in eye position): Ask the patient to "fixate" on the clinician's nose. Then ask the patient to glance back and forth between two horizontal or two vertical targets (clinician's nose and finger held approximately 20° eccentrically). Look for velocity, accuracy, latency, and conjugacy of the saccades. Peripheral vestibular defects do not impair saccades.

Increased *"latency"* is seen primarily with supratentorial cortical dysfunction (visual attention defects) or brainstem (initiation defect) whereas velocity changes, i.e., slowing of saccade—often accompanied by hypometric (undershoot) saccades occurs with "intoxication" or neurodegenerative diseases. Horizontal slow saccade occurs with pontine lesions (parapontine reticular formation) while slowing of vertical saccades indicates a midbrain lesion. Hypermetric saccades (overshoot saccades), identified by a corrective saccade back to the object, indicates lesions of cerebellum (vermis).

Pendular tracking test: Ask the patient to sit with head still and instruct him to follow with his eyes, the clinician's finger which is moved to and fro horizontally at a steady rate for 10 seconds. Keep the finger >1 meter away and do not move beyond 30° away from midline, on either side. Inability to carry smooth pendular tracking movement indicates "central lesion".

Body balance and gait: A patient with peripheral acute vertigo often prefers to sit upright without lying down or prefers to lie still with the affected ear on the top, and prefers to avoid sudden or jerky movements. Also, in cases of peripheral vestibulopathy, a patient can stand and walk with assistance, will tend to lean or fall in one direction—generally toward the side of lesion (opposite to the direction of fast phase of any SPN observed). While in central lesion, patient is unable to stand or take a single step and direction of fall may be variable. (*Note*: In a patient with AVA, if he/she is unable to sit/stand or walk without assistance, think of a stroke.)

Romberg test: The patient is made to stand with feet close together and arms folded across to chest, eyes open for 30 seconds and then eyes closed for 30 seconds. If the patient is able to stand stable with eyes open but not with eyes closed, Romberg's test is positive and is seen in lesions of dorsal spinal tract, severe proprioceptive defects (peripheral neuropathy) and acute vestibular defects.

Miscellaneous tests: Fukuda's stepping (Unterberger's) test—The patient is made to step knee high in place for 50 steps with arms extended in front of the body and eyes closed. Progressive turning is observed to one side by >30° is taken abnormal, indicative of unilateral vestibular lesion of same side. In central vestibular lesion, the sway (side-to-side movement while stepping) is abnormally high.

Gait: Ask the patient to walk as straight as possible with 10 steps heel-to-toe beyond the first two starting steps. Compare the results of this heel-to-toe test with eye closed (WOFEC—walk on floor with eyes closed) with that of eyes open (WOFEO). Also look for cerebellar ataxia, shuffling gait in Parkinson's disease.

Fukuda vertical writing with eyes closed (blind folded vertical writing test): The patient is asked to write 4 or 5 capital alphabetical letters such as ABCDE are written vertically on graph paper. Each letter should be as large as 3 × 3 or 5 × 5 cm.

This test is first done with eyes open and next in similar way with the eyes blind-folded. The greatest deviation of written letters is measured in degrees from a line drawn vertically from the middle of the top letter.

If a deviation of more than 10 degrees is found solely in the letters written during the blind-folded test, unilateral labyrinthine lesions may be indicated. A patient with cerebellar ataxia may write unrecognizable letters instead of letters showing a definite slant.

Past-pointing test: The patient is made to sit on the chair with his one hand palm down on his knee and index finger stretched out. He is then asked to raise his arm and touch the examiner's finger held in front of the patient. The test is performed first with eyes open and next with eyes closed, the deviation of patient's finger from the examiner's to either side is assessed. Past pointing in a labyrinthine lesion will affect both arms while, in a cerebellar lesion it may be present on the affected side only.

Note: Many authors have emphasized the importance of a three-step bedside oculomotor examination (HINTS: head impulse-nystagmus-test of skew) in acute vertigo syndrome and found it more sensitive for stroke than an early magnetic resonance imaging (MRI) [with diffusion-weighted imaging (DWI)], thereby it has been reported that finding one of three dangerous subtle oculomotor signs, normal head impulse, horizontal nystagmus that changes direction in eccentric gaze or skew deviation is more sensitive than the combined presence of all other traditional neurological signs for identifying stroke as cause of acute vertigo syndrome.

Mnemonic INFARCT (impulse normal, fast phase alternating nystagmus, refixation on cover test for skew deviation) is important to remember.

Laboratory Tests

These include:

Audiometry: Pure tone audiometry (PTA), speech audiometry, special test like short increment sensitivity index (SISI), tone-decay and alternate binaural loudness balance (ABLB) (*Note:* acute auditory symptoms usually manifest with strokes in the AICA territory and presumed secondary to labyrinthine artery infarction, cochlear nucleus involvement or both).
- Impedance audiometry with stapedial reflex decay.
- Brainstem electric response audiometry (BERA) and electrocochleography (ECoG).

Complete hemogram: To look for anemia and total and differential leukocytic cells.
- Erythrocyte sedimentation rate (ESR) and rheumatoid factor
- Blood sugar, thyroid profile, and tests for syphilis
- Urea, creatinine, and serum cholesterol
- Urine examination for albumin, sugar, pus cells, and erythrocytes.

Radiology: Depending upon the condition of patient and necessity of test.
- X-ray cervical spine [anteroposterior (AP) and lateral view]
- X-ray chest [posteroanterior (PA) view]
- X-ray mastoid (both Law's and Towne's view) for ear pathology
- X-ray internal auditory meatus for any widening of the meatus
- X-ray skull, in cases of suspected intracranial space occupying lesions.

CT/MRI scan: Indications of imaging in cases of acute vertigo are:
- Acute vertigo with normal HIT
- Single-sided or asymmetric sensorineural hearing loss
- Other brainstem or cerebellar symptoms apart from vertigo
- Factors that may predispose to stroke (e.g., diabetes, hypertension, and history of ischemic heart disease) and acute onset associated with neck pain
- Any signs/symptoms indicating that vertigo may be of central origin as discussed later in "management".
- Direction changing SPN
- Sudden onset of new symptoms such as severe headache (especially occipital), facial palsy, and numbness
- Inability to stand or walk.

CT scan (high resolution) is indicated in suspected lesions in the temporal bone, temporal bone fractures, complications of cholesteatoma, e.g., erosion into the SCC, patients with conductive hearing loss with vertigo, superior canal dehiscence syndrome, labyrinthine ossification, etc.

MR imaging (with gadolinium enhancement) is the gold standard for imaging the eight cranial nerves, cerebellopontine angle area, cerebral hemisphere, brainstem and posterior fossa for neoplastic, and vascular and demyelinating lesions. MRI is indicated mainly in "complicated vertigo", especially when a central etiology like a stroke or transient ischemic attack (TIA) is suspected. MRI also detects subtle changes in the water content of the grey and white matter and therefore demonstrates tumors and MS plaques in a better detail. Cerebral infarction is also detected early by MRI within hours of the event. Magnetic resonance angiography (MRA) is helpful in suspected cases of vascular occlusion or anomaly (VBI). (*Note:* Initially MRI may be falsely negative up to 48 hours in 10–15% cases of posterior circulatory stroke).

Electroencephalogram (EEG) and transcranial Doppler study in cases with history suggestive of seizures and vertebrobasilar artery insufficiency (VBI).

Vestibular function test: Following are the main laboratory tests recommended for assessment of a vertigo patient after the acute attack is over: (1) pure tone audiometry (PTA); (2) impedance; (3) routine blood tests; (4) radiology; (5) ENG; (6) craniocorpography (CCG); (7) computerized dynamic posturography (CDP)—for postural instability; (8) rotational chair—for VOR; and (9) vestibular evoked myogenic potential (VEMP).

- *Electronystagmography:* It is a test to ascertain the functioning of the VOR system in which the nystagmus can be studied, both quantitatively and qualitatively and helps to localize a lesion in the vestibulo-ocular system. The usual battery of tests for ENG includes calibration, pendular tracking, SPN (both with eyes closed and eyes open—SNEC and SNEO), gaze nystagmus, positional nystagmus, bithermal caloric test (to find canal paresis, directional preponderance—CP and DP), OKR test, and rotational test. ENG being noninvasive and documentary test of vestibulo-ocular system is recommended in all patients but has its own limitations of being poor in sensitivity and limited in the assessment of vestibular connections and in inability to assess the vestibulospinal system.
- *Craniocorpography:* It is photographic recording of patient's head and the body movements during "Unterberger's stepping test" and "Romberg's test" and useful in assessment of VSR. It has an inherent limitation in its inability to detect the lesion in the "proprioceptive or visual input" system.
- *Computerized dynamic posturography:* It is useful in documenting the patterns of sensory organization and motor control during various visual and support-surface challenges. It incorporates separate protocols for assessment of sensory (afferent) and motor (efferent) pathways. The sensory path (input) is called sensory organization test and any defect in sensory input can be individually detected, i.e., visual, proprioceptive, or labyrinthine input. Additionally, this test studies whether CNS can select the most accurate input when contradictory information is sent through the visual-vestibular-somatosensory systems. In this test, these three

inputs are individually and also collectively manipulated and the ability of the subject to maintain balance under these manipulated conditions is then assessed by a computer.

The test for *motor output system (motor coordination test)* reveals whether the reflex motor activity for the maintenance of balance is being and effectively executed after the sensory information from the somatosensory, visual and vestibular inputs have been received and integrated by the brain. CDP test is highly sensitive in detecting the central vestibular pathologies and nonvestibular brain pathology.

- *Rotational chair testing (RCT):* It is available in only selective centers. It assesses the VOR and visual-vestibular interaction throughout a broad frequency and velocity range and is helpful mainly in cases of bilateral vestibular loss, central lesions, or a poor compensation following a unilateral loss.
- *Vestibular evoked myogenic potentials:* It is a short latency muscle reflex evoked by labyrinthine stimulation due to sound or vibration. Cervical VEMP (cVEMP) is recorded from sternocleidomastoid muscle due to activation of vestibulocollic pathway, i.e., otolith organ saccules, vestibular nerve, VN, medial VST to the sternocleidomastoid muscle, then accessory nerve and accessory nucleus. It tests ipsilateral saccule and inferior vestibular nerve.

Ocular VEMP (oVEMP) recorded from extraocular muscle (inferior oblique) is a part of VOR. It tests the contralateral superior vestibular nerve and predominantly utricle.

Vestibular evoked myogenic potential like caloric test does not indicate any specific disease. A large VEMP with abnormally low threshold is characteristically seen in presence of third mobile window, e.g., superior SCC dehiscence or large vestibular aqueduct syndrome.

■ MANAGEMENT

After taking detailed history and performing relevant examination and available laboratory tests, one must try to find out whether the AVA is because of peripheral labyrinthine (8th nerve disease), central vestibular disease, or a diffuse lesion. If the AVA is because of labyrinthine, whether it is unilateral or bilateral pathology and whether the attack is an acute isolated or acute recurrent attack.

■ COMMON DIFFERENTIAL DIAGNOSIS FOR AVA

- Vestibular neuritis (dizziness only)
- Labyrinthitis (dizziness + hearing loss or tinnitus)
- Brainstem or cerebellar (infarction/hemorrhage)
- Multiple sclerosis (very rare).

The distinctive "peripheral vestibular pathology" is unique and it is easy to differentiate between peripheral and central vestibular pathology. BPPV, vestibular neuritis, Meniere's disease, and migraine are the most encountered peripheral vestibular causes. Less common diseases include vestibular schwannoma, PLF, labyrinthine trauma, autoimmune inner ear disease, and sudden sensorineural hearing loss (SSHL) with acute vertigo among others. In central vestibular lesions, on the other hand, there are always symptoms and signs of CNS because of disruption of connection along the pathways from the VN to the cortex. Commonly encountered central vestibular pathologies are vascular insufficiency, head trauma, demyelination, tumors, and degenerative diseases.

If the "AVA" is because of labyrinthine lesion, unilateral/bilateral involvement must be assessed for treatment and better prognosis, e.g., Meniere's disease. If bilateral, hearing conservation therapy is the main concern.

Also, "AVA" whether isolated acute or recurrent acute, helps in determining treatment protocol. "Vestibular neuritis", being most common isolated acute attack needs only symptomatic treatment while BPPV and Meniere's disease, both with recurrent acute attacks need different management protocols.

■ RED FLAG SIGNS

- Any neurologic deficit
- Total ipsilateral hearing loss
- Rapid evolution of symptoms and signs and presence of associated risk factors
- *Character of SPN:* Direction changing (gaze evoked nystagmus) or purely vertical nystagmus, sustained or nonfatiguing positional nystagmus, dissociated/disconjugate nystagmus, and failure to suppress SPN with optic fixation
- Sudden onset of new symptoms such as severe headache, facial palsy, and numbness
- Impaired smooth pursuit/abnormal saccades/deranged optokinetic nystagmus
- Associated focal motor deficits
- *Deadly Ds*: Dysphagia, dysphonia, dysarthria, diplopia, dysesthesia, drop attacks, and down-up distortion (room tilt illusion)
- Horner's syndrome on examination
- Loss of superficial sensation on one side of the face or on the other side of the body
- Intractable hiccups
- Abnormal sitting posture, inability to stand straight or walk unsupported, and severe ataxia.

TABLE 1: Important oculomotor signs in central vertigo.

	Peripheral	Central
Head impulse	Impaired	Normal
Direction changing nystagmus	–	+
Skew deviation	–	+

The *HINTS to INFARCT* approach is useful to diagnose patient of stroke with AVA.

Three important oculomotor signs in central vertigo are mentioned in **Table 1**.

■ MEDICAL TREATMENT

Acute vertigo attack is usually a severe clinical entity followed by nausea, vomiting, and other neurovegetative symptoms involving transient physical disability requiring urgent hospitalization.

The treatment planning involves symptomatic relief, i.e., the drugs to take care of acute vertigo with nausea and vomiting.
- Strict bed rest in a quiet room and administration of vestibular suppressants and antiemetics.
- Intravenous antibiotics (broad-spectrum) in suspected infective pathologies.
- Intravenous fluids and electrolyte replacement.

Drug Therapy

- *Acute vertigo with spontaneous nystagmus and nausea/vomiting:*
  - Intravenous fluids as per patient's clinical condition.
  - Diazepam 10 mg intramuscular or intravenous together with combination of dimenhydrinate 50 mg or diphenhydramine 15 mg.
  - Diazepam intravenous in 3–5 minutes provides most rapid relief of symptoms (intravenous line in a large vein to avoid venous thrombosis). More drug can be added to the intravenous bottle and infused slowly if severe symptoms recur and dose can be titrated by observing its effect on the nystagmus, turning both the nystagmus and vertigo sensation on or off by slowing or quickening intravenous rate. Always have resuscitation equipment ready if using intravenous diazepam because of its respiratory depressive effect. For the accompanying nausea and vomiting, intravenous "droperidol" is highly effective (2–5 mg intravenous every 3 hourly maximum three doses only). It also needs cardiopulmonary monitoring because of respiratory depressive effect.

- *In refractive vertigo with nausea/vomiting:* Promethazine 25–50 mg intramuscular is used instead of dimenhydrinate. Ondansetron can also be used to control persistent vomiting.
- "Promethazine hydrochloride" 25–50 mg, intramuscular or per-rectum or prochlorperazine 12.5–25 mg intramuscular or per-rectum can also be used as vestibular suppressants as well as antiemetic.
- Ondansetron, a serotonin antagonist specific for 5HT3 receptor found in chemoreceptor trigger zone (CTZ) and vomiting center, is useful to control nausea and vomiting. The recommended doses are 8 mg per orally twice daily or a single intravenous dose of 8–32 mg (0.15 mg/kg) given slowly over 15 minutes. "Glycopyrrolate" is another available anticholinergic drug which has mild vestibular suppressant effect, given in dose of 0.1 mg/kg/intravenous. Steroids can be administered to enhance the antiemetic and antivertigo effect of certain drugs (dexamethasone 4 mg intramuscular).

Note: Dimenhydrinate, diphenhydramine, and promethazine are antihistaminics, so only one should be used at a time and not more than one should be administered concurrently due to possibility of potentiation of side effects. It is also necessary that an 8-hour safe window period is required before administering another antihistaminic dose.

- *In cases of acute vertigo with positioning vertigo:* In addition, rehabilitative techniques depending on the SCC involved can be initiated.
  - Epley or modified Epley for posterior semicircular canal (PSC)-BPPV
  - Semont is an alternative maneuver for PSC-BPPV
  - Geotropic and horizontal SC (HSC)-BPPV is treated by log roll exercise
  - Gufoni maneuver is indicated in apogeotropic HSC-BPPV
  - Yacovino maneuver is indicated in AC-BPPV.

Maintenance Therapy

Maintenance therapy is given once the acute phase is over. "Diazepam" is generally given on a short-term basis (2, 5, or 10 mg, 6–8 hourly), depending on the severity of the patient's symptoms and level of anxiety. "Meclizine" in dose of 12.5–25 mg, 6–8 hourly or "dimenhydrinate" in dose of 50–100 mg, 6–8 hourly can be used. All these drugs have "sedation" as the most encountered side effect. Promethazine 25 mg 6–8 hourly and prochlorperazine 5 mg 8 hourly oral or by rectal suppository at 25 mg BD dosage are also useful for control of nausea and vomiting on an OPD basis.

Certain drugs can be prescribed to accelerate vestibular compensation which include *calcium-antagonists* (cinnarizine 25–75 mg, 8 hourly), *"betahistines"* (8–16 mg, 8 hourly), and *"gangliosides"* (Ginkgo biloba extract), the former two groups have an additional action as vestibular sedatives. "Cinnarizine" has additional benefit of improving cerebral circulation, maintaining red blood cell (RBC) flexibility, and reducing blood viscosity. "Ginkgo biloba" has antiplatelet aggregation effect, improves arterial and venous tone in hypoxic areas, inhibits oxygenated free radicals, and increases turnover of norepinephrine in the brain, given in dose of 1 tablet BD. Domperidone, 15 mg with cinnarizine 20 mg is a good combination which can be safely advised for management of vertigo associated with nausea and vomiting on outpatient department (OPD) basis.

In cases of *"Meniere's disease"*, potassium-sparing diuretic therapy with sodium restriction (1–2 g/day) is the recommended regimen. "Betahistine" (8–16 mg hourly or 24 mg BD) is also used with added benefit of sparing of vestibular compensation. Meclizine and diazepam are used only for acute recurrent attacks and not in between spells. Transtympanic low-dose gentamycin is preferred by some authors for unilateral Meniere's disease.

Benign paroxysmal positional vertigo patients should not be treated with vestibular sedatives. Rather, canalolith repositioning therapy (Epley's maneuver) is recommended in such cases.

Steroids

Steroids are used in certain inner ear disorders like SSHL with sudden onset vertigo, vestibular neuronitis, autoimmune causes, and Meniere's disease. Dexamethasone 4–6 mg bid or prednisone 1 mg/kg body weight/day is given for 10 days and then dose is tapered off in next 5–10 days.

The various vestibular suppressants drugs used in treatment of vertigo have been tabulated in **Table 2**.

Surgical Therapy

Only a small fraction (<5%) of all dizzy patients require surgical intervention which present with recurrent AVAs from unilateral disease and refractory to conservative management as discussed earlier. Surgical procedures can be ablative/nonablative with hearing preserved/hearing destroyed.

Ablative procedures are transmastoid labyrinthectomy and vestibular nerve section and transtympanic gentamycin therapy. Nonablative procedure includes endolymphatic sac decompression, and posterior canal occlusion (refractory case of BPPV). The details of these surgical procedures are beyond the scope of this chapter and must be looked into relevant books.

■ ACUTE CENTRAL VERTIGO

Prevalence of cerebrovascular disease in patient reporting to ENT emergency with acute dizziness is approximately 3–6%. Posterior fossa stroke accounts for estimated 25% of AVA and up to 90–96% are ischemic strokes. CT scan has low sensitivity for acute ischemic stroke. MRI, even with DWI can miss up to

TABLE 2: Vestibular suppressants drugs (VSDs).

Drug	Dosage	Frequency in day	Pregnancy category
Dimenhydrinate	50 mg	4–6 hours	B
Diphenhydramine	25–50 mg	4–6 hours	B
Meclizine	25 mg	8 hours	B
Cinnarizine	25 mg	8 hours	C
Betahistine	8–16 mg	8 hours	B2
Antiemetics			
Domperidone	10–20 mg	6–8 hours	B
Metoclopramide	5–10 mg	6 hours	A
Ondansetron	8 mg	12 hours	B
Prochlorperazine	5–10 mg	6 hours	C
Benzodiazepines*			
Alprazolam	0.25–0.50 mg	8 hours	
Clonazepam	0.25–0.50 mg	8 hours	
Diazepam	5–10 mg	12 hours	
Lorazepam	1–2 mg	8 hours	

- Pregnancy category A—adequate and well controlled studies have failed to demonstrate a risk to the fetus.
- Pregnancy Category B—animal studies show no risk to the fetus.
- Pregnancy Category C—no controlled studies have been conducted in animals or humans).

*Most benzodiazepines belong to category D and hence avoided in pregnancy.

TABLE 3: HINTS plus. HINTS plus is an important bedside examination for a suspected acute central lesion.

1.	*Head impulse (HI):* Look for corrective saccade. Its absence is indicative of central pathology
2.	*Testing nystagmus (NT):* If nystagmus is direction changing/vertical/torsional, it suggests central lesion
3.	*Skew deviation (S):* Its presence is indicative of a central pathology
4.	*General neurological examination (brainstem and cerebellar testing):* Any neurological component indicates central lesion
5.	*Gait:* Inability to sit/stand/walk unassisted indicates central pathology
6.	*Bedside hearing assessment (bone conduction) for SNHL:* • Mainly peripheral except vestibular neuritis • SNHL can be seen in central lesion (AICA, labyrinthine stroke)

(AICA: anterior inferior cerebellar artery; SNHL: sensorineural hearing loss)

20% of strokes in AVA during first 24–48 hours. HINTS plus **(Table 3)** is more useful in clinical setting as a bedside tool.

The main causes include vascular disorders (stroke, TIA, and VBI); vertebrobasilar migraine, MS, tumors, seizures, and Arnold–Chiari malformations. TIA can present with dizziness/attack of vertigo. Approximately 5% of TIA suffer stroke within 48 hours; therefore, requires prompt diagnosis and treatment.

Acute central vertigo manifests as marked vertigo, nausea, and vertical nystagmus, along with additional neurologic symptoms (headache and gait ataxia). Hearing loss is rare and in some cases nausea may be absent. In severe cases, level of consciousness may be depressed. Because central lesions have more profound consequences, aggressive work-up and treatment are recommended:

- Intravenous fluids to rehydrate the patient
- Complete bed rest
- Parenteral medicines for symptomatic relief
- Always have a high level of suspicion in the presence of risk factors (advanced age, atrial fibrillation, diabetes, hypertension, and history of previous cerebrovascular accident) even if the symptoms are mild.
- Get neurologist/neurosurgical opinion. Consider neurologic imaging (MRI preferred over CT scan).
- In presence of acute neurologic deficit, it is often difficult to distinguish intracranial hemorrhage from ischemic infarct. Avoid administration of anticoagulants including aspirin, until intracranial hemorrhage has been ruled out by an indicated imaging modality, as hemorrhage in the cranium can cause rapid compression and compromise the vital medullary function due to herniation of medullary tonsils and obstructive hydrocephalus.
- In cases of *"acute ischemic stroke"* (clinically and radiologically proven), consider thrombolytic therapy and seek an urgent neurologist's opinion. (Thrombolytic therapy is contraindicated in patients who underwent major surgery in last 10 days, severe uncontrolled hypertension, evidence of acute hemorrhage or edema on CT scan of head, and rapidly improving symptoms.)
- Lethargic patients or those with altered level of consciousness require close clinical monitoring, electrocardiogram (ECG), pulse oximetry, and should be kept in "neuro-ICU" as they may need emergent intervention to minimize intracranial swelling and brainstem compression. They may also need an endotracheal intubation to protect the airway, control breathing, and allow therapeutic hyperventilation. Elevation of the head end of bed, perform diuresis with mannitol or furosemide, and administration of parenteral steroids may help to reduce brain edema.
- Always obtain "neurologic consultation" for all patients with central vertigo and "neurosurgical consultation" for all patients with space-occupying lesions or hydrocephalus. Suboccipital craniotomy or ventriculostomy may be lifesaving in patients with hemorrhage, brainstem compression, or edema.

- To palliate the symptoms of vertigo and/or ataxia, benzodiazepines (lorazepam, clonazepam, and diazepam) are useful but can cause psychological addiction and physical dependence. Gabapentin (100 mg BID to 600 mg TID) is useful to suppress SPN. Meclizine (25–50 mg BID to TID) and prochlorperazine can also be used. Non-responding acute vertigo may be managed with ondansetron. Carbamazepine and oxcarbazepine have also been tried in patients with epilepsy, or brief paroxysmal symptoms, micro-vascular compression or intrinsic brainstem lesion.
- Patients with VBI and evidence of small vessel cerebrovascular disease benefit from low dose aspirin (75–150 mg every day) or more potent antiplatelet agents or anticoagulant if TIA persists. Pentoxifylline (400 mg TID) may be used to reduce the viscosity.
- Pyritinol (Encephabol) 300 mg once daily is useful in head trauma patients (concussion vertigo) and acts by increasing uptake and utilization of glucose and oxygen in the CNS.
- For headache, especially in vertebrobasilar migraine, verapamil (120–240 mg sustained release) or amitriptyline (10 mg nightly, gradually increasing to 25–50 mg), or beta-blockers may be tried.

Follow-up

All patients need proper follow-up, especially in "vertigo clinic" staffed by team of otologists, neurologists, cardiologists, and physiotherapists. It is important to stop or modify medication used in acute stages of vertigo after assessment of symptom improvement, especially in acute vestibular conditions. Medications such as antihistaminics and steroids should be used only for a brief period for symptomatic relief. Some of these medications, are labyrinthine sedatives and may interfere in recovery of vestibular system during rehabilitation. Patients who have stable peripheral or central vestibular lesion, are advised rehabilitative therapy (various head and neck exercises, Cooksey Cawthorne exercises for vestibular compensation and Epley's maneuver and Brandt Daroff exercises for BPPV) to enhance central compensation. Dietary modification (avoidance of salted meat and fish, condensed milk, cheese, caffeine), healthy lifestyle habits, abstinence from alcohol, smoking and yoga. Meditation is also advised in the subsequent follow-up. Physical therapy, emphasizing effective use of appliances such as canes, walkers and footwear is also useful. It is also important to emphasize on maintenance of good eye sight as vision compensates for lack of vestibular function.

The major differences between acute peripheral vertigo and acute central vertigo have been outlined in **Table 4.**

Common Disorders Causing Acute Vertigo

- *Benign paroxysmal positional vertigo:* It is diagnosed by Dix–Hallpike maneuver and clinically presents with episodes of rotational vertigo

TABLE 4: Acute peripheral/acute central vertigo.

	Acute peripheral vertigo	*Acute central vertigo*
Onset	Sudden	Sudden (may be gradual)
Severity of vertigo	Severe, disabling	Less severe and less disabling
Change of head or body position	Vertigo increases	No remarkable change
Associated autonomic features (nausea, vomiting, pallor, diaphoresis)	Prominent	Less severe, may be absent
Nystagmus	• Horizontal or torsional (never vertical) • Always unidirectional with fast phase away from affected ear. Jerk nystagmus tends to follow Alexander's law, which states that in peripheral jerk nystagmus, the intensity of nystagmus increases on looking to the side of fast component • No effect of change in direction of gaze • Suppression with visual fixation • Fatigable with repeat testing • Latency from stimulus to onset	• Pure horizontal/vertical or rotatory • Unidirectional/multidirectional and may change direction with changes in direction of gaze (gaze evoked) • May increase with direction of gaze towards affected ear • No effect on intensity with visual fixation • Nonfatigable • No latency from stimulus to onset
Hearing loss, tinnitus	May be present	Very rare
Visual suppression	Yes	No
Direction of Romberg fall and past pointing	Opposite to the direction of fast phase of nystagmus	Same as that of fast component of nystagmus if unidirectional
CNS symptoms/signs	Absent	Present
Gait	• Mild to moderate ataxia • Sway/tendency to fall towards the side of lesion (opposite the nystagmus fast phase)	• Moderate to severe ataxia • Inability to walk or tendency to fall to either side
Head thrust (Halmagyi) test	Positive (corrective saccade present)	Negative (no corrective saccade)

(CNS: central nervous system)

lasting less than a minute, upon sudden changes of head position, especially on lying down and turning the head toward the affected ear. The cause is mechanical, either cupulolithiasis or canalolith formation. Symptomatic relief of acute attack is achieved by benzodiazepine, meclizine, diphenhydramine, or cinnarizine. Epley's canalith repositioning maneuver helps in treatment of 85–95% cases.

Central positioning vertigo/nystagmus: It is due to lesion of semicircular canals and their connection in vestibular nucleus and cerebellum; mostly caused by vestibular imbalance due to disinhibition of vestibular reflexes. Common causes are:
- Cerebrovascular disorders
- Spinocerebellar ataxia
- Multiple sclerosis
- Arnold-Chiari type 1 malformation
- Tumors of brainstem and cerebellum
- Some drugs.

Features usually mimic BPPV in terms of latency, course and direction of nystagmus, fatigability, vertigo, and vomiting. Important clinical differentiating point is—presence of pure vertical positional nystagmus which does not fatigue with repeated testing. MRI is a diagnostic test. The following clinical features are important for diagnosing central positioning vertigo:
- Persistent positional nystagmus
- Positioning-induced vomiting after single head movement without any clinically significant vertigo or nystagmus
- Positional/positioning vertigo with torsional/vertical nystagmus
- Positional/positioning nystagmus which does not correlate with the plane of semicircular canal stimulated by the head positioning.
  (*Note*: Positional nystagmus beating toward the upper most ear or lasting longer than 1 minute is no longer considered a reliable indicator of central pathology as both occur with the cupulolithiasis variant of BPPV.) **(Table 5)**

- *Labyrinthitis:* It commonly follows otitis media, URI, meningitis or drug toxicity. Clinically, patients have acute vertigo, hearing loss, nausea, vomiting, and fever. Suppurative labyrinthitis may also follow bacterial invasion via PLF, cochlear aqueduct, or internal auditory canal. Patient needs intravenous antibiotics and surgical treatment of otitis media (cholesteatoma).

Labyrinthitis secondary to otitis media (acute/chronic): Clinically, three types of labyrinthitis may present in ENT emergency as AVA.
1. *Circumscribed labyrinthitis (labyrinthine fistula):* Patient presents with brief periods of imbalance, dysequilibrium or vertigo, and Tullio phenomenon (loud sound provoked brief imbalance). Clinically,

TABLE 5: Difference between BPPV and central positioning vertigo/nystagmus (CPV).

	BPPV	CPV
Latency	Up to 30 seconds	Nil
Duration of nystagmus	Up to 10 seconds	>30 seconds
Direction of nystagmus	• Torsional/vertical (P, A canal) • Horizontal (H canal)	Pure vertical or torsional unrelated to any canal axis
Fatigability	Seen	No
Vertigo	+	−
Nausea	+++	+
Vomiting	Variable	Variable
Additional neurological signs	Nil	±

(BPPV: benign paroxysmal positional vertigo)

fistula test is positive in 55–70% of lateral SSC fistula. But if present, it is single most indicator for surgical exploration. High-resolution computed tomography (HRCT) is also helpful for diagnosis. Management is canal wall up/canal wall down mastoidectomy and management of fistula. If fistula is small, cholesteatoma matrix can be easily elevated. If fistula is large, it is advisable to leave fistula covered with matrix.

2. *Diffuse serous labyrinthitis:* Defined as reversible nonpurulent inflammation of inner ear. Clinically, patient has vertigo, nausea, vomiting, and spontaneous nystagmus (beating toward involved ear) with some element of sensorineural hearing loss. If untreated, complicates into suppurative labyrinthitis. Management is with hospitalization, bed rest, intravenous fluids, intravenous antibiotics, and labyrinthine sedatives. Surgical intervention includes myringotomy and cortical mastoidectomy in ASOM and while patients with CSOM require modified radical or radical mastoidectomy.

3. *Diffuse purulent labyrinthitis:* It defines the stage when inflammation yields pus formation in inner ear. Tinnitus and dizziness rapidly grow to manifest as whirling vertigo, pallor, diaphoresis, nausea, and repeated vomiting.

Initially, spontaneous nystagmus (irritative) beats toward the infected ear, soon to be replaced by paralytic nystagmus beating toward normal/opposite ear. This determines the preference of patient to lie on healthy ear. After 2–3 weeks, CNS compensation results in near-normal/normal body balance. Tinnitus may continue but patient has complete nerve deafness. Treatment is same as serous labyrinthitis.

- *Vestibular neuronitis:* It is acute unilateral vestibulopathy, presenting with a paroxysmal and prolonged single attack following a nonspecific viral illness, with no cochlear symptoms. Treatment is mainly symptomatic along with steroids. The role of antiviral is controversial.
- *Meniere's disease:* It is an idiopathic inner ear disorder presenting with acute vertigo, fluctuating sensorineural hearing loss, tinnitus and aural fullness, which occur because of endolymphatic hydrops. Nystagmus is of horizontal type with rotatory component with slow phase toward the side of affected ear. Patient feels comfortable to lie down with affected ear up and avoids looking to the normal side. Electrocochleography (ECOG) is a test to diagnose endolymphatic hydrops but with a specificity of only about 40%. Low salt diet and diuretics are main stay of medical treatment along with vestibular suppressants (cinnarizine or betahistine). In refractory cases, surgery may be advised or chemical ablation with transtympanic gentamycin injection is indicated.
- *Vertebrobasilar insufficiency and brainstem stroke:* Vertebrobasilar insufficiency refers to TIA affecting the posterior circulation (supplying labyrinth, brainstem, cerebellum, and occipital lobes). When significant vascular compromise lasts longer than several minutes, an infarction results (known as stroke or cerebrovascular accident). The presentation of "brainstem stroke" is acute vertigo along with neurologic symptoms (visual alteration, impaired muscle strength, coordination, and altered sensation). While VBI presents as acute vertigo with other brainstem symptoms or visual dysfunction (drop attack, mental status change, limb ataxia, dysarthria, inversion of environment, loss of consciousness, tinnitus, perioral numbness, focal sensory or motor dysfunction, visual loss, and diplopia), along with nausea and vomiting.

  Most common central cause of vertigo is *Wallenberg's syndrome (lateral medullary infarction)* **(Fig. 1)** caused due to ischemia in the distribution of posterior-inferior cerebellar artery (PICA), i.e., dorsolateral medullary plate and portion of posterior medial cerebellum (uvula, nodulus, paraflocculus, and nucleus ambiguous). The patient presents with acute vertigo, spontaneous nystagmus, facial and limb numbness, disequilibrium, dysarthria, dysphagia, unusual visual illusion and incoordination, decreased facial sensation ipsilaterally, "dissociated" sensory loss to pain and temperature contralaterally, Horner's syndrome (with ptosis and anisocoria), ipsilateral limb ataxia, and gait ataxia. Vocal cord palsy, decreased gag and palatal reflexes, and skew deviation are the pathognomonic findings.

  Pontine syndrome (mixed central-peripheral lesion): This is because of anterior-inferior cerebellar artery (AICA) **(Fig. 2)** involvement, which supplies the lateral pons, part of middle cerebellar peduncle and facial and 8th cranial nerves via internal auditory artery and 6th nerve nucleus.

Acute Vertigo

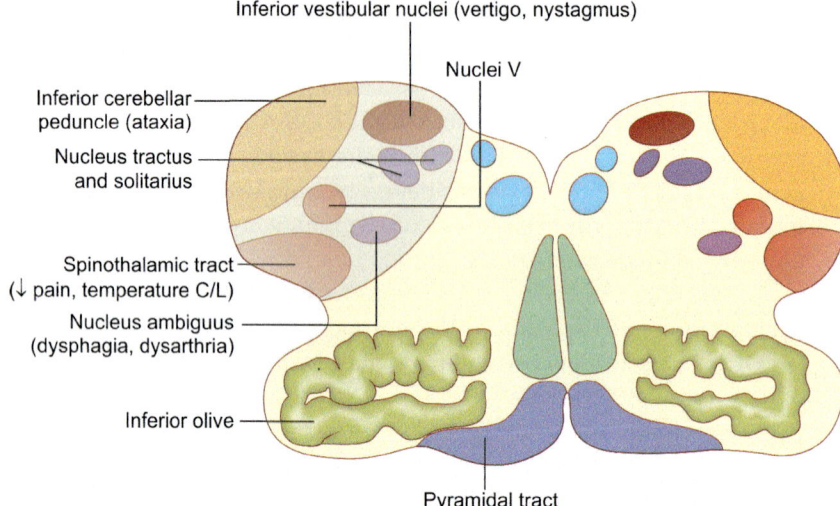

Fig. 1: Lateral medullary syndrome of Wallenberg (PICA).

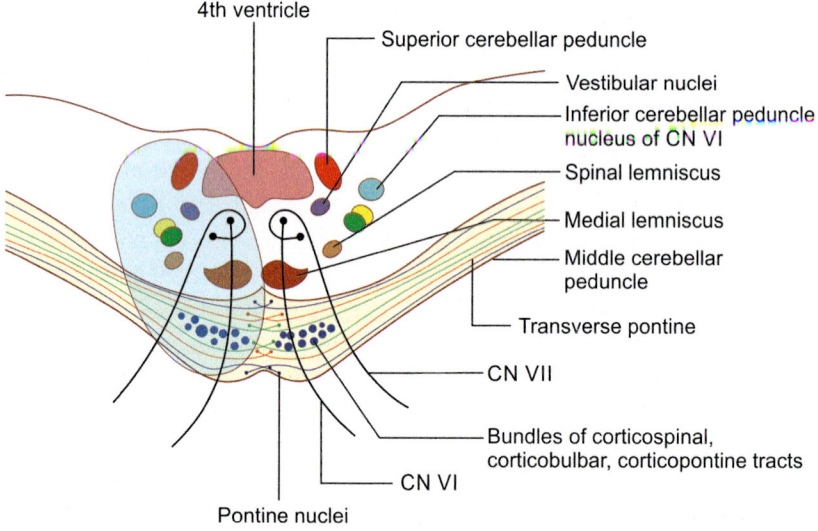

Fig. 2: Pontine hemorrhage.

The clinical presentation of peripheral lesion that includes hearing loss, *screaming* tinnitus, acute vertigo, direction-fixed nystagmus, and facial palsy in a patient with vascular risk factors should make one suspicious of central pathology. The signs of brainstem involvement include: dysarthria, paresthesia, Horner's syndrome, gait and cerebellar ataxia, ipsilateral facial hemianesthesia, and contralateral hemibody sensory loss.

Typical of AICA syndrome:
- Tinnitus, hearing loss, and facial weakness
- Gaze palsy
- Ipsilateral reduced response on caloric testing.

Typical of PICA syndrome:
- Hoarseness
- Skew deviation
- Vocal cord palsy on fiberoptic laryngoscopy
- Saccadic lateropulsion

Features seen in both AICA and PICA syndrome (due to damage of 5th nerve nucleus, spinothalamic tract and vestibular nuclei):
- Vertigo.
- Facial and limb numbness
- Dysphagia
- Vestibular nystagmus
- Horner's syndrome
- Ipsilateral limb ataxia
- Ipsilateral facial decreased sensation
- Contralateral dissociated sensory loss to pain and temperature.

Cerebellar hemorrhage: It presents clinically with vertical or gaze evoked direction changing nystagmus, not suppressed with visual fixation (in contrast to unidirectional spontaneous nystagmus accentuated with gaze in the quick phase direction, in acute labyrinthine lesion). Patient is unable to stand unassisted (*Note:* In a patient with acute vertigo with a sudden headache and inability to ambulate, suspect cerebellar hemorrhage until proven otherwise, even in the absence of other neurological signs).

Investigation in VBI-induced lesions includes "transcranial Doppler" and MRI angiography. Treatment of VBI includes reduction of risk factors and antiplatelet therapy along with urgent neurologist/neurosurgical opinion.

- *Acoustic neuroma (vestibular schwannoma):* It usually presents with unilateral hearing loss or tinnitus. But 5% of cases may present with paroxysmal attacks of vertigo (mimicking Meniere's disease), 16% may have momentary vertigo on sudden head movements and 8% may suffer acute vestibular failure with or without hearing loss. MRI of the internal acoustic meatus (gadolinium enhanced) is gold standard diagnostic test.
- *Perilymph fistula:* Intermittent vertigo, fluctuating sensorineural hearing loss, tinnitus, dizziness, and motion intolerance are the observed clinical features. Management includes bed rest for 1-2 weeks and to avoid any straining action. Surgical repair may be indicated in severe cases of PLF.
- *Superior semicircular canal dehiscence (SSC):* It usually presents with episodic dizziness, pulsatile oscillopsia, Tullio phenomenon (vertigo and nystagmus induced by loud sound), and Hennebert's sign. In addition, patient has pulsatile tinnitus, mixed hearing loss, and autophony. HRCT scan (Pöschl view) and VEMP are diagnostic.
- *Multiple sclerosis:* Vertigo can be paroxysmal, positional or may persist for long duration. Pendular nystagmus and internuclear ophthalmoplegia

are common. If demyelinating plaque occurs at the roof of entry zone of vestibular zone or nucleus, clinical presentation is similar to vestibular neuritis, i.e., true vertigo, vomiting, horizontal—torsional nystagmus with fast phase toward healthy side with visual suppression. If auditory nerve is involved, sudden nerve deafness occurs, if only vestibular nuclei are involved, all features typical of peripheral lesion are seen except optic fixation does not suppress the nystagmus.

If central vestibular structure such as vestibular nuclei, cerebellar peduncles, or cerebellum is involved—severe ataxia, cranial nerve palsies, central type nystagmus, intention tremor, and pyramidal tract dysfunction along with vertigo are presenting features.

- *Vestibular migraine*: It presents with recurrent attacks of various combination of vertigo, cervical muscle spasm, ataxia of stance and gait, photophobia, phonophobia, brainstem symptoms, accompanied or followed by head pressure, pain, nausea, or vomiting. In addition, memory disturbance and fear are also seen. Treatment is similar to migraine with aura, including beta-blockers, calcium channel blockers, serotonin reuptake inhibitors, valproic acid, or topiramate. Tricyclic antidepressants are prescribed for prophylaxis. During an acute attack—aspirin and antiemetics are offered.
- *Motion sickness:* It is an acute clinical syndrome, arising during passive transportation in moving vehicle because of mismatch between vestibular-visual stimuli. Nausea and vomiting develop within minutes to hours associated with dizziness, physical discomfort, tiredness, periodic yawning and pallor, as well as slight vertigo (subjective and objective, both). Facial pallor, cold sweats, increased salivation, hypersensitivity to smells, pain in occipital region, and pressure feeling in upper abdomen are the other features. Spontaneous amnesia occurs in hours to 1 day after the end of the stimulus and if stimulus continues, relief occurs within 3 days because of centrally mediated adaptation (habituation). Motion sickness develops in closed vehicle or while reading on the back seat of a car. Treatment includes keeping head position supine with head in direction of movement (in cars), close the eyes to avoid optical-vestibular conflict, and antivertiginous drugs such as dimenhydrinate or belladonna alkaloids (0.5 mg scopolamine transdermal patch), diazepam 2-5 mg TID as advised. Cinnarizine 20 mg and domperidone 15 mg are also recommended in the dose of one tablet, ½ to 1 hour prior to onset of journey and can be continued as ½ tablet (children <7 years) or 1 tablet TID (>7 years of age) for longer trips.
- *Post-traumatic vertigo:* Dizziness post head injury is reported in 25–90% cases and has a significant medicolegal importance. Any trauma to head, neck, or craniocervical junction or temporal bone fracture can result in peripheral or central vestibular dysfunction, clinically

TABLE 6: Clinical test: localization value.

Hemogram and blood sugar	Anemia, hypoglycemia.
Cardiac examination, electrocardiogram (ECG) with rhythm strip	Cardiac arrhythmia, e.g., atrial fibrillation (may be source of embolic stroke)
Hyperventilation	Anxiety/psychogenic
Ear examination	External and middle ear pathology
Fistula test	Labyrinthine fistula
Romberg's test	Proprioception, vestibulospinal tracts
Tandem gait test	Body balance system assessment
Spontaneous nystagmus	Vestibular lesion
Upbeat/downbeat/disconjugate nystagmus	Brainstem involvement
Dix-Hallpike maneuver	BPPV/central positional vertigo
Cranial nerves	Brainstem, cerebellopontine angle (CPA)
Cerebellar test	Central lesion
Oculomotor test (saccade, pursuit, fixation)	Central pathology

(BPPV: benign paroxysmal positional vertigo)

presenting as short-lasting symptomatology to severe disabling vertigo with vomiting.

Early vestibular syndrome occurring within 24 hours of trauma (due to falls, road traffic accidents, assault, and contact sport) include BPPV, labyrinthine concussion, traumatic labyrinthine dysfunction, and PLF (due to rupture of oval or round window membrane), and sudden SNHL. Early central vertigo is due to dysfunction of the brainstem or the cerebellum caused by a direct concussion of these structures or secondary to ischemia caused by a traumatic dissection of a vertebral artery. Trauma or concussion or hemorrhage along the central vestibular pathway can also lead to acute central vertigo.

In general, the common causes of vertigo can broadly be localized from the relevant clinical tests (**Table 6**). Other causes such as cervical vertigo, syphilis, and metabolic disorders are beyond the scope of this chapter and relevant books may be referred. The management algorithm of acute vertigo attack is summarized in **Flowchart 1**.

■ ACUTE VERTIGO IN CHILDREN

Acute vertigo in children is mostly benign and can be treated effectively with favorable prognosis. Most common causes include:

- Vascular—migraine and benign paroxysmal vertigo of childhood (BPVC)
- Infective—acute/chronic otitis media, viral labyrinthitis, and vestibular neuritis

Flowchart 1: Management algorithm of acute vertigo attack.

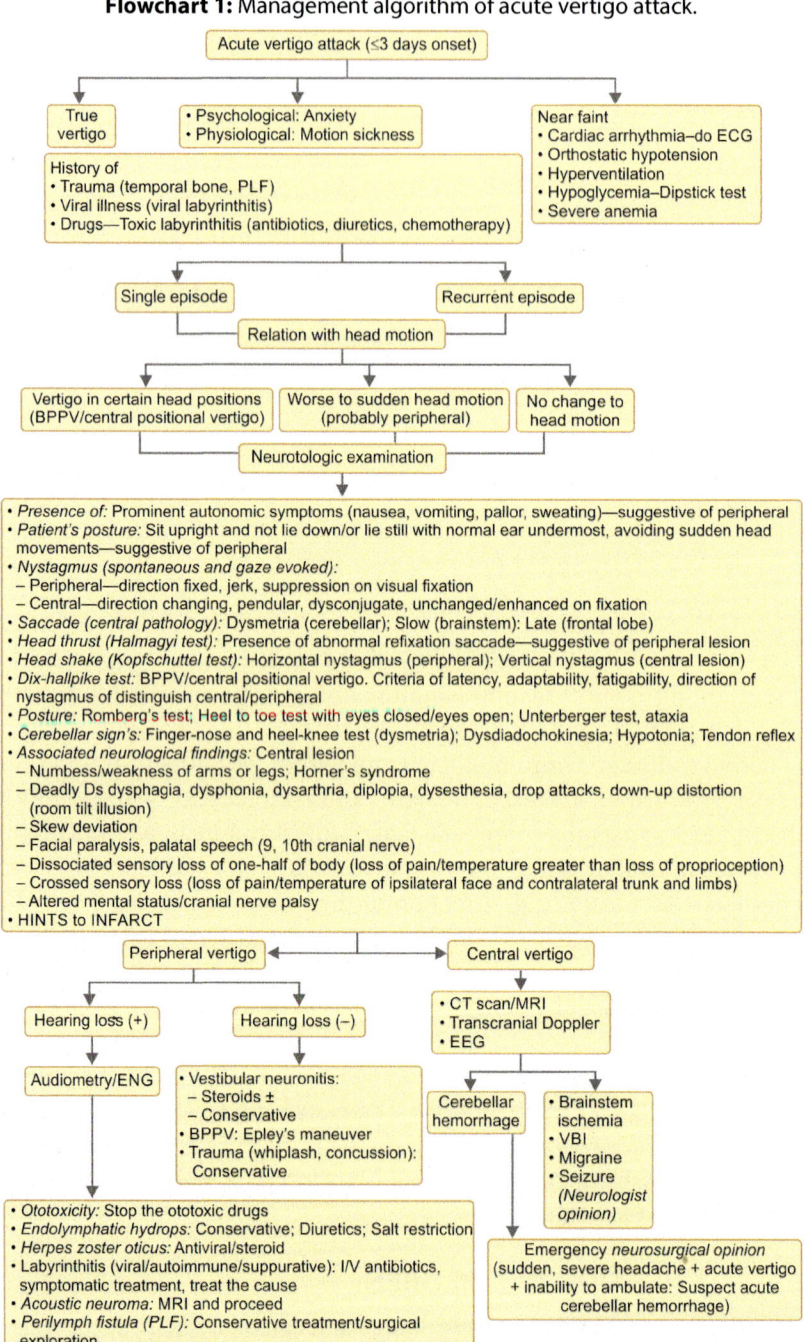

(BPPV: benign paroxysmal positional vertigo; CT: computed tomography; ECG: electrocardiogram; EEG: electroencephalogram; MRI: magnetic resonance imaging; PLF: perilymph fistula; VBI; vertebrobasilar insufficiency)

- Meniere's disease
- Miscellaneous—ototoxicity, psychogenic seizure/syncope, and congenital malformations.

"Acute vertigo in pediatric age group" is very difficult to manage because of difficulty in proper history taking and getting various investigations done. A dizzy child is unable to explain properly the sequence of events, precipitating or inducing factors, and any abnormal sensations perceived. Moreover, the parents blame the school premises, peer pressure, various mobile apps, social networking, or other behavioral problem for acute dizziness.

It is important to perform a detailed otological examination and rule out a middle ear infection or cholesteatoma of middle ear as cholesteatoma can be aggressive in children with cellular mastoid and occasional involve bony labyrinth resulting in vertigo of acute onset. This is particularly important as the management options are completely different for this subset of patients.

In the management of a child with acute onset vertigo, try to elicit detailed history from the parents or child including:
- Nature of symptoms
  - Acute/paroxysmal
  - Pure rotational sensations/blackout
  - Associated hearing loss/tinnitus
  - Change in symptoms with head positions
- History of vomiting, headache, head injury, concussion, and trauma
- Ask for provoking factors such as change in body and head position, cough, and sneezing
- Look for anxiety, depression, and level of sensorium
- Look for sleep deprivation, psychosocial stress, and history of drug intake
- Ask for family history of hearing loss, vascular headache including migraine, and seizures
- Conduct full neurological and otological examination.

Investigations

Magnetic resonance imaging is indicated to exclude encephalitis, congenital malformations, and space occupying lesions. Pure tone audiometry, activated brainstem response, nystagmogram, rotational testing, and other specific vestibular tests have limited role and may be useful only in otherwise cooperative child thus helping to differentiate peripheral from central pathology.

Head impulse test has been found to be more reliable than various laboratory tests.

Important Causes

- *Migraine associated vertigo:* It is most common diagnosis and presents with frontal or periorbital nonthrobbing headache usually <2 hours which

may precede, follow or occur simultaneously with dizziness. Associated features may be nausea and photophobia.
- *Benign paroxysmal vertigo of childhood:* It is regarded as migraine equivalent. BPVC is usually seen in <4 years of age to up to 8 years. Child appears frightened and feels a spinning sensation. Typical findings are: episodic vertigo of seconds to minutes associated with nystagmus in a frightened child who is unable to stand without support, vomiting, tinnitus, pallor, and diaphoresis, is seen. Important finding is absence of loss of consciousness and complete recovery after the attack. Caloric test may be normal or abnormal (complete unilateral or bilateral canal paresis). EEG and MRI brain are normal. In acute attack, betahistine is prescribed and for prophylaxis, propranolol 5 mg OD and magnesium supplementation is given.

  Diagnostic criteria:
  - Vertigo occurring without aura, maximal at onset and resolving spontaneously after minutes to hours with no loss of consciousness.
  - Associated with one or more of the following: Nystagmus, ataxia, vomiting, pallor, and fearfulness
  - Neurological, audiometric, and vestibular function normal
  - Absence of any significant medical history.
- *Motion sickness:* It is mostly seen in 4–10 years age group. Children <2 years are resistant because they do not use visual system for dynamic and spatial orientation. Drug prophylaxis—dimenhydrinate (1–2 mg/kg) 1 hour prior to travel is indicated.
- *Perilymph fistula:* It is more common in children than adults. Attack is provoked by cough, sneeze, weight lifting, loud noise, and air travel. HRCT temporal bone is indicated.
- *Vestibular paroxysmia:* It is acute vertiginous attack provoked by head movements, probably because of nerve vessel compression of 8th nerve root entry zone to brain stem. MRI can diagnose the anatomical fault. Treatment is low dose carbamazepine.

General Guidelines for Treatment of Acute Vertigo in Children

- Intravenous fluids
- Diazepam (intravenous 0.05–0.15 mg/kg/dose, 0.12–0.8 mg/kg/dose by oral route)
- Meclizine 25–100 mg/dose/day by oral route
- Prochlorperazine 0.05–0.15 mg/kg/dose by intramuscular route, oral 0.4 mg/kg/dose by oral route in 3–4 doses
- Diphenhydramine 5 mg/kg/day by intravenous or intramuscular route in 3–4 divided doses
- Antibiotics for otitis media/labyrinthitis

- Antiviral for herpes zoster—acyclovir 3–5 mg/kg/day
- Steroids for autoimmune and viral neuritis
- Oxcarbazepine (4–8 mg/kg/day)/carbamazepine (2–6 mg/kg/day) for vestibular paroxysmia
- Betahistine, diuretic for Meniere's disease
- Betahistine for BPVC
- Paroxysmal positional vertigo-positioning maneuvers
- Early mobilization for central compensation
- Parents counseling—explain the benign nature of disease
- Psychogenic vertigo—psychiatric counseling
- Balance rehabilitation on follow-up
- *Lifestyle modifications*:
  - Avoid lack of sleep, excessive exposure to sunlight, loud sounds, strong smells, bright lights, etc.
  - To keep same schedule of meals, sleep routine, and daily activities

■ FURTHER READING

1. Brandt T, Strupp M, Dieterich M. Five keys for diagnosing most vertigo, dizziness, and imbalance syndromes: an expert opinion. J Neurol. 2014;261(1):229-31.
2. Desmond AL. Vestibular Function: Evaluation and Treatment. New York: Thieme Medical Publishers, Inc.; 2004.
3. Halmagyi G, Cremer P. Assessment and treatment of dizziness. J Neurol Neurosurg Psychiatry. 2000;68(2):129-34.
4. Lampert T, Olesen J, Furman J, Waterston J, Seemungal B, Carey J, et al. Vestibular migraine: diagnostic criteria. J Vertib Res. 2012;22(4):167-72.
5. Uemura T, Suzuki JI, Hozawa J, Highstein SM. Neuro-otological examination with special reference to equilibrium function tests. Igaku Shoin Ltd. Tokyo 1977.

CHAPTER 3

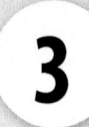

Acute Facial Palsy

Subirendra Kumar, Ajit Man Singh, Monica Manhas

■ INTRODUCTION

Acute facial palsy (AFP) is a difficult problem to manage, both from diagnostic and therapeutic perspective. The patient presenting with AFP suffers not only the functional consequences of impaired facial motion, but also the psychological impact of asymmetrical facial appearance. Data collected from recent studies does clarify and explain the etiology and pathogenesis of many facial disorders, but no clear consensus has yet emerged on many aspects of their evaluation and management.

Table 1 lists numerous disorders with unilateral facial palsy. Two percent of patients with AFP, present with bilateral involvement and may indicate an underlying systemic disorder with multiple manifestations **(Table 2)**.

The most important of AFP include:
- *Bell's palsy*: It is an acute, "idiopathic" unilateral paresis or paralysis of the face with rapid onset and evolution (<48 hours), with features of peripheral 7th cranial nerve dysfunction. It may be associated with acute neuropathies affecting the other cranial nerves (hypesthesia or dysesthesia of 9th cranial nerve, trigeminal nerve, hypesthesia of C2, vagal motor weakness, trigeminal motor weakness, facial or retroauricular pain, hyperacusis, dysgeusia, and decreased lacrimation). Recurrence of Bell's palsy occurs in 7–12% of patients. Of the 12% of recurrent Bell's palsy, 8% recur on the same side and 4% on the other side.

    The proposed causes of Bell's palsy include microcirculation failure of the vasa vasorum, viral infection [herpes simplex virus-1 (HSV-1)], ischemic neuropathy, and autoimmune reaction. Of these, the viral hypothesis is most widely accepted, relying on clinical observations and changes in viral antibody titers. However, no virus has been isolated from the serum of these patients.
- *Herpes zoster oticus*: It is a syndrome of acute otalgia with varicelliform lesions. When the facial nerve is involved, the whole picture is termed as "Ramsay Hunt syndrome" (accounts for 10–15% cases of AFP). Clinically, skin vesicles are seen on the pinna (concha), retroauricular area, ear canal, face or tongue, larynx, buccal mucosa, and soft palate.

TABLE 1: Acute facial palsy (AFP) (unilateral).

1.	Polyneuritis	• Bell's palsy, herpes zoster, encephalitis, poliomyelitis (type I), mumps, and mononucleosis • Guillain–Barré syndrome, Lyme disease, human immunodeficiency virus (HIV), and Kawasaki disease
2.	Otitis infections	• Acute otitis media and chronic otitis media (cholesteatoma) • Malignant otitis externa
3.	Trauma	• Temporal bone fracture and barotrauma • Facial injuries and basilar skull fractures • Birth trauma (molding and forceps delivery)
4.	Neurological disorders	• HIV and meningitis • Cerebrovascular disorder—central/peripheral • Opercular syndrome (cortical lesion in facial motor area) • Millard–Gubler syndrome (6th cranial nerve palsy with contralateral hemiplegia—lesion in base of pons) • Benign intracranial hypertension
5.	Autoimmune	Autoimmune syndrome of temporal arteritis, polyarteritis nodosa, and vasculitis
6.	Metabolic	Diabetes mellitus, hyperthyroidism, pregnancy, hypertension, and alcoholic neuropathy
7.	Neoplastic	Acoustic neuroma, leukemia, facial nerve neuroma, and metastatic lesion (from breast, kidney, stomach, lung, larynx, prostrate, and thyroid)
8.	Toxic	Tetanus, diphtheria, and lead intoxication
9.	Idiopathic	Sarcoidosis, Melkersson–Rosenthal syndrome, and multiple sclerosis
10.	Iatrogenic	Otologic, skull base, parotid surgery, local anesthesia, etc

TABLE 2: Bilateral facial palsies.

1.	Polyneuritis	Bell's palsy, infectious mononucleosis, postvaccination neuropathy, poliomyelitis, and Guillain–Barré syndrome
2.	Traumatic	Skull base fracture
3.	Neurological	Meningitis, malaria, bulbar palsies, multiple sclerosis, and Parkinson's disease
4.	Autoimmune	Polyarteritis nodosa
5.	Metabolic	Diabetes mellitus
6.	Infective	Lyme's disease
7.	Miscellaneous	Leukemia, syphilis, sarcoidosis, and myasthenia gravis

Sensorineural hearing loss (SNHL) (10% case), dysacusis, and vertigo (40% cases) indicate involvement of 8th cranial nerve (cochleosaccular dysfunction). Cranial nerve (V, IX, and X) and cervical branches of C2,

C3, and C4 having anastomotic communication with facial nerve, may be involved in some cases. The natural history of herpes zoster oticus differs from Bell's palsy in the following ways:
- Bell's palsy recurs in 12% of cases while herpes zoster oticus rarely recurs.
- Acute phase of infection is 5-10 days with Bell's palsy but 10-14 days in herpes zoster oticus.
- 84% of patients with Bell's palsy will have satisfactory recovery as compared to less than 60% with herpes zoster oticus, thereby indicating poor prognosis with latter.

- *Melkersson-Rosenthal syndrome (MRS):* It is a rare neurological disorder often presenting with recurrent, long-lasting swelling of the face (edema), particularly of one or both lips (granulomatous cheilitis), facial muscle weakness, and a fissured tongue. Most affected individuals present with only one or two features although all three may also be present. All ages may be affected, but most commonly young adults. The presentation varies and these individuals may present with facial paralysis, unilateral or bilateral that may get better or remain permanent. The cause of this is unknown but infection due to viruses, allergens, hormonal influences, and also familial inheritance have been proposed. There is no cure for MRS, but symptoms can be treated with anti-inflammatory agents, antihistamines, corticosteroids, and in some cases surgery, especially in refractory cases of facial paralysis.

■ EVALUATION

When a patient presents with clinical features of facial nerve palsy (asymmetrical face, widened palpebral fissure, inability to close the eye, and eye ball turning up and out, i.e., Bell's phenomenon, difficulty in chewing, dribbling of saliva from angle of mouth, epiphora, occasional noise intolerance due to stapedial paralysis, and altered taste), the examiner should attempt to ascertain whether the lesion is peripheral or central. In *unilateral central lesion*, forehead movement is spared because of bilateral cortical representation (crossed and uncrossed fibers). *Peripheral lesions* involved both upper and lower face ipsilaterally. Also, emotional facial movements and tone of facial muscles are also retained in central lesion.

Signs of possible tumor involvement are facial twitching, associated other cranial nerve involvement, SNHL, recurrent episodes of facial palsy and mass in middle ear, external ear canal, digastric region or parotid gland, facial weakness with conductive hearing loss, unilateral eustachian tube dysfunction, prolonged otalgia, or facial pain.

On examination:
- Look for typical vesicular eruptions in pinna, ear canal, face, and oral cavity.

- Look and ask for any blunt/penetrating trauma in face, ear, temporal bone, head injury, and skull base fracture. *Battle's sign* may be seen with longitudinal or transverse temporal bone fractures, and is probably due to extravasation of blood along the posterior auricular artery or an emissary vein.
- Ask for symptoms of acute and chronic otitis media, accompanying vertigo, altered taste sensation, otalgia, hyperacusis, tinnitus, decreased hearing, and numbness in middle and lower face. Look for any nystagmus.
- Relevant medical history of diabetes mellitus (DM), alcoholic neuropathy, hyperthyroidism, and hypertension.
- Look for signs of corneal irritation (redness, itching, foreign body sensation, and visual blurring) to avoid exposure keratitis.
- In routine otoscopy, look for "red chorda" sign, hemotympanum, any evidence of cholesteatoma, and do the tuning fork tests.

LABORATORY INVESTIGATIONS

- Complete hemogram [hemoglobin (Hb), total leukocyte count (TLC), differential leukocyte count (DLC), erythrocyte sedimentation rate (ESR), and peripheral blood film].
- Renal function test, blood sugar, and thyroid profile in suspected metabolic etiology.

Pure Tone Audiometry

- Conductive hearing loss is a usual finding with middle ear trauma, cholesteatoma, and other middle ear lesion involving horizontal segment of facial nerve.
- Sensorineural hearing loss usually indicates acoustic neuroma, meningioma, congenital cholesteatoma, dermoid, facial nerve neuroma, etc., which may affect the nerve in cerebellopontine CP angle or internal auditory canal.

Radiology

It is usually not a part of diagnostic workup in a patient with acute facial nerve palsy. High-resolution CT scan (HRCT) and gadolinium-enhanced MRI (Gd-MRI) are two main radiological investigations to exclude neoplasm and assess other pathological processes along the intracranial, intratemporal, and extratemporal portions of the facial nerve.

High-resolution CT scan (without contrast), both coronal and axial cuts, is useful in assessing detailed bony anatomy of the temporal bone (mastoid and middle ear spaces) and course of facial nerve from internal auditory canal to the stylomastoid foramen. It can detect lesions, >5 mm. Its main use is in "traumatic" facial nerve palsies.

On the other hand, MRI provides the most sensitive method of imaging the intratemporal segment of facial nerve, entire intracranial (pontine, cerebellopontine angle and intracanalicular), and extratemporal segments of the nerve. MRI is the investigation of choice for inflammatory, neoplastic and other nontraumatic causes.

Facial Nerve Testing

It is important for prognosis, i.e., recovery of facial function which is often the most important and relevant concern of the patient. Early determination of the prognosis for recovery may permit intervention to minimize nerve injury and optimize regeneration.

- *Topographic testing*: It helps in determining the level of facial nerve injury.
  - *Schirmer's test*: It is a method to assess parasympathetic innervation of the lacrimal gland via the greater superficial petrosal nerve (place 5 mm paper strips in the conjunctival fornix of each eye and compare the length of paper moistened by tear flow over a 5 minutes period). 25% reduction of the involved side compared with normal side or <25 mm bilateral lacrimation indicates abnormal Schirmer's test.
  - *Stapedial reflex*: Abnormal recording by impedance audiometry reflects impairment above the stapedial motor branch from the facial nerve trunk distal to the second genu.
  - *Chorda tympani functions*: These are assessed by submandibular gland secretion and taste testing. Dysgeusia and decreased salivary gland flow indicates the level of injury above the branch point of the chorda tympanic nerve from the vertical segment of the facial nerve.

More proximal the level of dysfunction, higher is the risk of degeneration and incomplete recovery. But due to unreliable topographic test results and presence of "skip lesion" of the nerve, "electrophysiological test" are accepted as the most reliable means of assessing nerve conductivity and risk of nerve fiber degeneration.

- *Electrophysiological test*: These are:
  - *Nerve excitability test (NET)*: A 1 ms square wave electrical pulse is applied, over both the affected and uninvolved facial nerve and threshold for "minimal" facial muscle response are recorded and compared. A 3–4 mA or greater difference indicates impending degeneration (Limitation: It is inaccurate during first 72 hours after onset of paralysis because it takes 3 days for Wallerian degeneration to occur). Patients with >3.0 mA difference need surgical intervention.
  - *Maximal stimulation test (MST)*: In contrast to NET, MST uses "maximal" electrical stimulation at a level sufficient to depolarize all motor axons underlying the stimulator. The results are recorded as a subjective account of difference in facial movements between normal

and involved side. If responses are symmetrical during first 10 days of paralysis, complete recovery will occur in 90% of the cases. If the response completely disappears within first 10 days, recovery will be incomplete with significant sequelae.

- *Blink reflex*: This is an electrodiagnostic test that evokes the corneal reflex and evaluates the integrity of trigeminal and facial nerve. In this reflex, afferent arm is constituted by supraorbital division of trigeminal nerve, while as motor fibers of facial nerve form efferent arm of the reflex. Blink reflex is more sensitive than clinical examination as subtle contraction is also detected.

  Procedure: The subject is placed supine and is asked to stay relaxed, with eyes open or gently closed. Active electrode (E1) is kept over inferior aspect of orbicularis oculus while as reference electrode (E2) is placed either over the bony prominence of zygomatic arch or the nose. Ground electrode (G) is kept over forehead or under the chin. Using a prong stimulator, each supraorbital nerve is stimulated and response from orbicularis oculi is recorded bilaterally **(Fig. 1)**.

  It is important to prevent habituation, by allowing a rest period of few seconds between successive stimuli.

  Interpretation: Normally, the ipsilateral electrical stimulation of trigeminal nerve will produce an eye blink bilaterally as seen with corneal reflex.

  This test is indicated in facial palsy, acoustic neuromas, stroke or tumors of brainstem, multiple sclerosis, and polyneuropathies like Guillain-Barré syndrome (GBS).

- *Electroneuronography (ENoG)*: It is also known as evoked electromyography (EEMG). It measures and compares the amplitude

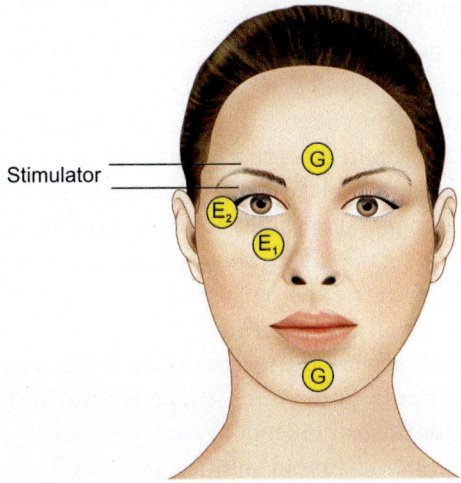

Fig. 1: Placement of electrodes in blink reflex.

of the muscle summation potential that are elicited when a supramaximal level of electric stimulus is applied over the main nerve trunk on normal and paralyzed side. The compound muscle action potential (CMAP) can be displayed, printed, and the waveform responses thus elicited are analyzed to compare peak-to-peak amplitudes between normal and paralyzed sides. An evoked summation potential of 5–10% compared with normal side indicates approximately 90% degeneration and is indicative of need for intervention.
- *Electromyography (EMG)*: It is useful in AFP because it determines the muscle action potential rather than the nerve activity, generated by spontaneous and voluntary activity. Denervated muscle being hyperirritable, produces spontaneous electrical potentials known as fibrillation potentials, can be readily picked up by EMG. Degeneration potential is seen 10 days after onset of paralysis, therefore, have limited value in prognostic workup. Loss of voluntary motor units (EMG) within first 3–4 days of paralysis suggests a poor prognosis. Its main role is in decision making for nerve crossover/transfer. Reinnervation potentials are indicative of regeneration and indicate to withhold nerve anastomosis.
- *Nerve conduction velocity (NCV)*: It is measured between stylomastoid foramen and mandibular branch of facial nerve. Normal facial NCV is 37–58 m/s. NCV between 20 and 30 m/s have 50% chance of significant residual paresis or synkinesis and those with <10 m/s have poor prognosis.

■ MANAGEMENT

It involves medical, surgical, and rehabilitative aspects.

Medical Treatment

Medical treatment involves:
- Broad-spectrum antibiotics in presence of acute infective (bacterial) pathology such as acute, acute on chronic otitis media, and meningitis.
- Antibiotic-steroid cream for herpetic vesicles.
- Care of eye to protect against exposure keratitis. Prescribe artificial tears four to five times/day. Ophthalmic lubricant can be applied to the eye, followed by patching or taping the eyelids shut at night. Use of glasses and/or moisture chambers helps to protect against wind, foreign bodies, and drying.
- Ophthalmologic opinion regarding temporary tarsorrhaphy or gold weight to facilitate eye closure for those who develop exposure keratitis.
- Analgesics for acute pain relief, especially in herpes zoster oticus (pregabalin in the dose of 150 mg/day may be given).
- Topical otic, antibiotic-steroid solution in cases of secondary bacterial otitis externa.

- *Steroids*: These are useful because of their anti-inflammatory action in addition to the facilitatory action on the neuromuscular junction. The treatment of AFP is centered on timely administration of steroids despite its controversial role in herpes zoster cases.

Steroid Therapy in Bell's Palsy
- May help to reduce risk of denervation
- May prevent or lessen synkinesis
- May prevent progression of incomplete to complete paralysis
- May hasten recovery
- May prevent autonomic synkinesis and crocodile tears

Studies have revealed that acute/active phase of inflammation in inflammatory neuritis peaks in 5-10 days in Bell's palsy and 10-14 days in herpes zoster oticus. Therefore, oral prednisolone is prescribed in the dose of 1 mg/kg/day for 7-10 days and then the daily dose is tapered to zero over the following 10 days. The important side effects of steroid are hyperglycemia, central nervous system (CNS) changes (psychotic reaction), fluid shifts, electrolyte disturbances, and gastrointestinal irritation. The risk of steroid-induced viral dissemination is important while treating AFP of viral origin, but this risk is significant with steroid therapy beyond 1 month. Some studies have pointed that steroid can ameliorate postherpetic neuralgia, relieve acute pain and reduce vertigo in cases of herpes zoster oticus.

Antiviral Therapy
Viral etiologies are suspected to play a major role in most forms of idiopathic facial palsy (Bell's palsy), but their role in treatment of Bell's palsy is controversial. Whereas, antivirals are drugs of choice in herpes zoster oticus. Acyclovir (800 mg 5 times/day) or valacyclovir (1,000 mg twice daily) are most preferred antiviral drugs.

Poor prognostic indicators in acute facial palsy are:
- Hyperacusis and decreased lacrimation
- Age >65 years
- Presence of comorbidity such as DM, hypertension, and human immunodeficiency virus (HIV)
- Presence of vesicles (herpes zoster)
- Immediate onset facial palsy, post-traumatic
- Radiologically complete disruption of fallopian canal
- Presence of transverse fracture on HRCT temporal bone
- Poor response to electrophysiological testing

(*Note*: Presence of SNHL is not considered to be a poor prognostic feature.)

Surgical Treatment

Surgical intervention depends upon the etiology of facial nerve lesion. These include:
- *Surgery of ear*: Myringotomy and tympanomastoidectomy
- *Surgery of facial nerve*: Nerve decompression and nerve anastomosis

Otologic Surgery

- *Myringotomy*: It is indicated in patients of acute suppurative otitis media (ASOM) presenting with AFP. Parenteral antibiotics are also prescribed. Some authors recommend 10 days course of steroids in addition to the antibiotics.
- Cortical mastoidectomy is performed when antibiotics or myringotomy fails to render the patient afebrile after 24 hours or when facial nerve palsy persists for >1 week. Nerve decompression is not necessary except in cases of prolonged dysfunction.
- "Tympanomastoidectomy" is done in patients of chronic suppurative otitis media (CSOM)/cholesteatoma presenting with facial palsy, in which disease pathology is eradicated and nerve is decompressed without opening the perineurium.

Neural Surgery

Nerve decompression is recommended when total paralysis is present with evidence of extensive nerve degeneration. It is indicated when "ENoG results" reveal <10% of normal (tested before day 14 post onset).

Role of surgical therapy (nerve decompression) in Bell's palsy is controversial. Initially, the vertical segment alone was decompressed. Next decompression of the entire mastoid segment was recommended. The preferred procedure was then extended to include the tympanic and mastoid segments and most recently, the labyrinthine segment including the meatal foramen. As anatomic and electrophysiologic evidence of specific anatomic site of lesion in Bell's palsy has emerged, surgical procedures have focused on decompressing the meatal foramen and adjacent labyrinthine segment of facial nerve, which is the "physiologic bottleneck" or pressure transit zone in presence of neural edema. Both transmastoid extra labyrinthine posterior tympanotomy approach and middle cranial fossa approach has been described for those cases who will have poor prognosis for complete recovery with medical treatment alone. Current recommendation as per some authors is that surgery of Bell's palsy is an appropriate therapeutic measure in carefully selected patients using electroneurographic criteria (>90% degeneration on ENoG, some authors recommend >95% degeneration on ENoG) and electromyographic criteria (without voluntary EMG potentials within 2 weeks of onset of facial palsy). But there is definite risk of hearing loss (temporary or permanent) so surgery should be performed for very definite indications where chances of improving prognosis are there.

Nerve Anastomosis/Grafting

It is indicated for repair of a partial/complete transected nerve. If >50% of nerve is transected, it should be repaired.
- *Direct anastomosis*: It involves perineural repair, i.e., end-to-end approximation with 8-0 or 10-0 monofilament sutures, without putting tension on the anastomosis.
- *Nerve grafting (cable grafting)*: Nerve grafts from sural nerve or greater auricular nerve are useful if end to end anastomosis is not feasible or is under undue tension. Cross-innervation from the contralateral side is a difficult surgery to perform.
- Facio-hypoglossal anastomosis, where hypoglossal nerve is transected near the tongue and swung posteriorly to join the facial nerve.
- *Facio-masseteric nerve anastomosis*: It is a versatile, powerful early facial dynamic reanimation surgical intervention with almost negligible morbidity.

Physiotherapy

It includes heat massage and facial exercises, performed twice a day. Heat massage is done by keeping a hot Turkish towel on the face until the towel cools. Then facial cream is massaged into the skin around the eyes and mouth and over the midface for a few minutes, ideally using an electric vibrator. Facial exercises include raising the eyebrows, squeezing the eyes closed, wrinkling the forehead and nose, whistling, blowing out the cheeks, and grinning. Facial exercises help to maintain the muscle tone. Transcutaneous facial muscle stimulation can be utilized in facial exercise therapy this can prevent atrophy of the muscles and can restore the volume and function of muscles in chronic denervation. Some physiotherapists advice chewing gum as an exercise but it should be discouraged as masticator muscles are not supplied by facial nerve and it may also induce synkinesis.

Management of Associated Depression

Depression a commonly associated with facial palsy because of cosmetic problem and needs psychological counseling, antidepressants, and detailed explanation of the disease cause, prognosis, and management strategy.

The management of acute facial paralysis is summarized in **Flowchart 1**.

■ SPECIAL CONDITIONS

Temporal Bone Trauma

About 80–90% of temporal bone fractures are longitudinal with associated facial nerve injury in 10–20% of cases, with delayed onset paralysis being the

Flowchart 1: The management of acute facial paralysis.

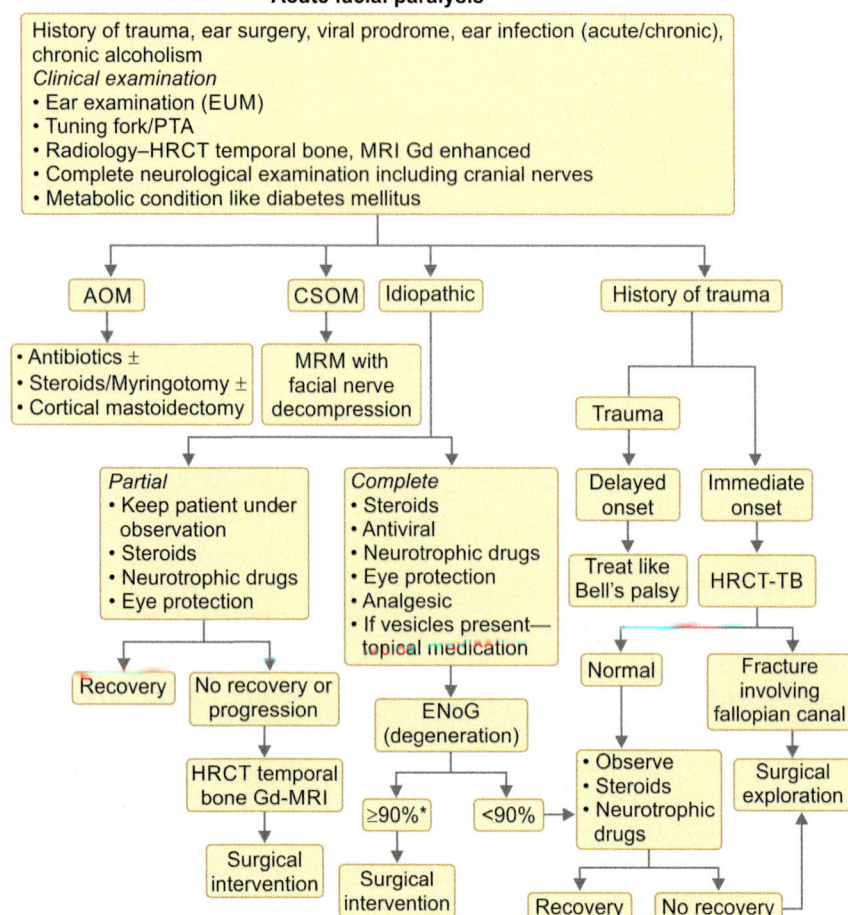

*Some authors recommend ENoG >95% as strong indicator for surgical intervention

(AOM: acute otitis media; CSOM: chronic suppurative otitis media; ENoG: electroneuronography; EUM: examination under microscope; Gd-MRI: gadolinium-enhanced MRI; HRCT: high-resolution CT scan; MRM: modified radical mastoidectomy; PTA: pure tone average)

most common. The most frequent site involved is in the geniculate ganglion region followed by second genu or vertical portion of the nerve. The most common injury being intraneural hematoma (50%), followed by disruption (30%) and an impinging bony fragment (20%). Other features are tear in bony external auditory canal, perforated drum, conductive hearing loss, cerebrospinal fluid (CSF) otorrhea (due to dural tear at tegmen tympani) with no evidence of vestibular injury, i.e., vertigo. The transverse fractures account for 15% of cases, will involve facial nerve in 50% of cases and frequently the palsy is immediate and complete, secondary to avulsion of the nerve or laceration by a bony fragment, usually in the geniculate ganglion region (especially the labyrinthine segment) and rarely in the intracranial segment in internal auditory canal. Other features are intact drum, presence of hemotympanum, severe neurosensory hearing loss, and vestibular injury (vertigo). In another classification of temporal bone fracture, the "otic capsule" involving fracture, has two times more chances of facial palsy as compared to the "otic capsule" sparing fracture.

Surgical intervention depends upon the time of onset, i.e., immediate onset, electrophysiological testing, evidence of nerve transection or impingement on HRCT (both coronal and axial), or penetrating trauma.

Surgical Procedure

- Postauricular incision.
- Cortical mastoidectomy
- Extended posterior tympanotomy
- Vertical segment exposure till stylomastoid foramen
- Removal of incus and malleus head to expose labyrinthine segment, first genu, and tympanic segment
- Removal of thin overlying bone over facial nerve by blunt elevator
- Slit opening of facial nerve sheath
- Drainage of intraneural or perineural hematoma and removal of any impinging bony spicule
- Surgical repair of facial nerve in cases of total transection (end-to-end anastomosis or cable grafting)
- Ossiculoplasty in presence of dislocated ossicles

More than 90% of temporal bone fractures with complete facial paralysis involve the geniculate ganglion region and this region should always be inspected when patient is surgically explored. Surgical exploration can be delayed up to 3 weeks after immediate onset facial palsy, to allow resolution of edema and hematoma resulting in a clearer surgical field. Some authors recommend the waiting period of up to 3 months before surgical intervention in complete facial nerve palsy, even in presence of poor electrodiagnostic prognostic factors such as ENoG and NET.

Penetrating injuries including gunshot in addition have involvement of dura, CSF leak, otic capsule injury, and vascular injuries. These patients need to be investigated with HRCT, carotid arteriography, facial nerve electrical testing for proper assessment, and further intervention. In cases of delayed onset facial palsy (most common cause of injury is traction from tethering of the facial nerve by the greater superficial petrosal nerve at the geniculate ganglion), medical management with steroids and electrophysiological monitoring is advised and if indicated, surgical exploration may be contemplated.

TABLE 3: House–Brackmann facial nerve grading system.

Grade I	Normal	Facial appearance and function normal, in all areas
Grade II	Mild dysfunction	• Normal symmetry and tone at rest • *Forehead:* Moderate to good function • *Eye:* Complete closure with minimal effort • *Mouth:* Slight asymmetry
Grade III	Moderate dysfunction	• *Asymmetry:* Obvious. Normal symmetry and tone at rest • *Forehead:* Slight to moderate movement • *Eye:* Complete closure with effort • *Mouth:* Slight weak movement with maximum effort
Grade IV	Moderately severe dysfunction	• Asymmetry and dysfunction obvious • *Forehead:* No motion • *Eye:* Incomplete closure • *Mouth:* Asymmetric with maximum effort
Grade V	Severe dysfunction	• Only minimally perceptible motion, asymmetry at rest • *Forehead:* No motion • *Eye:* Incomplete closure • *Mouth:* Slight movement
Grade VI	Total paralysis	No movement at any level and obvious asymmetry at rest

Pregnancy

Acute facial palsy may present in third trimester of pregnancy or immediate postpartum because of hormonal and fluid changes. Medical treatment with steroids is indicated which poses minimal risk to the developing fetus, especially in the third trimester.

■ HOUSE–BRACKMANN FACIAL NERVE GRADING SYSTEM

House-Brackmann facial nerve grading system is presented in **Table 3**.

■ FURTHER READING

1. House JW. Facial nerve grading systems. Laryngoscope. 1983;93:1056-69.
2. May M, Schaitkin M. The Facial Nerve, 2nd edition. New York: Thieme Medical Publishers; 2003.
3. Riodan M. Investigation and treatment of facial paralysis. Arch Dis child. 2001;84:286-8.
4. Tiemitra JD, Khatkhate N. Bell's palsy: diagnosis and management. Am Fam Physician. 2007;76:997-1002.

CHAPTER 4

Epistaxis

C Preetam Chappity, Vikas Gupta, Parmod Kalsotra

■ INTRODUCTION

Bleeding from nose ranks among the most common ear, nose, and throat (ENT) emergencies in all age groups, with a prevalence rate of 10–12%. Despite its high prevalence, the management of epistaxis is still debatable. Anterior epistaxis (AE) is more common in children and young adults while posterior nasal bleed is mostly seen in older patients with hypertension. Epistaxis is more common during hot dry climates with low humidity. In clinical practice, only few cases of epistaxis are due to a well-defined primary cause as listed in **Table 1**. In majority of patients, epistaxis is seen without any obvious causative factor and thereby known as idiopathic epistaxis. Nose-blowing, sneezing, coughing, straining, pregnancy, and upper respiratory tract infection, all can contribute to bleeding in an epistaxis prone patient by increasing the vascular pressure suddenly or induce mucosal inflammation making it more vascular and friable.

Trauma is the most common cause of epistaxis which may be blunt trauma to the nose or digital trauma (nose picking), the latter is the most common cause in children. In elderly patients, hypertension is a common cause. The arteriosclerotic vessels, lying under the delicate mucosa are unable to retract and clot easily when damaged and cause troublesome bleeding. Fear and anxiety due to bleeding and the pain associated with epistaxis management may further elevate the blood pressure (BP) causing a vicious cycle. Bleeding disorders may present clinically as epistaxis in children with leukemias, idiopathic thrombocytopenic purpura (ITP), von Willebrand disease, or chemotherapy-induced thrombocytopenia. In the end, it is worthwhile to mention that the tumors of nasopharynx, sinuses, nasal septum, lateral nasal wall, and nasal vestibule which may not be visualized until the bleeding has stopped and edema has subsided.

Various sites of bleeding from the nose are as follows:
- *Anterior nasal septum:* Venous bleed from the anterior nasal septum from the retrocolumellar vein.
- *Nasal septum:* Kiesselbach's plexus (Little's area), at the anteroinferior part of septum, has a rich blood supply from the anterior ethmoidal

TABLE 1: Causes of epistaxis.

A. *Local causes*		
	(a) Idiopathic	Spontaneous bleeding from artery of epistaxis (Little's areas) by slight trauma or atmospheric drying leading to crusting (Little's area/Woodruff's plexus)
	(b) Traumatic	• Simple abrasion • Compound/internal trauma of nose and PNS, base of skull • Foreign bodies including rhinoliths • Reactionary or secondary bleeding after nasal operation • Nose picking in childhood and old age • Septal spurs
	(c) Inflammatory	• Acute and chronic rhinitis • Adenoids causing congestion of nasal mucosa • Rhinitis sicca, atrophic rhinitis • Sinusitis
	(d) Neoplastic (benign/malignant)	In nose, PNS or nasopharynx
	(e) Environmental	High altitude having drying effect and also lower atmospheric pressure
	(f) Endocrinal	Vicarious menstrual bleeding
	(g) Drugs/inhalants	Cocaine, tobacco, heroin, wood-dust, cannabis, etc.
B. *General causes*		
	(a) Raised arterial pressure	Hypertension (atherosclerosis) and excitement
	(b) Raised venous pressure	• Cardiac causes • Pulmonary causes: Whooping cough, pneumonia
	(c) Diseases of blood and blood vessels.	Leukemia, hemophilia, sickle cell anemia, vitamin C and K deficiency, liver disease, von Willebrand disease, familial hemorrhagic telangiectasia, and bypass surgery
	(d) Thrombocytopenia	Bone-marrow aplasia, hypersplenism, DIC
C. *Specific diseases of nose/PNS*		
	(a) Granulomatous disease	Lupus, tuberculosis, leprosy, syphilis, Stewart's and Wegener's granuloma
	(b) Fungal	• Rhinosporidiosis • Blastomycosis • Coccidiomycosis
D. *Tumors*		• Nasopharyngeal angiofibroma • Inverted papilloma • Malignancy of nose and PNS

Contd...

Contd...

E. Hormonal	- Puberty, pregnancy - Granuloma gravidarum - Vicarious menstruation
F. Miscellaneous	- Uremia, hypothyroidism - Exanthematous fever: Measles, mumps, typhoid
G. Drugs	Aspirin, anticoagulants, immunosuppression, alcohol, chloramphenicol, chemotherapy, oral contraceptives

(DIC: disseminated intravascular coagulation; PNS: paranasal sinus)

artery (AEA) and sphenopalatine artery (SPA) (via the posterior nasal artery branch); anastomosing with branches from the greater palatine and nasolabial artery (branch of facial artery). 90% of AE arise from this site, also known as epistaxis digitorum; bleeding polyps of septum arise from here (also bleeding can occur behind a spur).
- *Inferior turbinate* and nasal floor.
- *Naso-nasopharyngeal plexus (Woodruff's area):* In the posterior part of lateral wall, below the posterior end of inferior turbinate is Woodruff's plexus formed by the anastomosis of the sphenopalatine, the posterior nasal, and the ascending pharyngeal arteries. It does seem, however, that there is a venous component of Woodruff's plexus which is situated on the lateral wall of the nose at the posterior end of the inferior turbinate. Bleeders in this region are difficult to visualize due to their location under the posterior end of the inferior turbinate. Other posterior bleeders may arise from the lateral nasal wall, posterior choana, or posterior septum.
- *Above middle turbinate:* Isolated spontaneous bleeding from AEA is rare and usually seen in hypertensive patients, trauma associated with skull bone fractures, or intraoperative injury.
- *Middle meatus:* Spontaneous bleeding from polypoidal swelling which may be neoplasia.
- *Diffuse* (both from septum and lateral nasal wall): It is seen in bleeding diathesis or general systemic dysfunction.
- *Nasopharynx:* Seen in angiofibroma and carcinoma of nasopharynx.
- *Sinuses*: Rarely spontaneous bleeding occurs from the vessels of maxillary antrum or ethmoidal sinuses.

■ CLASSIFICATION
- *Anterior epistaxis* is the term most often used to describe the bleeding from Little's area on the septum. Sometimes, AE may also originate from anterolateral nasal wall. Practically, epistaxis controlled by anterior nasal

packing (ANP) is known as AE. Anatomically any epistaxis anterior to piriform aperture is classified as AE.
- *Posterior epistaxis (PE)* usually describes the bleed from Woodruff's plexus. Again, any epistaxis which fails routine ANP is termed as PE. Anatomically, if the source is posterior to pyriform aperture, it is classified as a posterior nasal bleed.
- *Refractory epistaxis (RE)* is the continued bleeding occurring with anterior and posterior nasal pack in situ or shortly after the removal of both.

■ MANAGEMENT

It includes a history taking regarding excess alcohol intake, chronic pulmonary disease, bleeding tendencies (history of prolonged bleeding after trauma, dental extraction or bruising, etc.), hypertension, and cardiovascular diseases, which can cause epistaxis or increased morbidity or mortality in compromised patients. History of trauma, site of bleed, recurrent attacks of sinus infection, sinonasal surgery, or any drug intake (aspirin and anticogulants) is obtained. The examination of patient includes monitoring of vital signs, also look for signs of purpura, bruising, and swollen joints. Intravenous line is indicated in patients who give a history of profuse bleeding or previous serious illness, e.g., ischemic heart disease and cerebrovascular accident (CVA) in elderly or hypertensive patients. Blood products are also arranged. The laboratory tests include a complete blood count, bleeding and clotting time, platelet count, and Hess test. Deficiencies in clotting factors are less common and are screened with prothrombin time (PT) and partial thromboplastin time (PTT). PT measures the extrinsic clotting system and PTT measures the intrinsic clotting factors, especially the factor VIII, IX, XI, and XII. Specific factor assays of all the known clotting factors can be performed when indicated. In the presence of the deficiencies of clotting factors, attention should be to replace or replenish these factors as local measures in nose may not be very helpful. Liver and renal function tests are also undertaken, if indicated. After a posterior nasal pack is placed, arterial blood gas (ABG) analysis is advisable.

The *management of epistaxis* at any age group is done by resuscitating the patient, identifying the site of bleed, stopping the bleeding, and treating the cause. In young, resuscitation is uncommon and therefore pinching of nostrils bilaterally with firm pressure by the thumb and forefingers for 5–10 minutes is a time-honored method of stopping the venous bleed from the caudal end of the septum. Unilateral pressure may be applied with the thumb on the ala nasai of the affected side and the middle finger behind the angle of the jaw on the opposite side. This allows the patient's one side of the nose and the mouth for respiration. Patient is asked to sit down with head and neck leaned slightly forward because lying supine will cause the blood to drain into the pharynx and result in spitting of the blood or swallowing and subsequent vomiting, creating more anxiety, increasing the BP, and thereby causing more bleeding. Ice packs or damp clothes on the forehead or back of the neck have no role to play. After these initial measures, nasal examination is performed, which includes anterior and posterior rhinoscopic examination and flexible and rigid endoscopy.

In the absence of any obvious local disease, attention is turned to the septum which will often reveal an engorged vein, a microaneurysm or only prominent vessels in the Little's area itself. Cotton pledget soaked in topical anesthetic agent with vasoconstrictor (2 or 4% xylocaine with 1:10,000 adrenaline) is placed against the bleeding site for approximately 4-5 minutes which stops or slows the bleeding to a trickle. Chemical cauterization of the bleeding site is done with 10-20% silver-nitrate-soaked cotton-tipped applicator or by fused bead of chromic acid. Occasionally, 5% trichloroacetic acid (TCA) can also be used. Chromic acid bead is made by picking up a crystal of chromic acid at the end of a metal probe and heating the metal in a spirit lamp close to the crystal which melts and fuses into a smooth bead. The applicator is placed firmly against the area to allow the chemical to work without the blood washing away the chemical cautery and sometimes suction can be used along with it to keep the area clean. Care must be taken not to touch the skin, which causes smarting, but if it happens, thick paste of sodium bicarbonate should be applied (Note: Repeated chemical cautery at the same site can cause "septal perforation", especially with chromic acid. Septal perforation has also been reported when chemical cautery was applied on both sides of septum at the same site). In case of failure of chemical cautery, electrocautery (preferably with bipolar forceps) is used, in which repeated applications are made to the adjacent areas because of the presence of submucosal excursions of small arterioles with anastomotic connection in Little's area, which are taken care of. Afterward, the nose is loosely packed with an ointment-impregnated pack which can be safely removed after 1-2 days. Whichever method is adopted, patient is instructed to keep the area moist with antibiotic ointment or Vaseline. Instructions are given to the patient to avoid nose-blowing, digital manipulation, and physical strain for at least 1 week. Gentle sniffing may be allowed which is less traumatic.

Diagnostic nasal endoscopy (DNE) is indicated:
- To locate bleeding point
- For targeted hemostasis using insulated hot wire cautery or bipolar cautery.

Note: Monopolar cautery not used because of rare complication of blindness due to transmitted current to optic nerve.

In cases of *major AE*, oxycel pledgets, tampons, or ANP **(Fig. 1)** is indicated. Oxycel pledgets are packed when bleeding site is identified under

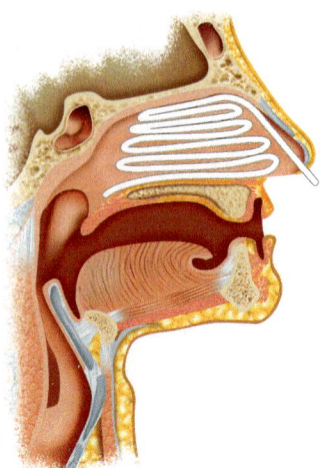

Fig. 1: Anterior nasal packing.

the inferior or middle turbinate and oxycel is packed from the floor of nose, tightly under the turbinate, thereby obviating the need of total anterior nasal pack. Nasal tampons are simplest way to pack the nose which consist of a desiccated, compressed sponge, which when inflated with any water-based fluid, expand dramatically. Insertion is quite simple. Lift the tip of the nose and slide the lubricated tampon into the nasal cavity along the floor of nose and inflate it with water or saline. Tampon is secured with a stitch passed through it, which is then taped to the face. Anterior nasal bleeding can be taken care of using *Merocel pack* which can be easily inserted and can be customized to put pressure on specific bleeding site. Merocel hemoX is made of low density, large-pore Merocel sponge with oxidized cellulose. This helps with maximum absorption and wicking of fluid while minimizing pain and rebleeding upon removal. When hydrated, it quickly swells, expands, and provides gentle, evenly distributed pressure to control the bleeding, while platelets aggregate on the surface of the pack to enhance clot formation.

Anterior nasal packing is indicated for bleeding from superior and inferior region of the nasal cavity that cannot be controlled by cauterization or if specific bleeding site cannot be identified. The nose is packed firmly on the side of bleed with petroleum-soaked gauze, or Vaseline gauze or bismuth iodoform paraffin paste (BIPP) pack. Packing is done in horizontal layers beginning along the floor of nose as shown in **Figure 1**. The pack should be 25 mm wide for adults, 12 mm wide for children, and 1 meter long. It should be prepared for each side, if both sides require packing. Topical anesthesia with 4% xylocaine is essential.

A Thudicum speculum is inserted and the gauze is placed in a layered fashion into the nasal cavity using Tilley's dressing forceps. The first 10 cm should be folded double and inserted along the floor of the nose and the nasal cavity packed, as tightly as possible and as far backward and upward as possible. This, being a painful procedure, should always be done in good light and as rapidly as feasible. It is recommended to pack nonbleeding side also simultaneously to support the pack kept in the bleeding side. Prophylactic antibiotics are advised to prevent infection and "toxic shock syndrome". Pack is removed after 48–72 hours. On removal of the pack, sometimes there is mild oozing due to irritation and the inflammatory response of the nasal mucosa which stops without any further treatment. If not, gentle application of a thin layer of oxycel pledgets controls it.

If significant bleeding occurs during pack removal, immediate reinsertion of fresh pack is done. If the free end of pack slides down to appear hanging behind the soft palate, it is better to remove and repack the nose rather than just cutting off the visible portion of the hanging pack.

In presence of severe deviated nasal septum (DNS) with ridge and/or spur, or if bleeding site is located behind the spur, the better option is immediate septal correction *[septoplasty/submucosal resection (SMR)]* with intranasal packing.

Humidification and the avoidance of further trauma from nose-blowing, picking, or scratching are mandatory for a week, heavy work and sports are avoided for 2 weeks after pack removal. ANP can cause respiratory compromise (nasopulmonary reflex), the genesis of which is still controversial. Many authors describe this pulmonic morbidity because of preexisting lung disease, aspiration, and sedation.

Posterior Epistaxis

When the bleeding is posterior (or both anterior and posterior) an additional posterior nasal pack is advisable, which may be a balloon catheter (e.g., Foley catheter). Foley's catheter is inserted along the floor of nasal cavity on the bleeding side until the catheter tip is just visible below the soft palate. The balloon is inflated with 15 mL of sterile water or saline and then withdrawn to impact on the choana. Foley catheter is useful in emergency because it can be manipulated under topical anesthesia. Deflation is prevented by an umbilical clamp or hemostat, which is kept over a dental bolster roll to prevent damage to the nasal ala or columella.

Bilateral ANP is done with it. In case of severe posterior bilateral bleeding, where bilateral Foley catheter is technically impossible, posterior nasal packing (PNP) is done **(Fig. 2)**. PNP *(classical posterior–Bellocq pack)* is also indicated in cases of skull-base fractures, tumors, and postadenoidectomy bleeding. It is generally done under general anesthesia. Topical anesthesia is used only in emergency situation. Anterior nasal and posterior oropharynx is anesthetized with 10% xylocaine spray. In children, general anesthesia is always preferred. Posterior pack is made by rolling a 4 × 4-inch gauze

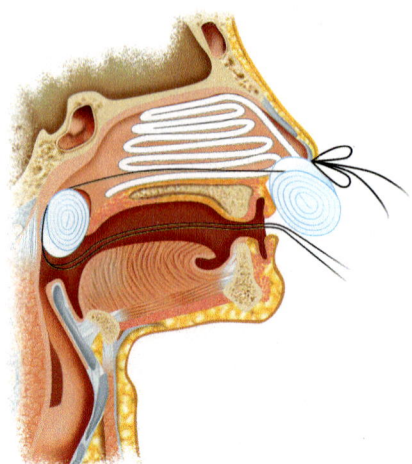

Fig. 2: Anterior and posterior nasal packing.

sponge into a 1-inch diameter pack and secured with three heavy silk sutures or umbilical cord tapes which are left long. A 10 French catheter is passed through each nostril from anteriorly backward into the oropharynx and grasped with a hemostat intraorally. One suture or umbilical tape is tied to each catheter, and the catheter is pulled back through the nose to deliver the pack through the mouth into the nasopharynx, which is guided by fingers of other hand until the pack goes behind the soft palate and snuggles against the choana. The third suture or tape is fixed on cheek via oral cavity and is used to retrieve the pack when it is to be removed. Posterior pack is secured by tying the two sutures or tapes over a dental bolster roll over the columella and a bilateral ANP is done. Purpose of nasopharyngeal portion of PNP, i.e., gauze tampon is usually not to put pressure on the bleeding site itself but serves as a buttress to prevent ANP from falling into the nasopharynx, providing more pressure on posterior bleeding sites. These patients usually require low flow oxygen therapy by face tent or mask to combat hypoxemia, and antibiotics to prevent infection. Patient should be hospitalized ideally with continuous oximetry and cardiac monitoring, which becomes mandatory if PNP is done.

Removal of posterior pack should be done under general anesthesia so that it can be reinserted in case of a persistent bleed.

The potential complications of PNP are hypovolemic shock, vaso-vagal reflex, hypoxia, hypoventilation, respiratory obstruction, local infection, bacteremia, toxic shock syndrome, inadequate oral intake, obstructive sleep apnea, cardiac arrhythmia, and/or ischemia, and aspiration pneumonia.

Nasal Balloon

Also, available with the bulbs, one for the postnasal space (can be inflated with 10 mL saline) and second bulb for the nasal cavity (Epistat, which can be inflated with 20–30 mL saline). The catheter incorporated with bulbs provides the airway. Efficacy is not much in controlling the severe epistaxis.

Surgical Intervention

The patient who continues to bleed every time the pack is removed or when bleeding persists with the pack in situ needs blood transfusion. Also, surgical intervention in the form of arterial ligation is considered, mainly the ligation of the external carotid system because of the fact that 90% of nasal mucosa is supplied through external carotid artery. This is also to be considered in patients with severe pulmonary disease, which can get exacerbated by the hypoxia and hypercarbia induced by nasal packing. The arteries which can be ligated are the sphenopalatine, internal maxillary artery (IMA), the anterior ethmoidal artery (AEA), posterior ethmoidal artery, and external carotid artery as a last resort.

- External carotid artery is ligated in the neck at the level of upper border of thyroid cartilage. The carotid bifurcation is identified and then external carotid artery is identified by its branches and also that it is oriented anteriorly, and the ligation is performed after the origin of its first branch, the superior thyroid artery. This allows the propagation of prospective blood clot from the ligated site into the branch than the internal carotid artery. External carotid artery ligation is least successful as it is very proximal and distant in relation to the actual bleeding site.
- AEA ligation is usually indicated in high lateral wall or high septal bleed, which is approached through an external ethmoidectomy incision (lynch incision). Other indication is RE after nasoethmoid fracture because of laceration of AEA. AEA is identified at a depth of 22–26 mm from anterior lacrimal crest along the frontoethmoidal suture line and posterior ethmoidal artery lies 10–12 mm posterior to AEA and only 4–7 mm anterior to the optic nerve. The rule of thumb is 24-12-6, average distance of AEA from anterior lacrimal crest, between anterior and posterior ethmoidal arteries and between posterior ethmoidal artery to optic nerve, respectively. AEA is secured with a Hemoclip/Ligaclip coagulated with bipolar cautery.

    Transnasal Endoscopic Anterior Ethmoid Artery Ligation (TEAEAL): In this, we perform the maxillary antrostomy and anterior ethmoidectomy on the side of epistaxis, define the lamina papyracea and ethmoid roof for identification of AEA canal, make a small opening in lamina papyracea below the AEA canal (using small curette) and unshell the bony fragments off the AEA adjacent to the lamina papyracea, elevate the tissue posterior and anterior to the AEA (for clip placement), and place small clip across the AEA next to the orbital periosteum. Apply clip very gently otherwise one can enter skull base as it is the thinnest area of the skull base. Unipolar suction cautery can be applied to cauterize the artery, but should be avoided. Note: AEA runs across the fovea ethmoidalis at a 45° angle from lateral to medial and mostly found behind the upward continuation of the bulla ethmoidalis. In the presence of suprabullar recess, AEA will be in the frontal recess. In 14–43% cases, AEA may lie in a mesentery suspended from the skull base.

- *Internal maxillary artery ligation:*
  - *Seiffert's operation (transantral approach):* It can be performed under local or general anesthesia as per patient's status and feasibility. After performing Caldwell-Luc maxillary antrostomy via sublabial approach, the posterior maxillary sinus wall is identified and removed (15 × 15 mm) using operating microscope (300 mm focal length objective lens). The periosteum is opened via cruciate incision. IMA and its three major branches are carefully explored in the pterygomaxillary fossa (taking care that the neural structures are always in the deeper plane) and vascular clips are applied to IMA, SPA, pharyngeal artery, and descending palatine artery (to prevent collateral flow). The Caldwell-Luc incision is closed.

    This procedure is best suited for intractable bleeding, because the ligation occurs close to the bleeding point. In cases of atypical origin of the ophthalmic artery from the middle meningeal artery (0.1%), ligation of the IMA may induce a reflex spasm of the ophthalmic artery, leading to sudden blindness.
  - *Transoral ligation* of IMA is achieved through buccal fat pad that too in presence of sinus fracture or chronic sinusitis where transantral ligation is not possible. The ligation is achieved proximally as compared to transantral route. Also, the patient complains of postoperative trismus and cheek swelling which may take up to 3 months to resolve.
- *Posterior ethmoidal* artery ligation is not routinely recommended, because it may be absent in many patients. Also, the procedures aimed at only the IMA or SPA and AEA ligation are more than sufficient.
- *Transnasal endoscopic sphenopalatine artery ligation (TESPAL):* After the decongestion of nasal mucosa, the lateral insertion of the middle turbinate on the medial orbital wall is identified, lateral nasal wall incision posterior to the maxillary sinus is made. Mucosal flap is elevated off the lateral nasal wall and the middle turbinate basal lamella. *Ethmoid crest* is identified which marks the anterior limit of possible SPA. The SPA is identified and isolated as it exits the sphenopalatine foramen and a vascular clip is applied proximally along with cauterization of distal SPA. Mucosal flap is repositioned.

Some authors advocate AEA ligation through external ethmoidectomy approach or via TEAEAL along with TESPAL.

Despite the fact of mentioned advantages such as minimal hospitalization, low morbidity, or better visualization, the limitation in our setup remains, because of lack of instruments and lack of required expertise.

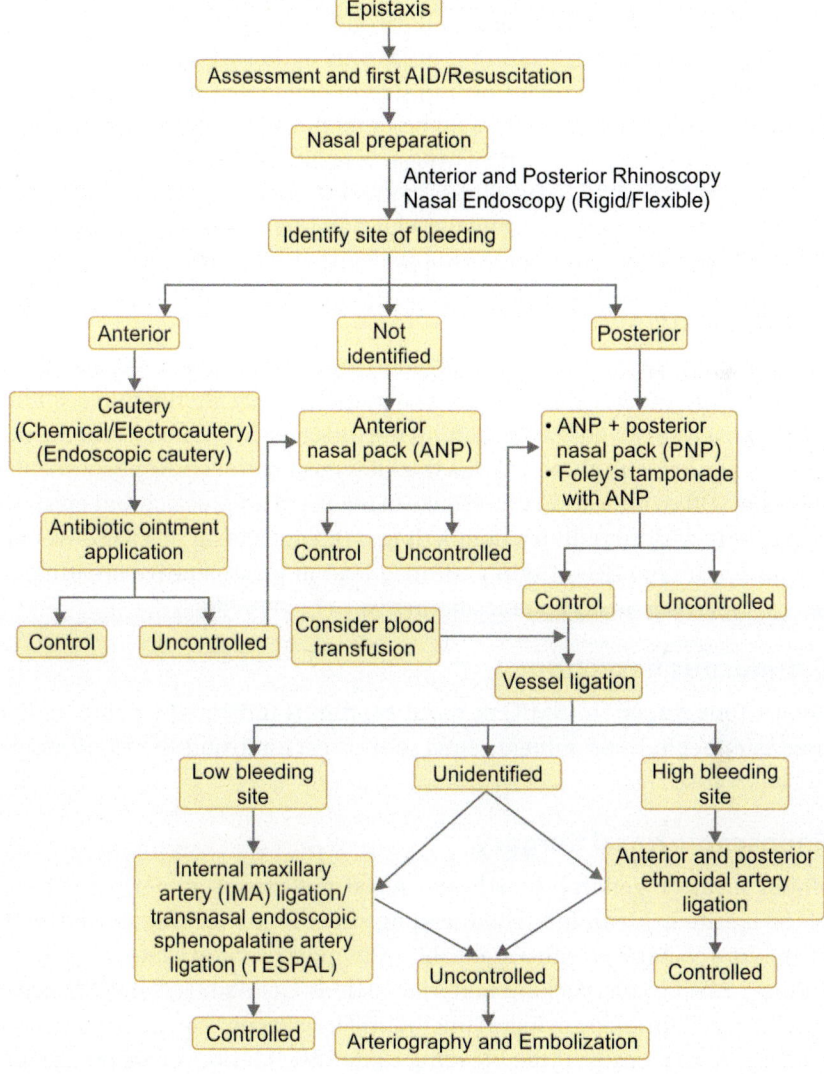

Flowchart 1: The management of epistaxis.

The indication probably remains in those patients who have persistent bleeding despite nasal packing in situ.

The management of epistaxis is summarized in **Flowchart 1**.

■ OTHER PROCEDURES

Internal Maxillary Artery Embolization

When neither packing nor surgical intervention controls epistaxis or epistaxis is due to congenital arteriovenous malformations, aberrant arterial vessels, nasal tumors, facial trauma and intractable cases of PE, angiography with gelfoam (temporary)/permanent embolization is indicated. IMA embolization is performed only with intravenous sedation in an institutional setup. Bilateral external and internal carotid angiography is performed via transfemoral route. Embolization of IMA using absorbable gelfoam and/or polyvinyl alcohol particles or tungsten or steel microcoils is performed. Ipsilateral facial artery should also be embolized to prevent recirculation. The procedure can be performed in case of recurrent epistaxis.

The drawback of this procedure is inability to check AEA bleed, its selective embolization is technically difficult with potential serious cerebrovascular complications. Also, the facility is not available at every hospital.

Dermoplasty

It is sometimes indicated in cases of recurrent epistaxis from Little's area, not controlled by conservative means. The pathologically altered mucosa from Little's area is removed leaving behind the intact perichondrium and the raw area is splinted with three-fourths thickness or full thickness postauricular skin graft. Other indication is presence of recurrent and recalcitrant epistaxis in patients with hereditary hemorrhagic telangiectasia or Osler–Weber–Rendu syndrome. Use of skin graft may lead to postoperative crusting, so buccal mucosa is an acceptable alternative.

Submucous Resection

Submucous resection (SMR) of nasal septum is indicated when bleeding originates behind a prominent septal spur, also it interrupts the blood supply to Little's area.

Endoscopic Nasal Surgery

Under local or general anesthesia, nasal endoscopy is performed and bleeding site is identified. The bleeding site and the feeding vessels in its vicinity are cauterized with a malleable monopolar suction cautery or bipolar cautery. Absorbable packing material such as Gelfoam (gelatin), Surgicel (oxidized cellulose), or Avitene (microfibrillar collagen) can be used if nasal endoscopy has localized the bleeding under the inferior turbinate. Placing the absorbable material between Merocel pack and bleeding site can reduce the chances of rebleeding on removal of the Merocel.

Laser

Recently, the use of lasers [carbon dioxide, argon, potassium titanyl phosphate (KTP), neodymium- doped yttrium-aluminum garnet (Nd-YAG)] has been reported for bleed control.

■ CONCURRENT MANAGEMENT

- Assess blood loss. Monitor BP and pulse.

- All patients with bilateral ANP and/or PNP should be admitted, intravenous line maintained, and given supplement oxygen.
- High-risk patients (elderly, debilitated, and alcoholics with liver disease) and unstable patients need constant monitoring.
- Bed rest with head elevation is advised.
- Humidification of the room along with low-flow oxygen by face mask for patients with posterior packing.
- Broad-spectrum antibiotics with adequate hydration.
- Complete blood profile and management of hypertension, if indicated.
- Blood cross-matched for transfusion, if required.
- Hematologist, physician consultation sought as and when the situation warrants.
- Vitamin C, vitamin K, and calcium supplementation.
- Absorbable packing (Gelfoam, Surgicel, or Avitene) or porcine strip packing (frozen salt pork) is useful in patients with blood dyscrasias or on chemotherapy where pack removal will reactivate the bleeding.

■ MEDICAL TREATMENT

Tranexamic acid and epsilon aminocaproic acid (EACA) (systemic inhibitors of fibrinolysis) are only indicated as adjuvant therapy or in recurrent or refractory cases. They are contraindicated in preexisting thromboembolic disease.

Topical hemostatic agents: Only indicated as additional tool for management of difficult/secondary bleed.

■ IN BRIEF

Epistaxis can be minimal or troublesome, dramatic, and life-threatening emergency. Treatment ranges from simply holding the nose for 10 minutes to ligation of IMA and/or ethmoidal vessels after failed posterior packing. The protocol of treatment is always dictated by the site and severity of the bleeding, as well as the experience of treating ENT surgeon. Therefore, it is worthwhile for treating ENT unit to set up its own protocol for management of epistaxis depending upon the infrastructure and available facilities.

Epistaxis tray should contain the following:
- Mask, gown, and eye protection gear (personal protection gear)
- Nasal speculums, kidney tray, and nasal suction tips (blunt end)
- Packing forceps and tongue blades
- Foley catheter
- Three hemostats, syringe, and cotton-tipped applicator
- Gauze packing (½ inch), gauze square (4 × 4 inch)
- Petroleum jelly saturated ANP

- Merocel
- Silk sutures (1-0) or umbilical cord tapes
- Two urethral red rubber catheters (10 French) for PNP
- *Medications:* Silver nitrate and carbolic acid
- Antibiotic ointment (avoid neomycin)
- Adrenaline ampules and decongestant nasal drops
- Head light (head mirror with bull's lamp), suction machine, and electrocautery
- Nasal endoscope zero-degree 4 mm in adults and 2.7 mm in pediatric age group for DNE along with camera and monitor is desirable.

■ FURTHER READING

1. Lin G, Bleier B. Surgical management of severe epistaxis. Otolaryngol Clin North Am. 2016;49:627-37.
2. Rosenfeld RM, Shiffman RN, Robertson P; Department of Otolaryngology State University of New York Downstate. Clinical Practice Guideline Developmental Manual. Third edition: a quality-driven approach for translating evidence into action. Otolaryngol Head Neck Surg. 2013;148(1):S1-55.
3. Sethi RKV, Kozin ED Abt NB, Bergmerh R, Gray S. Treatment disparities in the management of epistaxis. Laryngoscope. 2018;120:356-62.
4. Viducich RA, Blanda MP, Gerson LW. Posterior epistaxis clinical features and acute complication. Ann Emerg Med. 1995;25:592-6.

CHAPTER 5

Foreign Bodies

Arvind Kairo, Amit Manhas, Kapil Sikka

■ INTRODUCTION

The tendency of a child to accidently or intentionally lodge objects in the numerous orifices and cavities of the head and the critical physiologic importance of the upper airway, makes foreign bodies a subject of major importance when discussing the otolaryngological emergencies. Presentation of foreign body in ear, nose, and throat (ENT) area depends mainly on the age of the patient, the degree of obstruction that the foreign body produces and the inflammatory response it induces and the anatomical site that it is lodged in with, symptoms ranging from an absolutely normal patient with no symptoms to an acute airway emergency. Also, it is important to stress the possibility of multiple foreign bodies in same or different orifices, especially in mentally abnormal and psychotic patients. Same is true for prisoners who sometimes attempt to temporarily escape "justice", i.e., prison by inserting foreign bodies.

■ NOSE

Common organic foreign bodies are peas, beans, dried pulses, nuts, and cotton wool among others. Parts of metal and plastic toys, pebbles, and beads are also common. Button batteries may also be inserted in the nose. Animate foreign bodies include screw worms and their larvae, maggots and roundworm, leech, etc.

The *"inert foreign body"* may present with no symptoms at all and may be noticed usually while examining for other reasons or remain unnoticed in the nasal cavities for years. Others, like organic foreign bodies, however may generate an inflammatory response with the infection of the mucosa, leading to purulent, foul-smelling discharge often tinged with dark blood. These features are usually unilateral and in chronic cases a granulation tissue is formed around this inflammation with a resulting ulcerated mucosa that may rarely cause resorption of local bone or cartilage after many months. If a foreign body gets buried in granulation tissue or firmly impacted, it may act as a nidus for concretion and becomes a *"rhinolith"* which is usually seen near the floor of nose and is radiopaque **(Fig. 1)**. Maggots usually give rise to a severe inflammatory reaction and if untreated, may also involve the

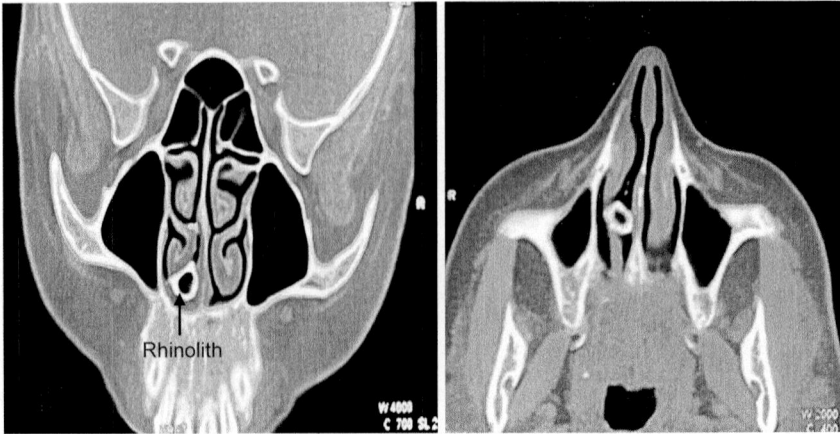

Fig. 1: CT showing radiopaque rhinolith.

adjoining paranasal sinuses, orbital cavities, skin, and skull base including the brain and its meninges.

With *inanimate* foreign bodies, any child with a unilateral, foul-smelling, and purulent nasal discharge should be examined for a foreign body until proven otherwise. Frequently, the foreign body is seen on anterior rhinoscopy or endoscopy after suction and application of vasoconstrictor nasal drops. Plain X rays are of limited use because most foreign bodies are radiolucent. CT scan (fine coronal and axial cuts) can be performed to detect small radiolucent and radiopaque foreign bodies. MRI is indicated in cases of confirmed nonmetallic foreign bodies (otherwise metallic foreign bodies can result in severe/fatal injury under MRI magnetic field). Management includes removal of the foreign body under controlled atraumatic conditions, in cooperative or anaesthetized patients. Instruments used to remove vary and while soft foreign bodies or those with a thin edge, can easily be grasped and removed with crocodile or Tilley's forceps, solid and round foreign bodies are maneuvered out using a bent Jobson Horne probe, by inserting the probe above and beyond the foreign body and then attempting to draw it slowly forward toward the external nostril. Presence of second concomitant foreign body in same nostril or another nostril is always ruled out. Otoscope or nasal endoscope can be utilized for this examination. Systemic antibiotics are advised to cover secondary rhinosinusitis. General anesthesia with cuffed tube is indicated along with the hypopharyngeal pack in children, uncooperative patients, and posteriorly placed foreign bodies because of risk of the foreign body getting pushed backward into the nasopharynx or chances of brisk hemorrhage.

Infestation with maggots and screw worms are managed by instillation of 25% chloroform solution or turpentine oil drops which suffocate the larvae and immobilize them allowing their manual removal with or without anesthesia. Other special animate foreign body is "leech" which is otherwise a painless foreign body. High index of suspicion is helpful in cases of epistaxis with nasal obstruction and itchy sensation, especially in leech season (May–September). Removal of leech requires special care and utmost gentleness because it attaches strongly with its suckers. Firm traction should not be applied to detach a leech, otherwise some part of it can be left at the site of its attachment causing persistent bleed and possibly infection. Removal is achieved after topical spray of xylocaine (4%) with 1:1,000 adrenaline followed by manual removal using forceps under local or general anesthesia.

■ EAR

Ear canals happen to be the most common site for foreign bodies in young children, who have a propensity to insert objects in them. Foreign body usually lodges just lateral to the narrowest part of the ear canal, the junction of bony-cartilaginous parts of external auditory canal, but can also get lodged in the isthmus of the ear canal, or may penetrate through the drum into the middle ear cavity. On examination, small smooth object especially pebble, bead, popcorn kernel is seen which is difficult to grasp and may be more than one. Usually, foreign bodies are asymptomatic but some cause secondary otitis externa, bloody-purulent discharge, and insects are the most troublesome. Obstructed foreign bodies cause decreased hearing.

Radiology has no role except in cases of penetrating foreign bodies to assess the depth of penetration, especially in the presence of inner ear damage. Diagnosis is usually straight forward with either the child complaining of otalgia or the parents being aware of foreign body insertion, bringing the patient to the ENT surgeon. Soft foreign bodies, e.g., cotton wool, and paper can be removed with crocodile forceps while solid foreign body like a bead can be rolled out with a curette or hook or Jobson Horne probe that can be passed beyond the foreign body and then gently pulled out while engaging the foreign body. Removal is also usually achieved by syringing with water at body temperature in cooperative children. In difficult cases or in those where removal cannot be performed in an awake patient, removal is done under general anesthesia using micro aural crocodile forceps or other micro hooks under microscopic/otoendoscopic guidance. In the presence of tissue reaction induced by the foreign body, subsequent treatment of otitis externa is required. Insects may be drowned with olive oil and then syringed out.

■ OROPHARYNX/HYPOPHARYNX

Sharp objects such as fish bones, fine copper wires, steel wools, and pins are prone to get lodged in palatine or lingual tonsils. Dental prosthesis or teeth may get dislodged accidently and get impacted, especially after a road traffic accident. Patient may give a history of initial gagging episode which may be absent in children. Other features are odynophagia, with correct side localization but level is poorly localized. Patient may complain of ipsilateral otalgia. Dysphagia and drooling are less common presenting features. A large foreign body impacted in hypopharynx will in addition cause obstruction of the airway leading to dyspnea (air hunger) and stridor (noisy breathing) on inspiration along with intercostal, suprasternal, and substernal retractions. Mostly foreign bodies are easily seen in oropharynx and tongue base. X-rays are helpful in metallic foreign bodies. Thin bones, nonferrous metal objects, and fish bones (cartilaginous) are usually not seen in X-ray film.

Removal can be achieved under local or topical anesthesia in cooperative patients. Otherwise, general anesthesia is preferred and direct laryngoscopic examination is done and removal achieved with forceps.

■ ESOPHAGUS

Over 90% of ingested foreign bodies pass through the gastrointestinal tract without any trouble. If a foreign body fails to pass through, hold up is most common in the esophagus. This lodging is common at four anatomically narrow sites in the esophagus that are the cricopharyngeal sphincter, the level of crossing of aortic arch, the crossing point of the left main bronchus, and the level of the diaphragmatic hiatus, with maximum impaction at cricopharyngeal level (80%) **(Figs. 2A and B)**. Other sites of pathologic narrowing, e.g., strictures, stenosis, tumors, and malignancies may also lodge impactions, when present. (*For button batteries ingestion, refer to chapter on caustic ingestion*).

Clinical features range from asymptomatic patient to obscure, unusual clinical symptomatology. There may be history of ingestion of foreign body and the patient may present acutely with coughing and choking with inability to swallow saliva, dysphagia, or vomiting. With chronic esophageal foreign

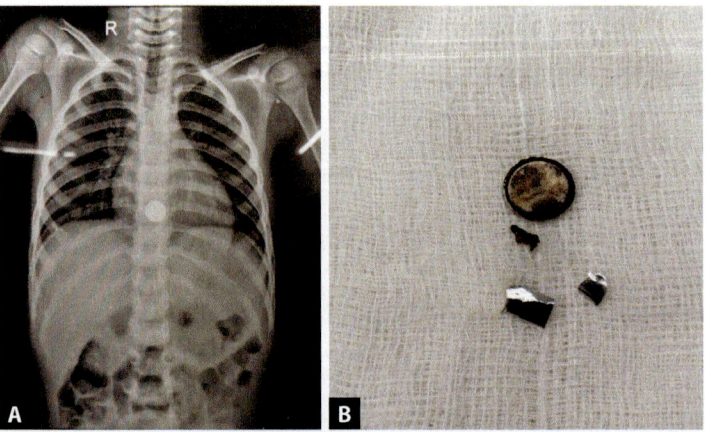

Figs. 2A and B: Foreign body button battery in esophagus and retrieved via esophagoscopy.

bodies, there is edema of tracheoesophageal wall, leading to tracheal airway symptoms like biphasic stridor. In some; wheeze, recurrent pneumonia, anorexia, blood-tinged vomiting, or pyrexia of unknown origin may be the presenting feature.

Diagnosis is confirmed on anteroposterior (AP) and lateral X-ray of the chest in radiopaque foreign bodies. In doubtful cases, barium esophagogram or CT scan may be required. Radiograph of neck and chest after swallowing small cotton ball soaked with barium, which may stick to the foreign body can help to localize the radiolucent foreign bodies.

Removal is done using direct esophagoscopy under general anesthesia. Sometimes, rounded objects can be dislodged by means of a Foley's balloon catheter. Button batteries deserve immediate attention because of the risk of erosion of esophageal wall. Underlying pathology like stricture or neoplasm is always looked for, especially in elderly patients.

Esophagoscopy Procedure

Explain the procedure to patient and/or attendants. Take written and informed consent. Esophagoscopy is generally performed under general anesthesia. Patient is placed in supine position and "sniffer" or "Boyce-Jackson" position is made (neck flexed on shoulders and head extended on the neck). Before passing the scope, the operator should ensure that a suitable range of grasping forceps is available. The appropriate sized esophagoscope (largest that is likely to be suitable) is selected. Surgeon stands on the "head end" keeping the esophagoscope in near-vertical position. The esophagoscope is inserted protecting the lips from injury with fingers of nondominant hand. It is introduced along the right side of tongue down to the posterior pharyngeal wall (lifting the tongue base, endotracheal tube, and arytenoid cartilages with its long bevel) to the right pyriform fossa, following the natural food passage. The thumb of the nondominant hand is used as fulcrum for esophagoscope to protect the teeth.

Esophagoscope is now directed toward the midline and "cricopharynx" is entered "without force" under direct vision. The esophageal lumen is looked at while applying steady pressure against the contracted cricopharyngeus and the tip of the scope is slowly advanced keeping the lumen in view. For further endoscopy, the surgeon has to "sit" and head end of the operating table has to be lowered below the horizontal. Esophagoscope is advanced gently following the lumen under direct vision and look/feel for aortic pulsations. Below the level of aorta/left branches, esophageal lumen may seem to disappear anteriorly which requires further lowering of head end of operating table to get proper visualization.

On further advancement of esophagus through the "hiatus" of diaphragm, the head end is lowered and moved horizontally to the right (to make the long axis of scope correspond to the axis of lower one-third of esophagus). With the deviation of lower end of esophagus to left and anteriorly, hiatus-lumen appears as anteriorly placed narrowing. The scope is gently advanced in the direction of "left anterior-superior iliac spine" and as the hiatus is passed, the stellate pattern of esophageal mucosa is replaced by deep red, velvety gastric mucosa with rugal folds (z line) at approximately 40 cm from incisors.

After visualization of the foreign body, appropriate forceps should be used to grasp the foreign body depending on the size and nature of foreign body. Large pieces should be grasped and impacted at the end of the scope, removing the scope and impacted material simultaneously. Soft material can be removed piecemeal through the lumen of the scope. Once foreign body is removed, always reinsert to look for a second foreign body, to rule out traumatic injury and predisposing factors such as tumors and strictures.

Sometimes the patient is aware of the foreign body in the esophagus and expressing discomfort, dysphagia, inability to swallow, neck tenderness, retrosternal fullness or blood-stained saliva but the endoscopy fails to indicate the presence of foreign body.

Impacted foreign body like denture/bone can be removed with the help of cutter or **lateral pharyngotomy approach**, while pointed foreign body (especially metallic wires/pins), can get lodged in surrounding soft tissues of neck or prevertebral space making lateral neck exploration (under C-arm guidance) **(Fig. 3)** a safe and effective alternative to esophagoscopy.

In **lateral pharyngotomy**, a transverse incision is made at the level of upper border of thyroid cartilage. Subcutaneous tissue and platysma

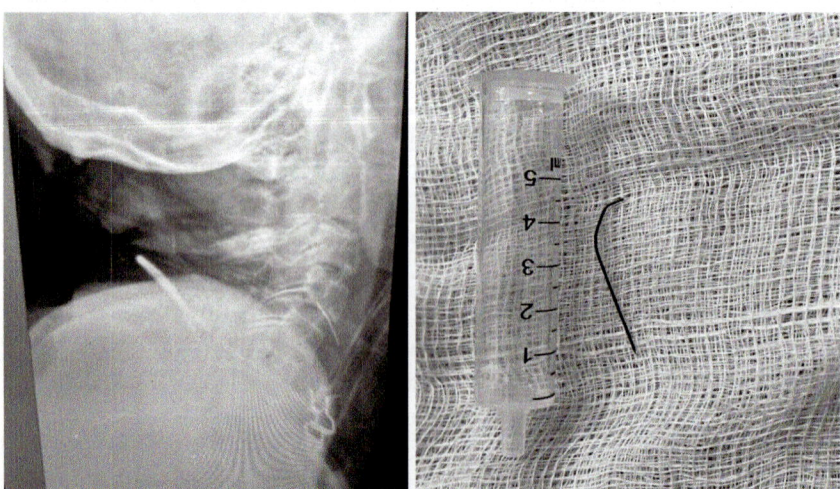

Fig. 3: Foreign body metallic pin migrated and lodged in the prevertebral space removed by lateral neck exploration.

are incised, strap muscles are retracted and right lateral border of thyroid cartilage is delineated followed by incising of mucosa of pyriform sinus.

Foreign bodies in thoracic esophagus can be lodged and get impacted, thus making esophagoscopy a difficult option. In all such cases, thoracotomy may be preferred.

Foreign bodies lodged in abdominal part of esophagus/GE junction require an exploratory laparotomy with a gastrotomy along the body of stomach near the fundus.

Complications of Esophagoscopy

- *Mucosal tears/lacerations:* Minor tears and lacerations do not require any intervention while those which appear significant can be managed by appropriate antibiotics and nasogastric tube and monitoring the patient carefully.
- *Esophageal perforation:* This is a surgical emergency with significant morbidity and mortality. Leakage of esophageal and gastric contents into the mediastinum leads to mediastinitis, sepsis, and multiorgan failure. It is suspected in case of chest pain, back and neck pain, odynophagia, dysphagia, tachycardia, tachypnea, pyrexia, crepitus, and signs of sepsis. This is managed by keeping the patient nil per mouth, nasogastric tube or parenteral feeding, broad-spectrum antibiotics, hemodynamic stabilization, and intensive monitoring and may even require surgical intervention.

■ AIRWAY FOREIGN BODIES

Airway foreign bodies are common in infants and toddlers and boys are more likely to aspirate than girls. The highest incidence of inhaled foreign bodies in infants and toddlers is due to tendency of the child to put objects in the mouth and when this object accidentally gets swallowed, upon reaching the pharynx, a startle response is elicited allowing the foreign body to enter into the larynx which is open during forced inspiration.

Further, high proportion of these young children are mouth breathers and also have a constant cough due to upper respiratory tract infections that allows the inhalation of food particles during the sharp intake of breath following a bout of cough.

Unlike in adults where most inhaled foreign bodies are lodged in right bronchus, in the young children, there is equal distribution of foreign bodies between both bronchi. This is mainly because of the anatomical differences between right and left bronchus are less pronounced. Rarely, these foreign bodies (<4%) may lodge in the larynx, especially when they are too big to pass through or if they have an irregular shape or have sharp edges resulting in their getting struck to the laryngeal mucosa, e.g., egg shells, glass fragments, or plastics.

Stridor is the most common feature seen which may be inspiratory (laryngeal) or biphasic stridor (indicating subglottic or upper tracheal impaction). Voice may be hoarse especially in glottic foreign bodies. Patient may also present with aphonia indicating complete impaction. Cough may be the presenting feature, especially in subglottic foreign bodies.

In case of foreign bodies in one bronchus, obstruction may range from none to partial or complete. Partial obstruction produces a check-valve effect that expands during inspiration but closes in expiration thus causing a hyperinflated lung distal to obstruction that can produce a mediastinal shift while complete obstruction produces atelectasis of distal lung.

There is commonly a definite history of choking, followed by an episode of coughing. After the initial paroxysm of reflex cough, the mucosa of tracheobronchial tree becomes tolerant to foreign body and the cough subsides, delaying the diagnosis. In about one-third, there is delay in diagnosis as the actual incident of aspiration is neither observed nor elicited in history and thus a high index of suspicion may reduce morbidity in such cases leading to increased morbidity. Other notifiable clinical features at presentation include unilateral wheeze and reduced breath sounds, unexplained persistent fever, and/or persistent or recurrent lobar pneumonia. Pain at the root of neck and an acute respiratory distress are seen in patients with laryngeal foreign body. The *classical "triad"* of unilateral wheezing, cough, and ipsilateral diminished air entry are observed in most cases of bronchial obstruction. Shifting of signs from one side to other is another important clue for inhaled foreign body. While "atypical asthma" not responding to usual treatment should make one think of a missed foreign body.

Prolonged impacted foreign bodies may complicate with bronchial suppuration, ulceration, and granulation tissue formation with a resultant bronchial stenosis, peribronchial and peritracheal lymphadenopathy with external compression of the bronchi and it may predispose to an infection of lung, collapse, obstructive emphysema, pneumothorax, and variable degree of airway obstruction.

Clinical diagnosis is supplemented with radiography of soft tissue neck and posteroanterior (PA) view of chest **(Figs. 4A to D)**. Plain X-ray chest is normal in most cases for first 24 hours in cases of tracheobronchial foreign body. Otherwise, the most common finding is obstructive emphysema on one side, collapse of the lower lobe on either side, consolidation or collapse of the lungs. Radiopaque foreign body is obvious on X-rays, while radiolucent foreign bodies are always suspected in patients with atelectasis or recurrent, prolonged, or migratory pneumonia. Inspiratory and expiratory chest X-rays are important in diagnosing obstructive emphysema. Also, the mediastinal shift is seen which is towards the side of lesion with atelectasis, away from the side of lesion in obstructive emphysema. In cases of uncooperative patients, right and left lateral decubitus X-rays are done where absence of volume

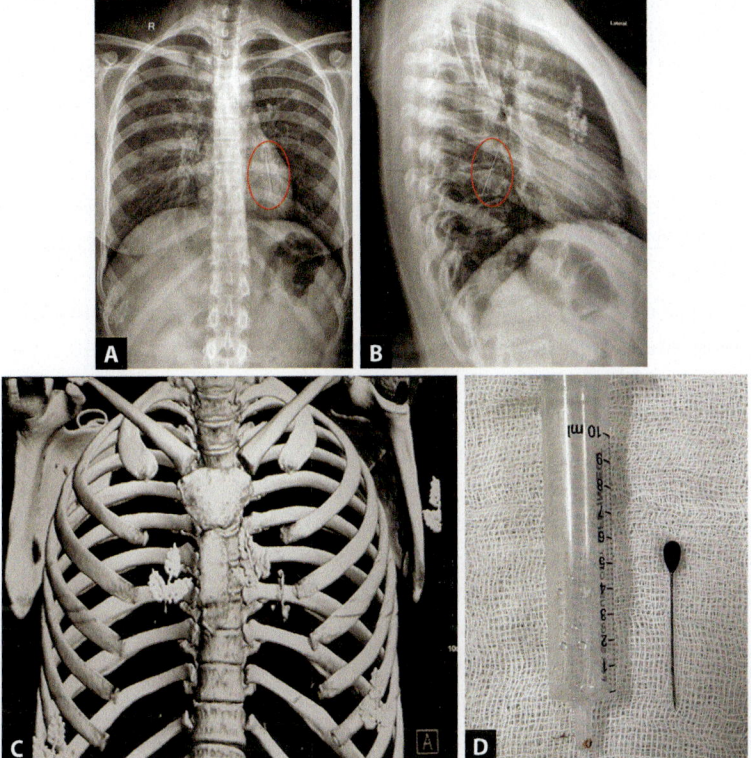

Figs. 4A to D: Metallic foreign body left bronchus.

loss on dependent side is seen with partially obstructive foreign body. Video fluoroscopy of lateral view of neck can be done in suspected cases.

Four types of bronchial obstructions have been described in the literature:
1. *Bypass valve:* Partial obstruction in both inspiration and expiration, causing aeration with normal X-ray findings, e.g., small, flat, or oblong organic foreign bodies such as watermelon or sunflower seed.
2. *Check-valve obstruction:* Air can be inhaled but cannot be exhaled, producing obstructive emphysema on the involved side and mediastinal shift to normal side.
3. *Ball-valve obstruction:* When a foreign body becomes impacted on inspiration, yet dislodges on expiration. It causes early atelectasis and collapse with mediastinal shift towards the involved side. It is seen in smooth round foreign body, e.g., whole peanut.
4. *Stop-valve obstruction:* Complete blockage by a large foreign body with no air passage on both inhalation and exhalation leading to consolidation of the involved segment with subsequent collapse.

For the removal of foreign bodies, open rigid endoscopy is the gold standard. Pounding the throat and Heimlich procedure can be counterproductive and may cause worsening of clinical situation with further impaction and a complete obstruction.

Indirect laryngoscopy (not possible in pediatric patients) and direct laryngoscopy without anesthesia are not of much help and value in a partially obstructed airway. ENT surgeon has to assess the airway obstruction on clinical parameters and should decide the urgency of endoscopy. In case of prolonged impacted foreign body, general condition should be assessed and pediatrician's opinion should be sought before deciding for general anesthesia.

In case of acute airway obstruction with or without cyanosis, airway establishment by intubation/tracheostomy or cricothyroidectomy is contemplated to save the life and then bronchoscopy is performed. In all doubtful cases, bronchoscopy should be done.

Laryngeal or large tracheal foreign bodies are treated as life-threatening emergencies and there should be facilities available for emergency tracheostomy for these cases. Sometimes, these foreign bodies may be too large to be delivered via rima glottidis and subglottis and may have to be recovered via tracheostoma. Laryngeal foreign bodies can be taken out by direct laryngoscopy under anesthesia with care, as induction may sometimes cause total obstruction due to dislodging of the foreign body necessitating an emergency tracheostomy or cricothyrotomy. Small tracheal and bronchial foreign bodies are removed using the rigid bronchoscopes under general anesthesia as emergency procedures in acute cases and as elective procedures with chronic obstruction or a stable patient. Rarely a bronchial foreign body may need an open exploration with a thoracotomy and bronchotomy.

Rigid ventilating bronchoscopes of different sizes (2.5–6 mm D) are used for rigid bronchoscopy. Tracheostomy set should be kept ready along with the regular bronchoscopy instruments such as various types of foreign body holding forceps, suction cannula, and cup-shaped biopsy forceps in the instrument trolley. Cardiac monitor and pulse oximeter is a must.

After endoscopic removal of foreign body, a *"second look"* bronchoscopy is a must to rule out second foreign body or remaining small fragments from the original foreign body like peanuts or beans, and to suck out any pus or mucus from the distal bronchus.

■ PROCEDURE OF BRONCHOSCOPY

After mask induction, vocal cords are anesthetized by topical lignocaine. A wet gauze piece or dental guard is kept on upper teeth to prevent any injury. Bronchoscopy can be done by directly passing the bronchoscope through glottis or can be done via laryngoscope wherein glottis is first exposed with the aid of a laryngoscope. An appropriate size bronchoscope is held in right hand in pen-like fashion. Fingers of left-hand help in guiding

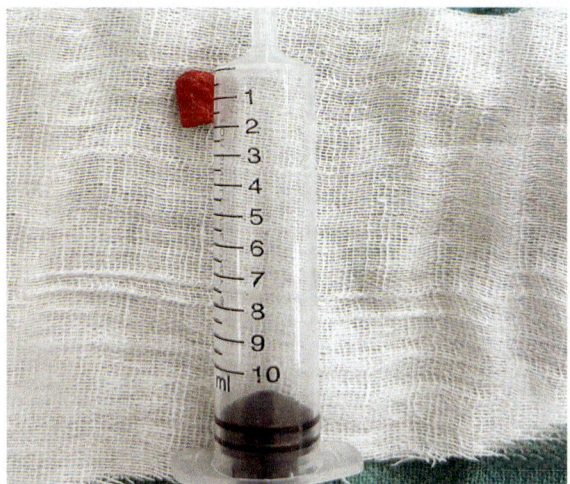

Fig. 5: Foreign body (chalk) retrieved by bronchoscopy from left bronchus.

the bronchoscope, which is then introduced into trachea via laryngoscope. Laryngoscope is then withdrawn once bronchoscope has crossed the vocal cords.

On reaching the glottis, bronchoscope is rotated 90° clockwise so as to align its beveled edge in the axis of glottis. As trachea is entered, bronchoscope is rotated back to original position.

Scope is guided further to look into carina, right, left bronchus, and segmental bronchi to visualize the foreign body. Different types of forceps are used for removal of foreign bodies depending upon their nature and size. **Figure 5** shows the foreign body retrieved by bronchoscopy from left bronchus using the forceps with double action jaws for soft foreign bodies. In case of sharp foreign body, grasp the sharp end and keep it within the tip of bronchoscope to minimize trauma to mucosa.

Complications

Various complications include laryngeal edema, pneumomediastinum, pneumothorax, and subcutaneous emphysema. Organic foreign bodies are associated with more complication rate as they are associated with more airway edema, secretions, and can cause chemical bronchitis.

■ FURTHER READING

1. Hunter TB, Taljanovic MS. Foreign bodies. Radiographics. 2003;23(3):731-57.
2. Kim JE, Ryoo SM, Kim YJ, Lee JS, Ahn S, Seo DW, et al. Incidence and clinical features of esphageal perforation caused by ingested foreign body. Korean J Gastroenterol. 2015;66(5):255-60.
3. Yao CC, Wu IT, Lu LS, Lin SC, Liang CM, Kuo YH, et al. Endoscopic management of foreign bodies in upper Gastrointestinal tract of adults. Biomed Res Int. 2015;2015:658602.

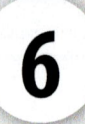

CHAPTER 6

Acute Upper Airway Obstruction

Amit Manhas, C Preetam Chappity, Rakesh Kumar

■ INTRODUCTION

A patient presenting to casualty/emergency with acute upper airway obstruction (AUAO) warrants a detailed physical examination along with relevant history of onset, duration, precipitating factors, etc. The important points during assessment of AUAO include:

- *Severity*: AUAO may be partial or complete (i.e., partial—respiratory difficulty with stridor, or complete—absence of any detectable airflow in and out of lungs). Occasionally, a patient may present with potential or impending airway obstruction because of a known anatomical or physical condition.
- *Stridor (noisy respiration)*: May be inspiratory (obstruction at the level of vocal cords and above), expiratory (distal obstruction) or biphasic (subglottic and extrathoracic trachea).
- *Hoarse voice/cry*: Laryngeal involvement
- *Breathy voice*: Vocal cord paralysis
- *Cough and choking* (aspiration)
- *Accessory respiratory muscles (i.e., strap muscles and sternocleidomastoid)*: Patient may be showing "air-hunger" with sweating and use of accessory respiratory muscles with suprasternal, intercostal, and supraclavicular retractions. Obstruction below the thoracic inlet generally does not cause suprasternal retractions although intercostal/subxyphoid retraction or epigastric indrawing may be seen.
- *Other associated findings*: Include local pain, restlessness, drooling of saliva, anxious look, pallor and if trauma is involved; bleeding, subcutaneous emphysema and loss of normal laryngotracheal landmarks.

Accurate history taking is important, especially in cases of inhaled foreign body. Prodrome of upper respiratory tract infection occurs in cases of "croup" [laryngotracheobronchitis (LTB)].

■ DIAGNOSIS

"Lateral X-ray soft tissue neck (STN)" (neck extended during inspiration) delineates supraglottic airway lesion while posteroanterior (PA) view depicts

the subglottic pathologies. "X-ray chest (PA view)" reveals the foreign body (radio-opaque) or pulmonic changes (collapse and emphysema) and mediastinal shift. *"Fluoroscopy"* is better option for visualization of mobile structure, e.g., pharynx in cases of suspected retropharyngeal abscess and mediastinal shift to the side of aspirated foreign body on inspiration.

"Endoscopy" is the definitive test for AUAO and includes nasopharyngoscopy (flexible fiber-optic nasopharyngoscope) for assessment of airway from nasal chambers down to vocal folds and subglottis, laryngoscopy, and bronchoscopy (rigid or flexible) is done for assessment of trachea and bronchi. These two combined can assess the anomalies of the entire upper airway. *"Sleep study"* (overnight polysomnography) is indicated for sleep disorders (apnea).

■ OPTIONS FOR INTERVENTION
- Medical management
- Heimlich maneuver and positioning maneuvers
- Nasopharyngeal/oral airway and intubation
- Surgical intervention

Medical Management
It is indicated when respiratory distress is because of edema secondary to injury, infective process, or in neoplastic conditions. It includes oxygen inhalation, steroids, and/or antibiotics.
- Oxygen administration to relieve hypoxia is the first and most important step in medical treatment of AUAO. Oxygen is given via a face mask using a humidifier, providing 50% inspired oxygen. A helium-oxygen mixture (80% helium and 20% oxygen) known as *heliox* can be used wherein low-density helium helps in transport of oxygen past the obstructing lesions of larynx, trachea, or bronchi. In transient cases of AUAO, heliox sometimes eliminates the need for intubation or tracheostomy.
- Epinephrine aerosols are useful in AUAO with an element of soft tissue edema (e.g., croup).
- Steroids (systemic and topical) in large doses have been advised to reduce edema. Parenteral hydrocortisone is given in dose of 100–200 mg stat and 50–100 mg every 8 hourly for 24–48 hours.
- Adjuncts in airway support (oropharyngeal/nasopharyngeal airways) prevent ventilatory obstruction due to tongue fall back/relaxation.
- A short course of antibiotics can be given in the dose of 1 million units of penicillin or any other broad-spectrum antibiotic every 6 hourly intravenous for 3–5 days.
- Humidification provides liquefaction of secretions.

Heimlich Maneuver and Positioning Maneuvers

Heimlich Maneuver

Acute airway obstruction by a food bolus or any foreign body is dislodged by Heimlich maneuver. The approach is from behind a standing patient. Sudden pressure is applied by rapid squeezing motion in the epigastrium, against the xiphoid region of sternum, with the clenched fist, thereby making the residual air in the lungs to expel the foreign body. Alternatively, in a supine patient, kneel beside the patient and apply the epigastric pressure with the palms of the hand. If the maneuver fails, proceed to cricothyrotomy in adult or tracheostomy in the young child. Forced ventilation in the form of mouth to mouth or Ambu bag often provides some ventilation to the lungs, while surgical intervention of the airway is being performed.

Positioning Maneuvers

These are useful in the unconscious patients who present with upper airway obstruction due to flaccidity of the tongue and pharyngeal muscles.

Lateral-prone position: In the absence of cervical spine injury, turn the patient on his side and place the head sideways and down without a pillow, allowing the tongue to fall away from posterior pharyngeal wall and secretions to drain by gravity from the mouth.

Head maneuver: It is performed by lifting up the back of the neck while gently pressing the top of the head back and toward the shoulder. This is not advisable in possible cervical spine injury. This position is for mouth-to-mouth respiration.

Jaw thrust maneuver: It is performed by placing the fingertips of each hand behind and beneath the angles of the mandible and lifting the mandible forward. This position is used for mask to mouth ventilation.

In case of *conscious patients*, who present with severe upper airway obstruction from the base of tongue or larynx, the following maneuver is performed to provide some temporary relief till a more secure airway can be established.

Patient is asked to sit up which improves the pulmonary function and decreases upper airway edema. Patient is also advised to lean forward from the hips and then extend the head from the upper neck so that chin comes up and forward which open the airway to its maximum extent, providing good pulmonary ventilation.

Airway and Intubation

Airway (Oral/Nasopharyngeal)

These overcome the problems related to the prolapse or relaxation of the palate and the base of the tongue and may provide a well-tolerated, fully adequate airway.

Nasal airway: It is better tolerated in the conscious or semiconscious patients or who have sustained a mild-to-moderate head injury with obstruction but with normal respiratory drive. Insertion of nasal airway is made easy by instillation of topical nasal decongestant drops and lubrication of the airway device.

Oral airway: It is curved and semirigid, and can be used to bypass obstruction in the nose or mouth. It is used primarily in the unconscious patient to help hold the tongue forward and can also be used in semiconscious intubated patient to prevent him from occluding the tube by biting it. It also facilitates suctioning of secretions.

Esophageal airway: This is inserted "blind" into the esophagus and a balloon is distended. Air is insufflated through the device into the hypopharynx with presumptive ventilation. Nowadays, this is not recommended because it can lacerate the esophageal mucosa and increase the supraglottic edema, thereby increasing the problem.

Intubation

In the patients where respiration has ceased but upper airway obstruction is not suspected, e.g., cardiopulmonary arrest, perform mouth-to-mouth or mask-to-mouth respiration, maintain effective cardiac output, and intubate the patient after he has been well oxygenated for several minutes.

Endotracheal intubation: Mask-to-mouth or mouth-to-mouth ventilation is performed till equipment required for intubation (laryngoscope, endotracheal tubes (ETTs) with stylet, and suction) are available. Patient is positioned in "sniffing position", i.e., lower chin and head are slightly extended. Laryngoscope is inserted with the left hand into the right side of the mouth so that the tongue is pushed to the left of the laryngoscope blade. The curved blade of laryngoscope is slid around the base of tongue into the vallecula which is lifted up and away from the operator. This maneuver lifts the epiglottis up and out and the glottic chink is visible. With the right hand, ETT with stylet is inserted into the mouth and through the vocal cords. As the tube passes through the cords, stylet is removed. Suction is used to clear the secretions. If the obstruction is considered to be lower down, then a rigid bronchoscope is passed to inspect the subglottic area and trachea.

In case of difficult intubation, do not struggle but ventilate the patient with a mask until oxygenation improves before attempting intubation again. In case of failed intubation, a laryngeal mask airway can be inserted.

Blind nasal intubation: This is indicated in presence of trismus, cervical spine injuries, severe mandibular injuries, distortion, or masses in the oral cavity. The patient should have good spontaneous respiration because the tube is guided by breath sounds. Being a blind procedure, it requires lot of expertise on the part of the performer. It can cause epistaxis, retropharyngeal mucosal laceration, and sinusitis.

Combitube: It can be used where skilled persons are not available. It can be inserted blindly.

Fiber-optic endotracheal intubation: It is the most direct and reliable method of securing the compromised airway. Intubation is aided in difficult patient (trismus, mandibular injury, cervical spine injury, obstructive oral cavity lesion, etc.) by passing a fiber-optic endoscope through the lumen of an appropriate size ETT, then guiding it into the laryngotracheal lumen under direct vision.

Transtracheal ventilation: It requires special equipment. Patient can be fully ventilated with this technique for a period of up to 1 hour, providing rapid control in the emergency setup till more definitive procedure can be performed.

Procedure involves palpation of cricothyroid membrane with index finger and infiltration of 1–2 cc of 2% xylocaine around the skin. A 14G/16G plastic sheathed intravenous cannula connected with a syringe containing few mL of xylocaine is introduced in the midline and directed downward and backward into the tracheal lumen with the application of slow negative pressure on syringe till air bubbles are seen. 1–2 mL of xylocaine is sprayed into the tracheal lumen to anesthetize the tracheal lumen and needle is withdrawn leaving behind the plastic sheet cannula into the tracheal lumen which is attached to the high-pressure oxygen (50 lbs. per square inch) by means of Luer lock connectors. Ventilation may be achieved with a jetting device and chest movements are observed till definitive procedure is performed.

Surgical Intervention

Surgical intervention by cricothyrotomy/tracheostomy reduces the anatomical dead space by approximately 50%, reducing the work of breathing thereby increasing the alveolar ventilation. Also, the patient is able to communicate and eat with a tube and is more comfortable as compared to the ETT.

Cricothyrotomy

This is a quick and straightforward way to establish the airway. It is recommended when a dire emergency exists. Also, in cases of severe head and neck trauma with compromised airway where unstable cervical spine fracture is suspected, cricothyrotomy is a safer option prior to planned tracheostomy.

Steps for cricothyrotomy:
- Identify and palpate sternal notch, thyroid cartilage, and cricoid cartilage.
- Use the non-dominant hand to stabilize the laryngeal skeleton.
- A vertical incision is taken in midline over cricoid cartilage and using the index finger of the left hand palpates the cricothyroid.
- A horizontal incision is taken in cricothyroid membrane while avoiding cricothyroid vessels.
- Insert a clamp/Trousseau dilator to separate the cartilages and increasing the vertical dimension of membrane.
- Insert small ETT/tracheostomy tube (5.0) and then rotate the dilator counter clockwise by 90°. ETT is secured and established.

Major delayed complication of this procedure is *subglottic stenosis*. Therefore, it is converted to definite tracheostomy as soon as the patient's condition permits, ideally within 48 hours. In children, it is avoided because of a high chance of subglottic stenosis; therefore, a tracheostomy using vertical incision is always performed.

Tracheostomy (Tracheotomy)

Indications for tracheostomy (**Box 1**) have been classified as per *5 R's* formula:
1. *Respiratory obstruction*:
    - Infections such as acute laryngotracheobronchitis and acute epiglottitis
    - Trauma—maxillofacial injuries and external injury to larynx and trachea
    - Neoplasms—benign and malignant neoplasms of larynx, pharynx, and tongue
    - Foreign body larynx
    - Congenital anomalies such as tetralogy of Fallot (TOF), laryngeal web, and cysts
    - Bilateral abductor paralysis
    - Edema larynx due to steam and irritants

BOX 1: Indications for tracheostomy.

- Prolonged intubation
- Facilitation of ventilation support
- Inability of patient to manage secretions including aspiration
- Excessive bronchopulmonary secretions
- Upper airway obstruction with any of the following:
  Stridor, breathlessness, signs of labored breathing like chest retractions, prominent accessory muscles of respiration, obstructive sleep apnea with documented arterial oxygen desaturation and bilateral vocal cord paralysis
- Inability to intubate
- Adjunct to major head and neck surgery
- Adjunct to management of major head and neck trauma

2. *Retained secretions*:
   - Inability to cough as in head injuries, paralysis of respiratory muscles, and spinal injuries
   - Painful cough as in chest injuries and multiple rib fractures
   - Aspiration of pharyngeal secretions as seen in bilateral laryngeal paralysis
3. Reduction of dead space
4. *Respiratory insufficiency*: Chronic lung conditions that impede gas exchange chronic bronchitis, atelectasis, and emphysema
5. Respiratory paralysis

Elective Tracheostomy

It is performed when the upper airway is potentially at risk. It is indicated for patients already intubated or as adjunct to management of major head and neck operative procedure, till swallowing functions improve. Other indications include mechanical respiratory insufficiency which occurs in drug intoxication, head and chest injuries, neurological diseases, chronic obstructive airway diseases, etc., which may require tracheostomy. Another important indication includes the patients requiring intermittent or continuous positive pressure ventilation.

The method used for tracheostomy is dictated by the degree of urgency in establishing tracheostomy whenever possible. The method to be used should be the one for the elective procedure. Old time teaching of *"the time to do a tracheostomy is when you think it may be necessary"* has no longer any strong footing and is quite controversial. It also holds true for fresh postgraduates to avoid "overenthusiasm" and aggressive attitude because potential complications of tracheostomy have minimal occurrence if the procedure is performed by experienced team under well controlled circumstances.

Steps:
- Calm the patient and explain the procedure to the patient and his attendants beforehand to reduce the anxiety.
- Written consent is to be taken. Inform the patient/attendants that the patient will not be able to speak till tracheostomy is closed or the cuff of the tube is deflated.
- If the time allows, inspect and palpate the neck to assess the laryngotracheal anatomy through:
  - Indirect and/or direct laryngoscopy
  - STN lateral view for laryngotracheal anatomy and X-ray chest (PA view)
  - Pulmonary function tests (PFTs), which may not be available at every hospital

- Can be performed under local or general anesthesia. Make the patient to lie supine.
- If patient is able to lie down, then supine position is the ideal position for tracheostomy. If not, perform the procedure in the semi sitting position.
- Place a shoulder roll under the patient's shoulder in order to extend the neck and keep the neck in the midline (imaginary straight line between chin and sternum).
- Anesthetize the neck midway between the cricoid cartilage and the suprasternal notch using 2% xylocaine with 1:100,000 adrenaline.
- Make a transverse incision 2 cm above suprasternal notch. In case of dire emergency, a vertical midline incision is safer.
- Anterior jugular veins are ligated; strap muscles are spread apart with a hemostat in a midline-vertical plane and retracted laterally. By staying in the midline and using blunt dissection, vascular structures can be avoided.
- Isthmus of the thyroid can be clamped with hemostats, divided and oversewn. But it is quicker and safer to retract the isthmus inferiorly or superiorly.
- Expose the trachea; make a horizontal incision with No. 15 scalpel blade in second or third tracheal space and excise a part of the tracheal ring (adult).

Pediatric Tracheostomy
- Do not over extend the neck.
- Preferably horizontal skin incision is given.
- Lateral stay sutures in trachea to stabilize the trachea and to prevent dislodgement of tracheostomy tube accidentally.
- Vertical incision in trachea is made.
- Avoid removal of tracheal cartilage.
- Stay sutures taped to chest with strict instruction to staff "not to remove" them.

Percutaneous Dilatational Tracheostomy
Percutaneous dilatational tracheostomy (PDT) is safe and rapidly conducted procedure in experienced hands and can be conducted on all patients except:
- Pediatric patients
- Presence of midline mass
- Presence of coagulation abnormalities
- Presence of cervical spine injury
- Patient with thick neck—landmarks are obscured

Technique: Mostly done blindly but video bronchoscopic guidance is preferable.
Extend the neck, palpate, and mark the laryngeal landmarks. Infiltrate with local anesthesia. Make a 2 cm incision from inferior border of cricoid

toward sternal notch and do blunt midline dissection with hemostat. Advance the video bronchoscope via ETT, withdraw the ETT till vocal cord, and pass 22-gauge seeker needle between the first and second/second and third tracheal ring and check the position with expiration of air.

Pass flexible J-wire through the needle into the airway, dilate with 14-F dilator and further enlarge the tract with tapered dilators. Load the tracheostomy appliance and introduce into the tracheal lumen under video bronchoscope control. Once airway is secured; guidewire, guiding catheter, and loading dilator are then removed.

Complications: Paratracheal entry of dilator, hemorrhage, and damage to posterior tracheal wall.

Emergency Tracheostomy

It is further classified as:
- *Emergent (slash trach)*: It is indicated in emergency airway distress when risk of death of a patient exists, i.e., when cricothyroidotomy (cricothyrotomy) is indicated. A slash trach is considered only when "cannot intubate/cannot ventilate/cannot perform a cricothyrotomy".
- *Urgent (awake)*: It is indicated in a patient in respiratory distress and needs immediate surgical intervention. It is best performed in operation theater (OT) or intensive care unit (ICU) using local anesthesia on an awake patient.

Steps:
- If there is no skilled anesthetist, local anesthesia is used.
- If the patient is able to lie down, then supine position with padding (shoulder roll) under the patient's shoulder is the ideal position. If not, perform the procedure in the semisitting position.
- Palpate the thyroid and cricoid cartilage between the thumb and index finger of the nondominant hand and a vertical midline incision **(Fig. 1)** is taken starting at the inferior aspect of thyroid cartilage and extending to the suprasternal notch. It is then extended deep down between the infrathyroid muscles.
- No time should be wasted to control the bleeding which may be sometimes heavy due to congested veins (because of increased respiratory effort).
- Feel the cricoid cartilage using index finger of nondominant hand while retracting the skin edge by pressure applied by the thumb and middle finger. In extreme emergency, a vertical incision is taken straight into the trachea, at the level of 2nd, 3rd, and 4th ring without regard for thyroid isthmus. The knife blade is rotated through 90° to open the trachea, any form of available tube is inserted into the trachea and blood and secretions are sucked out. Patient may cough violently with the entry of blood into trachea and may displace the scalpel kept inside tracheal

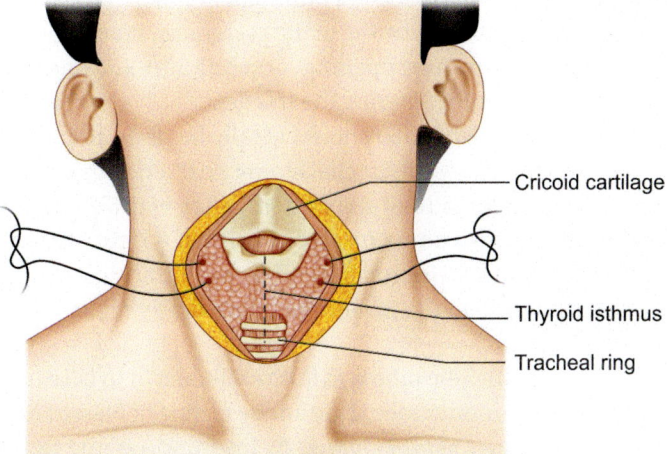

Fig. 1: Tracheostomy midline dissection.

lumen and operator must be extra careful at this juncture. After ensuring a safe airway, hemostasis is secured.

Care of tracheostomy tube includes:
- Proper fixation of tracheostomy tube by means of the tapes available, tie the tape in neutral neck position. Alternatively, it can be fixed to the neck skin to avoid dislodgement, especially when patient is on ventilator.
- A trained nurse, well acquainted with tracheostomy complications, sterile suctioning, humidification and change of tube should be in attendance. A especially created cubicle in the ward is much desirable with a bedside trolley having tracheostomy set, duplicate set of tracheostomy tube with introducer, laryngoscope, and oxygen cylinder with tracheostomy mask.
- Patient to be provided with a call-bell and a writing pad with pen to communicate.
- Children to be kept in ICU for first few days. Additional piece/segment of plastic tube can be inserted into the tracheostomy tube opening to avoid its obstruction by the "chin" of the child. X-ray chest (PA view) is done immediately after tracheostomy.
- Periodic suctioning of the tracheostomy tube, ideally every half to 1 hour in first 48 hours and thereafter every 4 hours by means of a smooth end disposable/sterile suction catheter with an external diameter less than half of internal diameter of the tracheostomy tube in situ, with all aseptic precautions.
- In case of tenacious mucus which is difficult to aspirate, isotonic saline or a mucolytic agent may be sprinkled through the tracheostomy tube by a fine nebulizer.

- Humidification by hot water bath, humidifier or nebulizer delivering cold droplets is done to avoid crusting of the secretions. Wet gauze can be kept over the tracheostomy tube opening for humidification and to avoid any flying foreign body from entering the trachea.
- Change of tracheostomy tube should ideally be done after 48 hours that too by putting the patient in tracheostomy position with a shoulder pad. By standing on right side of the patient, after withdrawal of old tube, place the fresh tube with its insertor in situ at a right angle to trachea and with 90° anticlockwise rotation movement, thus inserting it into the lumen following which the insertor is immediately removed to facilitate ventilation.
- Always check whether the tube is in tracheal lumen or in false tract anterior to the trachea, in anterior mediastinum by feeling of blast of expired air.
- *"Rail-road technique" of tube change*: By inserting a sterile catheter in old tube, withdraw the old tube over the catheter and new tracheostomy tube is threaded over the catheter into the trachea.
- In cases of metallic (double tube) tracheostomy tube, inner tube to be periodically removed and washed in sodium bicarbonate solution every 12 hours and cleaned off any crusts in the lumen.
- *Care of inflatable cuff*: Periodic deflation for 5 minutes every 2 or 4 hours to avoid ischemic changes to the tracheal mucosa. Low pressure cuffs or double cuffed tracheostomy tube can also be used.
- Breathing exercises by physiotherapist and regular sterile dressing all around the tracheostomy site.

Complications of Tracheostomy

Immediate:
- *Hemorrhage*: It can arise from anterior jugular veins or isthmus of the thyroid gland. It should be controlled at once by ligation or diathermy. If profuse, digital pressure and extension of the wound can be done to visualize the bleeding point.
- *Air embolism*: It can cause tamponade and death.
- *Apnea*: It occurs due to sudden discharge of pent-up carbon dioxide. Apnea is best avoided by carbogen (95% O_2 + 5% CO_2)
- *Cardiac arrest*: It can occur in anxious subjects, due to increasing alkalosis with rise in pH and hyperkalemia.
- Injury to *recurrent laryngeal nerve*.

Intermediate:
- *Surgical emphysema*: Most frequently caused by closure of skin tight around the tube and an improperly sized and fitted tracheostomy tube.
- *Dislodgement of tube*: Postoperative edema, hematoma, and emphysema enhance dragging of tube out of trachea.

TABLE 1: Various types of airways.

Airway	Indications	Drawbacks
Nasopharyngeal	Pharyngeal and/or base of tongue collapse in alert or semiconscious patients	Can cause epistaxis
Oral	• Obstructed or injured nasal airway • Unconscious patients	• Dislodged easily • Poorly tolerated by alert patients
Oral intubation	• Need for controlled ventilation • Failure of simple measures • Prevents aspiration	• Requires expertise and proper equipment • Potential injury to larynx and pharynx
Blind nasal	• Potential cervical spine injury with need for airway control • Massive oral cavity injury • Trismus	• Epistaxis • Requires expertise
Fiber-optic nasal	• Suspected cervical spine injury • Massive oral cavity injury	• Difficult to see if excess secretions or bleeding present • Requires expertise and expensive equipment
Cricothyroidotomy	• Failure of intubation • No laryngeal injury • Prior to definite tracheostomy	• Surgical procedure • Can cause acute and chronic laryngeal injury • Contraindicated in children
Tracheostomy	• Laryngeal trauma • Oropharyngeal obstruction not controlled by intubation • After cricothyroidotomy, preferably within 48 hours	• Difficult than cricothyroidotomy • Numerous potential complications • Safe in expert hands
Laryngeal airway	• Failure of intubation • Can be used without laryngoscope	Can cause aspiration in mask airway, full stomach patients

- *Infection*: Frequent change of local dressings around the tracheostomy tube prevents infection.
- *Dysphagia*: It is managed by Ryles tube feeding or by deflating the cuff of tracheostomy tube during feeds.
- *Pneumothorax*: It is caused by injury to a highly placed apex of the lung in the neck, especially in infants. Chest radiograph confirms the diagnosis.

TABLE 2: Size of tracheostomy tube.

Formula for size of tracheostomy tube	Age in years/4 + 4
Premature neonates < 1,000 g	2.5 mm
Premature neonates > 1,000 g	3.0 mm
Neonates or infants 0–6 months	3.0–3.5 mm

- *Tracheoarterial/tracheoinnominate fistula*: It occurs in 0.4% of tracheostomies with a mortality rate of 80–90%. It is usually due to erosion of innominate artery, especially in a low placed tracheostomy.
- *Scabs and crusts*: It is due to temporary loss of the movement of the ciliary blanket and continues dryness in trachea due to exposure via tracheostoma.
- *Tracheal necrosis*: It follows focal pressure secondary to infection.
- *Tracheoesophageal fistula*: Contributing factors are:
  - Overinflated cuff
  - Indwelling nasogastric tube in esophagus
  - Positive pressure ventilation

Late:
- *Difficulty with decannulation*: In long-standing tubes, granulations form resulting into tracheal strictures, causing difficulty in decannulation.
- *Tracheal stenosis*: Majority occurs from inflatable cuff of tracheostomy tube.
- *Tracheocutaneous fistula and scars*: A fistula causes continuous exposure of skin to secretions from the trachea that may result in skin irritation with recurrent and persistent infections and poor appearance.

■ VARIOUS TYPES OF AIRWAYS

Various types of airways are given in **Table 1**.

■ SIZE OF TRACHEOSTOMY TUBE

Table 2 presents size of tracheostomy tube.

■ FURTHER READING

1. Chan PW, Goh A, Lum L. Severe upper airway obstruction in the tropics requiring intensive care. Pediatr Int. 2001;43:53-7.
2. Chow CM, Cheung KL, Hon KL. Upper airway obstruction in children. J Paediatr Respirol Crit Care. 2005;1:5-9.
3. Sutherland GA, Lack HL. Congenital laryngeal obstruction. Lancet. 1897;2:653-5.

CHAPTER 7

Faciomaxillary Trauma

Gopika Kalsotra, Parveen Akhter Lone, Subirendra Kumar

■ INTRODUCTION

Faciomaxillary trauma is most commonly the result of road traffic accidents (RTAs) and physical combat. Facial injuries are considered different than any other injuries elsewhere in the body, because in facial trauma, restoration of esthetics and function are must otherwise a minor facial trauma leads to psychological impact due to serious problems.

■ INITIAL TREATMENT

Once the patient's general condition is stable, all necessary assessments should be carried out to derive a diagnosis and its treatment plan. This includes:
- History taking
- Physical examination
- Radiological examination
- Special investigation.

Important considerations in faciomaxillary trauma/fracture are:
- Check airway stability
- Check visual acuity in the middle third facial fracture (retrobulbar injury/neuritis)
- Tetanus prophylaxis
- Look for cervical spine injury association
- CT head and paranasal sinus (PNS) (facial bones) preferably with 3D reconstruction for extent of trauma.

Definitive management of these injuries is rarely emergent and other life-threatening injuries usually require greater priority for treatment. At the initial resuscitation, special care has to be directed to possible airway obstruction and risk of aspiration. The emergency resuscitation in any faciomaxillary trauma will include modified mnemonic *"ABCDE"* as explained here:
- Maintenance of an adequate *"airway"* and assess and establish "breathing" so that ventilation is effective.
- Adequate hemostasis to prevent *"blood loss"* and maintain the circulation.

- Inspect for and manage with appropriate stabilization of neck for an unstable *"cervical spine"* injury.
- Assess the level of consciousness and neurological *"dysfunction"*.
- *"Expose"* the other parts of the body of the patient to ensure all other areas have been inspected for injuries.

(In original mnemonic, "B" stands for establishing breathing and "C" for maintaining the circulation).

Definitive treatment of facial injury is always the second priority. In initial examination, always look for posterior displacement of tongue due to bilateral parasymphysis mandibular fracture, posterior-inferior displacement of the maxilla, inhalation of blood clot, vomit, thick mucus, teeth, bone dentures or foreign bodies, paradoxical chest movements due to flail chest segment, and laryngotracheal framework trauma. These all warrant establishment of a safe airway and effective ventilation by means of endotracheal intubation or tracheostomy.

Bleeding from nose or mouth in semiconscious/comatose patient will warrant timely intervention by means of nasal pack, balloons, catheters, sutures, or arterial ligation.

■ SCALP AND SOFT TISSUE INJURIES

In *scalp*, skull fracture and presence of any foreign body is looked for. Direct pressure application to the bleeding site controls most of the scalp hemorrhages temporarily. Large vessels are caught with hemostat and ligated. Scalp laceration with multiple points ooze is best controlled by using a 2-0 nylon running silk taking large, deep bites.

The wound is explored under local anesthesia (LA) or general anesthesia (GA) and copious irrigation with saline is done to remove the dirt and foreign matter. Nonviable tissue is debrided and wound is closed in layers. Antibiotics are given empirically and tetanus prophylaxis is advised as per the immune status (explained earlier in wound management chapter).

In cases of avulsions, small wounds are closed primarily while local flaps are used for other cases.

Soft Tissue Injuries

Type of soft tissue wounds:
- Abrasion
- Contusion
- Hematoma
- Lacerated wound
- Incised wound
- Penetrating and punctured wound
- Crushed wound
- Gunshot injuries (high velocity).

Treatment includes:
- Cleaning of wound
- Removal of foreign bodies
- Debridement
- Hemostasis
- Closure in layers (primary closure)
- Prevention of infection
- Pain control
- Follow-up.

In head and neck, soft tissue injuries generally heal well because of excellent blood supply. "Laceration" should be sutured at the earliest after the soft tissue wound is carefully explored, debrided, and cleaned off all dirt and foreign bodies (glass pieces, sand, dirt, plastics, etc.). Usually the laceration can be sutured under LA, after a local anesthetic has been injected into the edge of wound, soft tissue twigs having doubtful blood supply may be removed with sharp scalpel and local advancement flaps may be planned for proper approximation. In cosmetically/aesthetically important areas such as vermillion border of lips, eyelids, and nasal contour, the tissue replacement should be precise and by skilled surgeon.

A careful wound examination should be carried out in the depth of the wound to detect foreign bodies. Wound should be irrigated with copious amounts of saline solution. Lacerations of face and scalp may be masked due to blood crust and entangled hairs. Excellent healing of facial injury is a result of thorough wound cleaning and gentle handling with meticulous repair. Facial and scalp injury should be repaired at the earliest as soon as patients general condition allows in order to lessen edema and prevent formation of granulation tissue and infection.

During approximation, muscle and superficial layers are sutured in layers with absorbable (3-0/40) suture in such a way that the skin edges lie passively within 2 mm of their final position. The fine monofilament (5-0 or 6-0) suture is used to close the skin, avoiding the inversion of wound edges. Vacuum drain should be kept in the dead space.

Wound is covered by antibiotic ointment twice daily and broad-spectrum antibiotics are given. Alternate sutures are removed in 5 days and Ethistrips can be applied.

Facial Nerve Injury

It is encountered usually in lateral facial wound. If suspected in otherwise gross edema or in clinically evident ipsilateral facial nerve palsy, the wound should be explored. Proximal and distal flaps are raised in the relatively normal adjacent tissue to identify the severed nerve which may then be traced toward the laceration and its ends are approximated under the guidance of an operating microscope (8-0 to 10-0 fine monofilament sutures). Primary repair is always indicated but practically, it is extremely difficult in presence of otherwise edematous and damaged tissue. Sometimes, suture indicators can be left in wound for secondary repair but results are unsatisfactory.

Parotid Duct

Laceration of parotid duct usually accompanies the facial nerve injury. It is identified first by insertion of a small cannula in the parotid duct from Stensen's duct opening per orally, and cannulating till it presents at the wound site. The proximal end of parotid duct may then be identified from the site of the distal end marked by the cannula, and sutured end-to-end. Overlying tissue is sutured taking care to avoid displacement across the sutured ends of the duct and cannula can be left in situ till healing takes place. Some authors recommend side-to-side suturing of the Stensen's duct to avoid stricture of the duct.

■ NASAL FRACTURES

Trauma to nose will cause the damage depending upon the direction. In the frontal plane, the force of impact will determine the extent of injury. In *mild frontal trauma*, there is injury to the cartilaginous vault causing its separation and avulsion injury along with posterior dislocation of the septum. In *moderate frontal trauma, (also known as open-book fracture)* deviation of nasal bones with flattening and splaying along with deviation of a nasal septum is encountered. In *severe frontal trauma*, there is in addition the adjacent structural involvement such as frontal process of maxilla, ethmoid labyrinth, lacrimal bones, cribriform plate, and orbital plate of frontal bones. Collapse and telescoping of septal fragments may be seen. Lateral impact injuries are more common, causing depression of ipsilateral nasal bone, may also involve nasal process of maxilla and pyriform margin. Lateral displacement of contralateral nasal bone with fractured or dislocated septum is also seen.

Clinically, nasal fractures are classed into three types, depending upon degree of damage sustained with variable quantum/impact of force.

Type I: It is the depressed nasal fracture. In *"mild cases"*, there is unilateral nasal bone fracture with the fracture line running parallel to the dorsum of nose and nasomaxillary suture, joining at the junction point of the thin and thick part of nasal bone (i.e., upper one-third and lower two-thirds). Nasal septum is usually not involved. In *"severe cases" (Chevallet type)*, the fracture lines run parallel to the nasomaxillary suture on the fractured side and parallel and just below the dorsum on the contralateral side, connecting across the dorsum at the junction point of thin and thick parts of the nasal bone. The nasal septum is involved and fracture line involves both cartilaginous and bony parts. Clinically, type I fracture presents with edema of nose with no gross lateral displacement while depression of the fractured segment may be obvious or not. In pediatric age, the fracture is usually of *"greenstick"* type and the nasal deformity becomes obvious at puberty.

Type II (Jarjavay): This involves nasal bone, frontal process of maxilla and septum while ethmoid and orbit are spared. Frontal force causes comminution of nasal bones with gross flattening and widening of the dorsum. The lateral blow produces a high deviation of nasal skeleton. Septum is involved (both cartilaginous and bony parts) and may appear clinically as dislocation from maxillary crest. Clinically, "dislocated" caudal end of septum represents a Chevallet or Jarjavay fracture.

Type III (naso-orbito-ethmoid fracture): It results from high velocity facial trauma. Ethmoid being thin and full of air cells, forms a low resistance *"crumple zone"*, and thus allows the traumatic force to be dissipated, protecting the brain and optic nerve from the impact of injury. Nasal skeleton gives way and ethmoid labyrinth collapses or telescopes on itself. Ethmoidal perpendicular plate is rotated and the quadrilateral cartilage is pulled backward, resulting in "classical pig" like appearance of the patient with foreshortened nose facing forward. Clinically, telecanthus is seen and medial canthal ligament may be disrupted from lacrimal crest. Patient has mid-face retrusion and may result in epiphora due to involvement of lacrimal drainage.

Naso-orbito-ethmoid (NOE) fracture has been classified on the status of medial canthal tendon (MCT) and degree of comminution of the fragments of bone of its attachment **(Figs. 1 and 2)** (Markowitz et al. 1991).

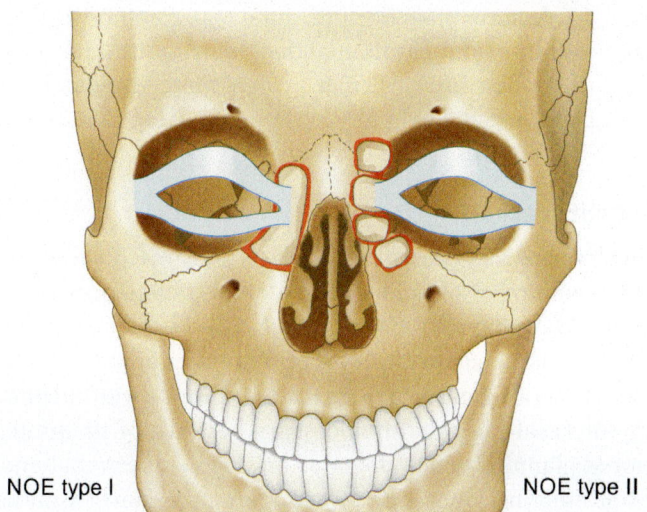

Fig. 1: Naso-orbito-ethmoid (NOE) type I (right) and NOE type II (left).

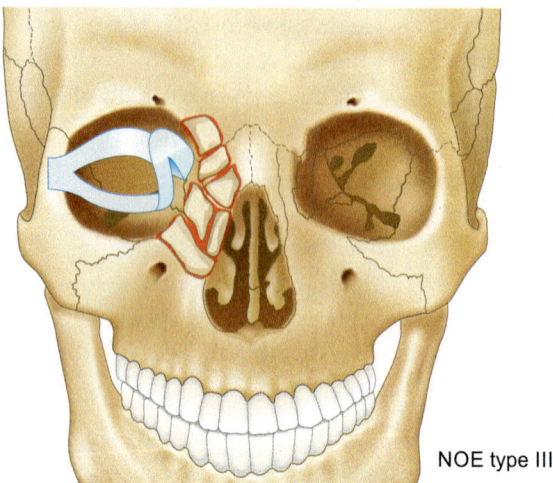

Fig. 2: Naso-orbito-ethmoid (NOE) type III.

Type I: The fracture line leaves a central segment of bone with MCT attached. It is simplest to reconstruct, by means of miniplating to the surrounding facial bones.

Type II: It involves comminuted fracture of the central segment but MCT remains firmly attached to a definable central segment of bone.

Type III: Severe comminuted fragmentation of central segment with disruption of the MCT insertion sites.

Type II and type III are difficult to repair and it would necessitate transnasal wiring of either MCT bearing bone fragments or the MCT. These injuries are difficult to identify clinically owing to soft tissue edema. Also, look for associated cribriform plate fracture, dural tear, cerebrospinal fluid (CSF) leak, pneumocranium and nasofrontal duct injury at its outflow in anterior ethmoid sinus. Ocular injuries such as hyphema, vitreous hemorrhage, dislocation of lens, and globe rupture may be seen in high force trauma which had caused NOE fractures.

Clinical Features

Nasal bone fracture may present clinically as an isolated nasal trauma or in combination with other injuries. Isolated nasal trauma presents with pain, tenderness, and swelling along with epistaxis and external nasal deformity. Careful history is necessary to differentiate recently acquired and old deformities and, if available, compare the nasal profile with old photographs. Radiology of nasal bones is unnecessary because of its limited role in management planning which depends on degree of external and internal deformity on anterior rhinoscopy. Most important reason of X-ray nasal bone is mainly for medicolegal purposes **(Fig. 3)**.

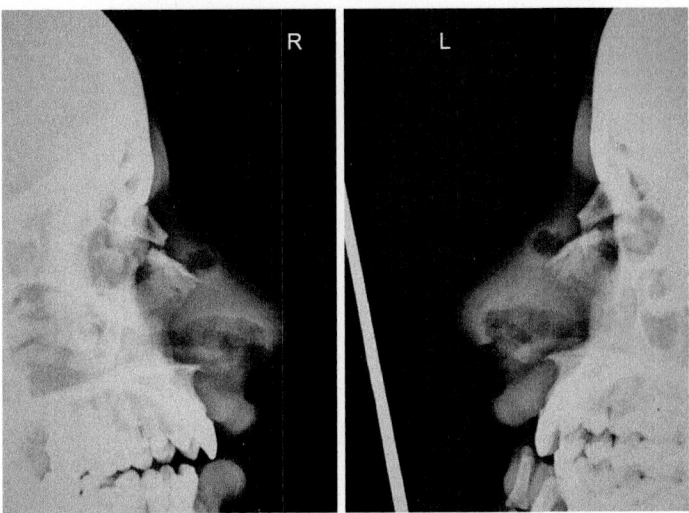
Fig. 3: Depressed nasal bone fracture.

Treatment

"Type I fracture" reduction is performed within 3–7 days in children and within 5–10 days in adults, when overlying edema has settled. Manual reduction is the easiest method of closed reduction, performed under LA or GA, where direction of reducing force applied is in reverse of causative trauma force. Bony nasal pyramid is reduced first followed by reduction and stabilization of septum. *"Walsham forceps"* is used to grasp and manipulate the nasal bones into correct position. *"Asch forceps"* is used to elevate the dorsum and disimpact the septum simultaneously. Anterior nasal pack is kept for 2–3 days which provides internal splinting. Dorsum is splinted with plaster cast or prefabricated splint which is removed after 1 week. An important problem with *"Asch"* and *"Walsham"* forceps is the possibility of "mucosal crush" injury and resulting hematomas. Alternatively, the *"Boies"* elevator can be inserted into the nostril deep to a displaced fracture, keeping thumb of oneself on the outside of the nose and gentle manipulation is done to raise or depress the misaligned bones to their original position.

"Type II fractures" are not managed properly with closed reduction because of displaced septal cartilages/or bone. Therefore, closed reduction of nasal bone is accompanied by an open reduction of septal deformity via Killian's incision approach.

In *"type III fractures"*, nasal collapse and telescoping of fractured segments require open reduction and internal fixation. Reduced frontonasal complex is supported by transnasal wires tied externally over either silicon or lead plates. Otherwise miniplates can be used to reconstruct comminuted bony fragments.

Sometimes, *"mild nasal trauma"* leads to *septal hematoma* only, especially in children because of bleeding in the subperichondrial planes, on both sides of the septum. It should be immediately evacuated or drained by means of hemi or full transfixation incision, followed by bilateral anterior nasal packing to prevent recurrence. If septal hematoma persists for 3–4 days, it can lead to irreversible damage to the septal cartilage because of ischemic necrosis leading to "saddle nose deformity" and retraction of columella.

In *"pediatric patients"*, nose is the most common site of fracture which is mainly of "greenstick" type because of cartilaginous nasal pyramid and unfused midline suture. Typically, pediatric nasal fracture presents as a *"splaying"* of the nasal bones over the frontal process of the maxilla. "Greenstick" fractures may go unrecognized because of extensive edema and absence of crepitus. X-ray of nasal bone also has limited role.

During examination, one must have high index of suspicion for "septal hematoma" and "CSF rhinorrhea". Also look for associated cosmetic and nasal obstruction.

Management in majority of pediatric patients is conservative. Closed reduction under GA is indicated for displaced nasal fractures, which may not be satisfactory in greenstick type fractures.

In cases of significant septal fractures, resulting in loss of support for the nasal dorsum, a conservative septorhinoplasty is indicated (minimal manipulation of septum), while nasal tip surgery is deferred till puberty.

■ EAR TRAUMA

Ear examination is usually missed as a part of polytrauma patients, but its morbidity is high, if neglected.

External Ear Trauma

- *Hematoma:* Hematoma of auricle is managed by aspiration or by incision and drainage. For incision and drainage, incision is made in the helical sulcus and hematoma is milked out. Some surgeons prefer not to close the wound, while some keep a drain routinely. Contours of pinna are packed with dental rolls or cotton soaked in betadine, or by using through and through mattress suture tied over a bolster in order to avoid dead space between skin and underlying cartilage, thus discouraging the formation of recurrent hematoma. Mastoid bandage along with broad-spectrum antibiotics against *Staphylococcus* are advised.
- *Laceration:* Laceration of the auricle is closed primarily after adequate cleansing and foreign body debris removal. Associated cartilage damage is repaired as per the clinical situation. Small pieces can be sacrificed, but a large piece of avulsed cartilage with intact perichondrium is placed in the wound and given soft tissue cover over it.

- *Avulsion:* If a piece of auricle is nearly avulsed but attached by a skin remnant, it is reapproximated primarily if the blood flow is adequate. If the blood supply is poor, the avulsed piece is sacrificed. Delayed repair is indicated if major portion of auricle has been avulsed or when there is significant exposed cartilage without any viable skin. In these patients, cartilage is buried into the postauricular pocket or abdominal pocket for 7–10 days and grafted at a later date. Broad-spectrum antibiotics are advised.

Middle Ear Trauma

It includes tympanic membrane perforation with or without ossicular disruption and occasionally associated with dizziness.

Most of the traumatic tympanic membrane perforations are seen in anterior-inferior quadrant of the pars tensa. If clean, they are managed conservatively and 95% of them heal spontaneously. Antibiotics and topical ear drops are avoided. The contaminated injuries are cleaned thus removing all foreign debris and advised oral as well as topical antibiotic drugs. No surgical intervention is required immediately and patient is advised to keep the ear dry. If perforation does not heal on its own, planned myringoplasty is done as a cold surgery.

Posterior-superior quadrant tympanic membrane perforations are usually associated with ossicular disruption (incudostapedial joint separation). Management is similar as described earlier and the hearing mechanism is investigated later with a pure tone audiogram and a CT scan of temporal bone, if necessary and repaired at a later stage as a planned surgery (ossiculoplasty or tympanoplasty).

Occasionally there is subluxation of incus on the stapes superstructure or displacement of the stapes into the vestibule, causing vertigo, nausea, and vomiting and nystagmus beating away from the injured side. Management includes the labyrinthine sedatives, antiemetics, and bed rest. Surgery is indicated if there is suspicion of fistula between inner and middle ear. High-resolution CT (HRCT) scan of temporal bone may be useful and help identify the fistula prior to surgery.

Inner Ear Injury

This is because of temporal bone fractures which may be *longitudinal* (due to direct trauma to parietal or temporal bone) or *transverse* (trauma directed at the occiput).

The longitudinal fracture results from the lateral blows to the head and the fracture line extends from external ear canal anteromedially along the anterior edge of the petrous apex to the foramen lacerum and foramen ovale. Conductive hearing loss is the most common presentation because of tympanic membrane perforation, hemotympanum, CSF in the middle ear, and/or ossicular disruption. Facial nerve injury occurs in 20% of cases, usually at the geniculate ganglion and horizontal portion of the nerve. The transverse fractures are typically caused by frontal or occipital blows to the skull and the fracture line extends from the jugular foramen through the internal auditory canal to the foramen lacerum leading to nerve deafness and associated facial nerve injury (50% cases). Management of facial nerve injury includes CT scan of the temporal bone (high resolution, both coronal and axial cuts) to locate the site of fracture, topodiagnostic tests to determine the site of injury and electrical nerve test to determine the physiologic status of facial nerve. Clinically, progression from partial to complete paralysis, loss of lacrimation, submandibular salivary flow rate <25% of normal, indicate unfavorable signs and warrant surgical exploration and nerve decompression and/or nerve repair at the earliest. The *"oblique fracture"* has been used to describe fractures that are neither longitudinal nor transverse and cross the petrotympanic fissure.

If facial nerve function does not recover after 1 year, facial-hypoglossal anastomosis, facio-masseteric nerve anastomosis or facial slings, is indicated.

Management of acute vertigo includes strict bed rest in a quiet room and administration of vestibular suppressants like diazepam (5–20 mg) in 3–5 minutes provides most rapid relief (in large vein in order to minimize the possibility of vein sclerosis). More drugs can be added to the intravenous bottle and infused slowly if severe symptoms recur and dose can be titrated by observing its effect on the nystagmus and vertigo sensation on or off by slowing or quickening the intravenous rate. For the accompanying nausea and vomiting, intravenous droperidol is very effective. Promethazine hydrochloride 25–50 mg intramuscular or prochlorperazine 12.5–25 mg intramuscular can also be used as vestibular suppressants as well as for the control of accompanying nausea and vomiting. Ondansetron (intravenous as single 32 mg dose over 15 minutes) may also be used to control nausea and vomiting.

Intravenous fluid and electrolyte replacement is another important aspect to be considered for the management of acute vertigo.

Maintenance therapy is given once the acute phase is over. Diazepam is generally given on short term basis (2, 5, or 10 mg 6–8 hourly), depending on the severity of the patient's symptoms and the level of anxiety. Meclizine in dose of 12.5–25 mg, 6–8 hourly or dimenhydrinate in dose of 50–100 mg, 6–8 hourly can be used.

Promethazine 25 mg, 6–8 hourly and prochlorperazine (5 mg 8 hourly) by oral or by rectal suppository (25 mg bid dosage) are also useful for the control of nausea and vomiting on an OPD basis.

Certain drugs can be prescribed to accelerate vestibular compensation which include calcium antagonists (cinnarizine 25–75 mg, 8 hourly), betahistine (8–16 mg, 8 hourly), and gangliosides (*Ginkgo biloba* extracts) of which the former two groups also act as vestibular sedatives. "Cinnarizine" has additional benefit of improving cerebral circulation and maintaining red blood cell RBC flexibility. Domperidone 15 mg with cinnarizine 20 mg is a good combination available which can be safely advised for management of vertigo associated with nausea and vomiting on outpatient department (OPD) basis.

Management of post-traumatic nerve deafness is unfortunately not possible because of permanent damage. Although there is some spontaneous recovery of the high frequency loss that often accompanies longitudinal fractures, there is little possibility of recovery of any useful hearing following transverse fractures. Only point to be stressed is to document the hearing loss (conductive, sensorineural, or mixed) on the case file, as per the tuning fork tests and pure tone audiometry (bed side if possible) from the medicolegal point of view.

Indications for Early Intervention in "Ear Trauma" Cases

"CLONE" mnemonic:
- C: Carotid artery injury (penetrating trauma)
- L: CSF leak
- O: Other intracranial findings (extra or subdural hematoma, temporal lobe injury)
- N: Facial nerve palsy—complete
- E: External ear canal fracture (significant displacement which might cause canal stenosis if left untreated).

■ MIDFACE FRACTURES

Middle Third

Middle third of face is the area which is bounded superiorly by a line drawn from frontozygomatic (FZ) suture on one side across the frontonasal suture and frontomaxillary suture to the zygomaticofrontal (ZF) suture on opposite side and inferiorly by occlusal plane of maxillary teeth but if patient is edentulous then upper alveolar ridge is taken as the inferior limit.

The region is demarcated posteriorly by sphenoethmoidal junction.

The area of middle face is complex and complicated anatomically so that fractures of this region are generally comminuted, especially bones of nasoethmoid (NE) complex and anterior maxilla.

The central midface comprises of several fragile bones that easily *"crumple"* when subjected to strong forces and this results in an inward crushing which causes typical dish-shaped deformity of the face. These fragile bones are protected by the surrounding peripheral thick and strong bones of the buttress system comprised by one strong frontal, maxillary, zygomatic, and sphenoid bones and their attachments to one another. This composite structure of rigid facial bones is so designed that it will withstand forces of mastication from below and provides protection to the vital structure (eye and brain, etc.). The buttress include: (1) vertical buttress: which are well developed primarily contributed by the medial nasomaxillary and lateral zygomaticomaxillary (ZM) buttress and also contributed by pterygomaxillary and vertical mandible buttresses and (2) horizontal buttress comprises of the frontal bone with its supraorbital rims (frontal bar), the nasal bones and inferior orbital rims with the maxillary alveolus, these connect to each other thus providing support for vertical buttress. The strong zygomatic bone at the lateral corner of midface acts as a bedrock to provide support to other facial bones. The maxilla is directly in contact with the frontal bone at the frontomaxillary suture and with the sphenoid bone posteriorly. The zygoma overlies and reinforces this lateral area of mid third face through its attachments to the underlying frontal, maxillary, sphenoid, and temporal bones.

"René Le Fort" (1901) devised a classification system for midface fractures by identification of patterns of fractures along three particular lines of weakness inherent in the design of the facial skeleton, in the cases with blunt trauma. Presence of pterygoid fracture is the key to establish the diagnosis and Le Fort fractures can be excluded, if CT scan does not reveal pterygoid fractures.

Le Fort I (low level/subzygomatic fracture): It is also called as *horizontal fracture of the maxilla or Guerin's fracture* **(Fig. 4)**. It is also known as *floating fracture,* as there is a complete separation of dentoalveolar part of the maxilla

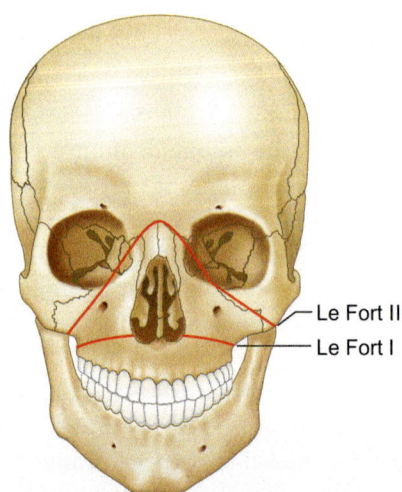

Fig. 4: Le Fort I and Le Fort II.

(pterygomaxillary dysjunction). The fracture line commences at the point of lateral margin of the anterior nasal aperture, passes above the nasal floor, and it passes laterally above the canine fossa and traverses the lateral antral wall, dipping down below the zygomatic buttress and then inclines upward and posteriorly across the pterygomaxillary fissure to fracture the pterygoid laminae at the junction of their lower third and upper two-thirds.

Le Fort II (pyramidal or subzygomatic fracture): It is a pyramidal-shaped fracture **(Fig. 4)**. Fracture line runs from thin middle area of nasal bones below frontonasal suture on either side, crossing frontal process of maxilla into medial wall of orbit, crosses lacrimal bone behind lacrimal sac within each orbit, and forward to cross inferior orbital margin slightly medial or through infraorbital foramen. It then runs downward laterally across lateral wall of maxilla below ZM suture and ends up dividing the pterygoid laminae about half way up.

Le Fort III (transverse or suprazygomatic fracture or high-level fracture): Fracture line extends from frontonasal suture transversely backward parallel with the base of skull along the medial wall of the orbit involving entire depth of ethmoid bone including cribriform plate **(Fig. 5)**. Deep in the orbit the fracture line passes below optic foramen into posterior limit of inferior orbital fissure. From the base of inferior orbital fissure line extends into two directions:
1. Posteriorly along the maxillary fissure and fractures the roots of pterygoid laminae.
2. Laterally along the lateral wall of orbit thus separating the inferior zygomatic bone from superior frontal bone.

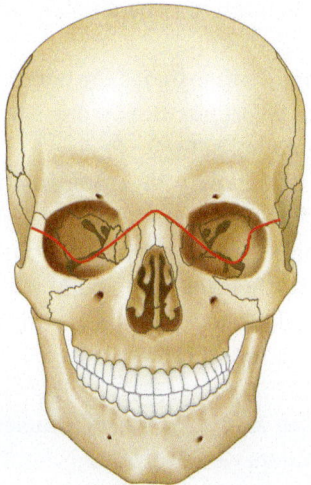

Fig. 5: Le Fort III.

TABLE 1: Modified classification system proposed by Marciani.

1.	Le Fort-I		Low maxillary fracture
		Ia	Low maxillary fractures/multiple segments
2.	Le Fort II		Pyramidal fracture
		IIa	Pyramidal and nasal fractures
		IIb	Pyramidal and nasoethmoid fractures
3.	Le Fort III		Craniofacial dysjunction
		IIIa	Craniofacial dysjunction and nasal fracture
		IIIb	Craniofacial dysjunction and naso-orbito-ethmoid (NOE) fracture
4.	Le Fort IV		Le fort II and III and cranial base fracture
		IVa	Supraorbital rim
		IVb	Anterior craniofacial fossa and supraorbital rim fracture
		IVc	Anterior cranial fossa and orbital wall fracture

Each Le Fort fracture pattern has at least one unique fracture. Only the Le Fort I fracture includes the lateral aspect of the pyriform aperture. Only the Le Fort II includes the inferior orbital rim and ZM suture line. Finally, only the Le Fort III involves the zygomatic arch and the lateral orbital wall.

A modified classification system is proposed by Marciani in 1993 to more preciously define Le Fort, NOE, and ZM fracture patterns **(Table 1)**.

Clinically, in a patient presenting with mid facial fracture:
- First always look at pterygoid plates. Presence of a bilateral pterygoid fracture indicates the presence of Le Fort fracture.
- As described earlier, involvement of the pyriform aperture, inferior orbital rim, and the zygomatic arch may be a telltale sign of underlying type of Le Fort fracture.
- Systematic inspection of other bones for fractures is essential because a patient might have a Le Fort fracture on one side and an isolated nasal or zygomatic fracture on other side.
- Always look for all three key indicators, fractures must be examined allowing each Le Fort level to be confirmed or ruled out, as there could be more than one Le Fort level fracture in same patient.
- On occasion, Le Fort fractures (especially with high energy fractures) extend to the anterior skull base via superior orbital fissure, thus extending across the orbital apex, and these are referred to as a Le Fort IV fracture by some authors.

Investigation includes X-ray paranasal sinuses, (submentovertex and occipitomental view) (Waters view and lateral view) and CT scan of head and PNS (facial bones), especially with 3D reconstruction.

Management of Middle Third Facial Fractures

Treatment plan includes:
- Skeletal fixation—internal/external
- Open reduction/closed reduction
- Type of maxillomandibular fixation required, i.e., arch bar, cap splints, gunning splints, etc.
- Reduction and fixation of other associated facial fractures (mandible, NOE, zygomatic arch, etc.)
- Stabilizing the occlusion.

Internal skeletal fixation: The middle third of facial skeleton can be stabilized using:
- Transosseous wiring
- Internal skeletal suspension:
  - Direct internal suspension to maxilla
  - Indirect internal suspension to mandible
- External skeletal fixation
- Transfixation with Kirschner wire or Steinmann pins
- Bone plate osteosynthesis.

Transosseous wiring—It includes direct wiring of mid face fractures at following sites:
- Frontonasal
- Frontomaxillary
- Frontozygomatic
- Maxillary-zygomatic
- Transpalatal.

Internal skeletal suspension—The underlying principle is to suspend a mobile fractured segment below to a firm stable segment above the fracture by means of subcutaneous wire **(Table 2)**.

External skeletal fixation—The primary aim of external skeletal fixation is to provide anteroposterior (AP) stability to facial skeletal (seen in case of concomitant bilateral condylar fracture of mandible).

Types/methods of external skeletal fixation:
- Plaster of Paris headcap
- Halo-frames
- Box frames
- Levant frame.

Bone plate osteosynthesis—Fixation with bone plates provides reliable fixation in all places obviate the need for any additional internal skeletal suspension or external skeletal fixation and need for maxillomandibular fixation.

TABLE 2: Different types of internal wire suspension.

Type of fracture	Type of internal wire suspension used
Le Fort I	• Zygomatic • Infraorbital • Pyriform aperture • Circumzygomatic
Le Fort II	Frontal: • Central • Lateral Circumzygomatic
Le Fort III	Frontal: • Central • Lateral
Gunning type splint	• Transnasal • Peralveolar • Circumpalatal

Transfixation with Kirschner wire—This method is simple and quick to perform and hence had been proved valuable in stabilizing middle third fractures, especially in battle fields and remotely located hospitals where adequate laboratory facilities were not available.

Indication:
- Le Fort II maxillary fracture without comminution
- Treatment of geriatric and severely ill patients
- Maxillofacial injury with associated skull fractures where use of halo frame or plaster of Paris headcap is contraindicated.

Contraindications:
- Severely displaced fractures of middle third face
- Le Fort I maxillary fractures.

Lacrimal apparatus: It gets involved in damage to eyelid and nasal bones in Le Fort II and III injuries. Because of gross edema and fractured bones, it is better not to attempt primary repair but to keep the patient under follow-up and if epiphora occurs, an ophthalmic opinion may be sought.

■ LATERAL MIDDLE THIRD FRACTURES

Zygomaticomaxillary Complex Fracture

The malar eminence of the zygoma is the most anterior projection of the lateral face. It is prominence, makes it vulnerable to trauma. Central zygomatic portion is sturdy and contributes to the vertical buttress and it is tough compared to its weak projections which help zygoma to articulate with the surrounding facial bones. This often results in fractures of zygoma at its line of attachment with the surrounding bones, classically labeled as a *"tripod fracture"* **(Fig. 6)**. These three sutures that form part of tripod include: the zygomaticofrontal (ZF), zygomaticotemporal (ZT), and zygomaticomaxillary (ZM) sutures. The zygoma has a deeper articulation site with the sphenoid bone, which is also fractured and radiologically five distinct fractures are seen involving the lateral orbital wall, orbital floor, anterior maxillary wall, lateral maxillary wall, and zygomatic arch. Patient presents with swelling over malar eminence, subconjunctival hemorrhage, localized tenderness, trismus because of coronoid process of mandible being trapped by depressed zygoma, malar eminence flattening on palpation, periorbital swelling and ecchymosis, and occasionally inferior rectus muscle entrapment leading to restricted upward gaze.

Diagnosis is confirmed by radiography, i.e., X-ray PNS (Waters view) but CT scan **(Figs. 7 and 8)** [noncontrast computed tomography (NCCT)

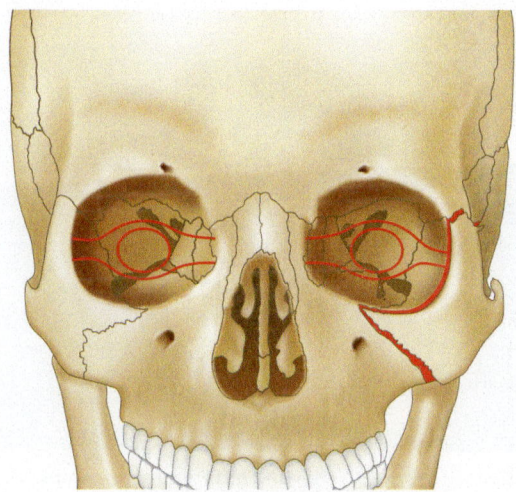

Fig. 6: Tripod fracture.

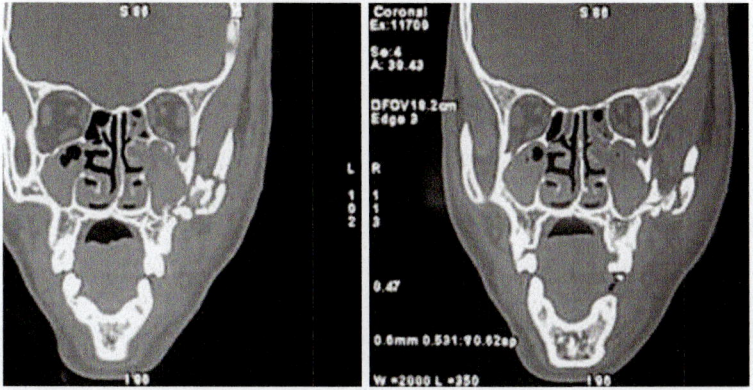

Fig. 7: Coronal section of CT showing left zygomatic complex fracture.

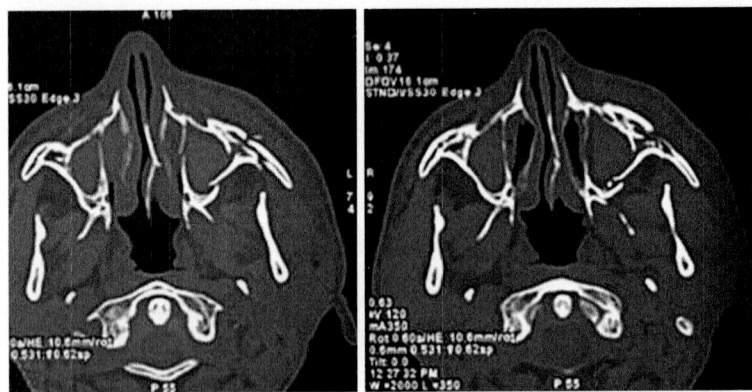

Fig. 8: Axial section of CT showing bilateral maxillary sinus wall fracture with hemosinus.

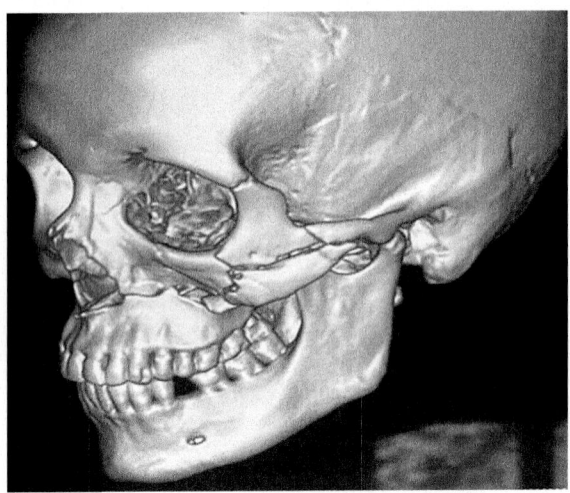

Fig. 9: 3D reconstruction showing left zygomatic complex fracture.

nose-PNS] and facial bones, especially with 3D reconstruction **(Fig. 9)** give accurate depiction of zygomaticomaxillary complex (ZMC) fractures **(Table 3)**. The malar eminence often gets displaced posteriorly, but this may be masked clinically owing to swelling in the surrounding soft tissues. The malar eminence tends to rotate internally or externally. Occasionally, the zygomatic arch fractures accompanying ZMC fractures may not be obvious radiologically and it is often useful to assess the curvature of the zygomatic arch with abnormal curvature being a discrete fracture.

Management is always open reduction by *"Gillies method of reduction"* where incision is made just behind the hair line anterosuperior to the pinna, deep to temporalis fascia, and passing *"Bristow or Rowe elevator"* deep to fascia to the zygomatic arch and elevating the depressed bone. Avoid undue pressure on the parietal bone.

TABLE 3: Classification of zygomatic complex fracture (Rowe and Killey 1968).

1.	Type I		No significant displacement
2.	Type II		Fractures of zygomatic arch
3.	Type III		Rotation around vertical axis
		a	Inward displacement of orbital rim
		b	Outward displacement of orbital rim
4.	Type IV		Rotation around the longitudinal axis
		a	Medial displacement of frontal process
		b	Lateral displacement of frontal process
5.	Type V		Displacement of complex en bloc
		a	Medial
		b	Inferior
		c	Lateral
6.	Type VI		Displacement of orbitoantral particular
		a	Inferior
		b	Superior (rare)
7.	Type VII		Displacement of orbital rim segment
8.	Type VIII		Complex comminute fractures

In case of *unstable fractures*, temporary fixation can be achieved by packing the maxillary antrum with bismuth-iodine-paraffin-paste (BIPP) packing via a Caldwell-Luc approach (maxillary sinus antrostomy) or by a Foley catheter inserted through an intranasal antrostomy. Open reduction along with interosseous wiring or plating is done.

Le Fort, nasal-orbital ethmoid complex and other facial fractures are frequent accompaniments of ZMC fractures. The importance in recognition of such additional coexistent fractures may lies in the fact that failure to identify such fractures may lead to malalignment of the ZMC with the displaced segment of the buttress system that is supposed to be aligned elsewhere, leading to postoperative cosmetic deformity.

Status of *"orbital apex"* is an important variable in ZMC fractures. Greater wing of sphenoid that forms the lateral wall of orbital apex houses optic nerve and lies in close apposition to internal carotid artery and cavernous sinus. ZMC fractures lead to displacement of greater wing of sphenoid and may result in number of serious injuries to the neurovascular bundle comprised of internal carotid artery and cranial nerves II, III, IV, V, and VI. In CT scan, the medial displacement into the orbital apex should always be looked for.

Status of orbital floor is another major variable affecting the surgical management of ZMC fractures. Zygoma forms both lateral and inferior orbital wall and their displacement results in increased volume of bony orbit causing post-traumatic enophthalmos. CT scan is most reliable method of making the decision of orbit exploration *(via subciliary or transconjunctival approach)*.

Radiological criteria for orbital exploration include severe comminuted fracture or displaced, displacement of more than half of the orbital floor with prolapsed orbital contents into the maxillary sinus, orbital floor fracture of >2 cm^2, and the fracture of both inferior and medial walls of orbit that predisposes to orbital content prolapse.

Orbital Wall and Floor Fractures

There are two main types of orbital fractures. The first type of orbital fracture is one or more of its bony walls. The inferior orbital rim is derived mainly from the zygomatic bone and is broken and displaced inward, and it follows zygomatic fractures frequently.

Second type of orbital fracture is commonly known as *"orbital blow-out"* fracture. This happens in injuries involving sudden increase in the intraorbital pressure (like a ball or a fist hitting the eye directly) where the orbital rim along the floor and the stronger inferior, lateral, and superior orbital rim remain intact, but the force of impact gets transmitted to the delicate bones of the orbital walls causing fractures in these bones without disrupting the continuity of rim of orbit. This leads to prolapse of orbital contacts into the maxillary sinus. It has high incidence of globe injury and always warrants ophthalmologist opinion. Patient presents with enophthalmos, diplopia due to inferior rectus entrapment or oculomotor nerve injury, subconjunctival hemorrhage, periorbital swelling, and ecchymosis. X-ray PNS (Waters view) and CT scan reveal *tear drop sign* due to orbital content herniation into maxillary antrum. Prior to discussing the management, it is important to assess and recognize other fractures so surgical planning encompasses all the injuries. The unique anatomical configuration of orbit is that orbit is like a cone with the apex posteriorly. It has its greatest diameter, i.e., 15 mm, behind the infraorbital rim, at a point behind which the walls of the orbit including the floor, the medial wall, and roof are convex. If this convexity is ignored during reconstruction, it may result in postoperative enophthalmos.

The main indications to treat "isolated orbital wall fractures" include:
- Fracture of orbital wall carries an inherent risk of extraocular muscle entrapment and this may lead to permanent damage and dysfunction with diplopia. CT scan can identify such entrapment and reveal the herniated extraocular muscle. In children, a green stick fracture involving the floor of the orbit may entrap the inferior rectus muscle in the fracture line. A coronal CT scan can identify this loss of inferior rectus muscle in the orbit indicating need for exploration.

- To prevent postoperative globe malposition and its resulting complications of diplopia or enophthalmos in the following situations:
  - Early clinical enophthalmos of >2 mm prior to resolution of the soft tissue edema. Due to herniation of orbital contents into the maxillary sinus.
  - Displacement of more than half of the floor of orbit.
  - Change in the orbit volume of >1.5 mL (5% of normal orbital volume).
  - Significant fat or soft tissue displacement.
  - Diplopia on upward/downward gaze and within 30° of primary gaze with a positive forced duction test.
- Lateral orbital wall (orbital plate of sphenoid bone) impacting into the orbital apex or middle cranial fossa for decompression of neural structures. Preoperative ophthalmologist opinion is always recommended.

Surgical management of orbital blow-out fracture is accomplished via the *subciliary or transconjunctival* approaches. It involves disimpaction of the prolapsed contents from the sinuses and repair of the orbital floor with silastic or cartilage graft. In the postoperative period, always assess the retinal blood vessels, visual acuity, or pupillary reflexes because central retinal artery may be compromised by retrobulbar hemorrhage.

■ FRONTAL SINUS FRACTURES

Frontal sinus fractures compromise about 5–15% of maxillofacial fractures. Frontal bone being the strongest of the facial bones, its fracture indicates a high force injury and one should search for other associated injuries. 55–85% of these patients have additional craniofacial injuries and 15–30% have associated CSF leak. Patient usually presents with pain, tenderness, swelling on the forehead, bilateral periorbital ecchymosis, and edema. The fractures are generally classified based on the involvement of the anterior table (wall), or posterior table (wall) and involvement of either the nasofrontal duct or anterior cranial fossa.

Anterior frontal wall is responsible for the shape of the forehead and the brows or the superior orbital rims. It also serves as one of the horizontal buttresses (frontal bar) and provides a strong foundation for the vertically oriented facial buttresses that support the forces of mastication.

In nondisplaced anterior wall fractures no surgical intervention is necessary. Displaced or depressed anterior wall fracture with severe comminution and mucosal injury requires bone grafting and frontal sinus obliteration, ideally performed within 10 days of the injury.

Posterior frontal wall forms the anterior wall of the anterior cranial fossa. Treatment of posterior wall fractures depends on extent of displacement, dural tear, CSF leakage, and presence of pneumocephalus.
- *Nondisplaced fracture with CSF leak*: Observe for 5–7 days with prophylactic intravenous antibiotics, avoiding nose-blowing, straining,

advise head elevation, and bed rest. If CSF rhinorrhea persists, frontal sinus obliteration is indicated.
- Displaced fracture may present with or without CSF leak.
  - If there is no leak and mild comminution on CT scan, osteoblastic flap and sinus obliteration is indicated.
  - If comminution is >30% of posterior wall (without CSF leak), a neurosurgeon's opinion for "cranialization" is indicated, i.e., posterior table removed and brain is allowed to expand into the frontal sinus.
  - *Displaced fracture with CSF leak:* Neurosurgical opinion regarding sinus obliteration or cranialization, depending upon extent of comminution is indicated.

In *"pediatric patients"*, these fractures are most common before age of 6 years. Since frontal sinus is not developed significantly till 5 years of age, fractures tend to be greenstick, do not communicate and fracture line may extend to the vertex of the skull or across the orbital roof. In displaced fracture, neurosurgeon opinion and intervention is required for bicoronal approach to repair the fracture and associated dural injuries. Inferiorly, displaced orbital roof fracture requires intracranial approach to reduce (with or without bone graft) to avoid encephalocele.

■ MANDIBLE FRACTURES

The weakest part of mandible being neck of condyle and is most common fracture, followed by the angle of mandible, body, and symphysis (mnemonic: CABS). Most important factor that determines the pattern of mandibular fracture is the direction and type of impact. The mandibular fracture may occur due to:
- Direct violence
- Indirect violence
- Uncontrolled muscular contraction.

The displacement of a fracture segment depends on the direction of line of fracture which in turn may be favorable or unfavorable, depending upon whether or not the line of fracture is in a direction to allow muscular distraction. The *"sling"* of the mandible that is the masseter and the medial pterygoid muscle, displaces the posterior jaw fragment upward and medially aided by the temporalis muscle. The opposing force is exerted by the suprahyoid muscles which displaces the anterior fragment forward. The line of fracture, which runs forward from lingual to buccal surface, resists medial displacement of the posterior segment and is termed as *favorable*. The fracture line running in posterolateral point to an anteromedial point known as reverse sagittal or oblique fractures can easily be displaced and is termed *unfavorable*.

Fracture of maxilla occurs with forces as low as 140 lb., whereas lowest tolerance level of mandible to frontal impact is around 425 lb. which consistently produces fracture of condylar neck. While a frontal force of 800–900 lb is required to produce fracture of symphysis and both condylar necks. The mandible is much more sensitive to lateral than to the frontal impact as latter is cushioned by opening and retrusion of jaw.

Clinically, patient presents with pain, malocclusion, anesthesia/paresthesia of the lower lip and chin (area supplied by inferior alveolar nerve), salivation and fetor of breath. Fractures involving symphysis, parasymphysis, and the body of the mandible, are also accompanied by the laceration to the gingiva of the teeth and hematoma in the floor of the mouth. On palpation, mobility of the fractures can be elicited. Trismus with inter incisor opening <35 mm is almost always seen (normally inter incisional opening is >40 mm). *Unilateral fracture* of condyle and condylar neck causes deviation of chin on mouth opening toward the fracture side and open bite on side opposite the fracture. Bilateral displaced neck condylar fracture produces symmetric anterior open bite.

Radiology includes panoramic view of mandible or plain X-rays of mandible (oblique view and AP view) as shown in **Figures 10 to 12**. CT scan **(Fig. 13)** is less reliable than plain X-rays for minimally displaced fractures.

Management includes securing the airway which may be compromised because of tongue base prolapse due to fracture mandible or excessive bleeding. Endotracheal intubation is always difficult and it is safer to perform temporary tracheostomy. Always check for associated laryngotracheal injury from blunt trauma to neck, which is causative of the fracture of mandible. Antibiotic prophylaxis is started at the earliest especially when fracture involves the tooth-bearing part of mandible (i.e., compounded into the mouth). Topical oral antiseptics are advised to minimize bacterial inoculum of the fracture site.

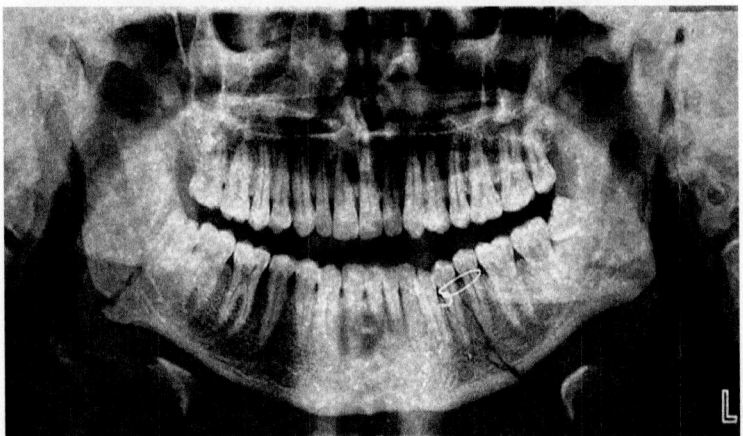

Fig. 10: Orthopantomogram (OPG) showing fracture of mandible.

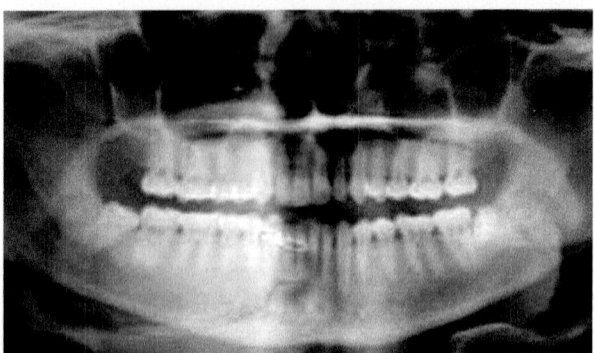

Fig. 11: Preoperative orthopantomogram (OPG) of mandibular right parasymphyseal fracture.

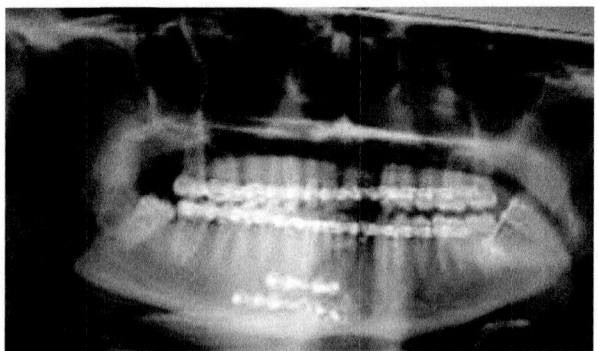

Fig. 12: Postoperative orthopantomogram (OPG).

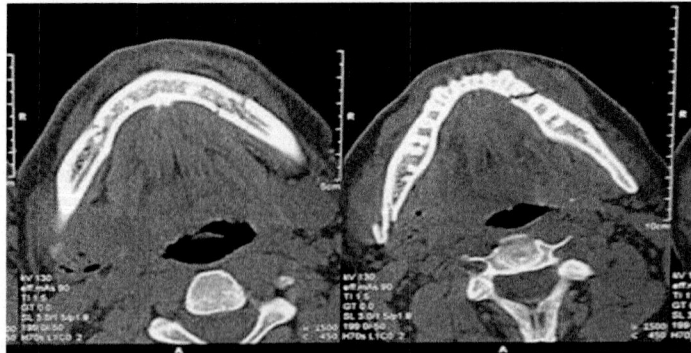

Fig. 13: Coronal section showing fracture of body of mandible.

The general principle of treatment of fracture of mandible includes:
- Reduction
- Fixation
- Immobilization.

Reduction allows restoration of functional alignment of the bone segments. In dentate mandible, teeth allow precise anatomical reduction of the fractured bony segments. Extensively comminuted or highly displaced fractures may require open reduction. If teeth/tooth is involved in a fracture line, a simple fracture gets converted to a compound one via open periodontal membrane. Reduction can be achieved via two ways, i.e., *open reduction and closed reduction.*

Closed reduction is alignment of fractured segments without direct visualization of fracture line. It includes intermaxillary fixation (IMF) with elastics or wires. It is indicated in nondisplaced favorable fractures, mandibular fractures in children, in case of significant loss of overlying soft tissues, fracture of coronoid process. IMF wires are used to position an arch bar on mandibular and maxillary teeth and then the teeth are fixed together in occlusion by attaching wires or rubber bands between the arch bars. IMF is kept for minimum of 4 weeks in children and 6 weeks in adults.

Open reduction is a method of surgically exposing the fractured segments through intraoral or extraoral incision and aligning the fractured bone segments together. This method avoids placement of IMF for long period of time as with closed reduction, hence patient can return to normal jaw function early.

Fixation allows the fractured bone segments to be fixed in their near anatomical position following adequate reduction. This method prevents displacement of the fracture during normal physiological movement of the bone. It is of two types:
1. Internal fixation
2. External fixation.

Internal fixation includes *rigid* (reconstruction plates, dynamic compression plates, and lag screws), semirigid (miniplates) or *nonrigid* (inter osseous wires).

Wire osteosynthesis require 0.35 mm stainless steel wire to secure the fractured segments. A small amount of movement of the proximal and distal segment occurs, causing healing with periosteal callus formation. Most rigid and some semi-rigid techniques obviate prolonged IMF and are useful among patients with epilepsy, diabetes, psychiatric disorders, or severe debility (who cannot tolerate IMF).

Rigid fixation **(Figs. 14A and B)** includes the use of either of the following:
- Lag screws across the fracture (oblique)
- Large compression plate [dynamic compression plate (DCP) or eccentric dynamic compression plate (EDCP)]
- Reconstruction plate with three screws on each side of the fracture
- Two miniplates with tension band in superior border
- One miniplate and one lag screw across the fracture.

Compression plates are applied to bone surface using screws which engages the inner cortical plate below the inferior alveolar canal.

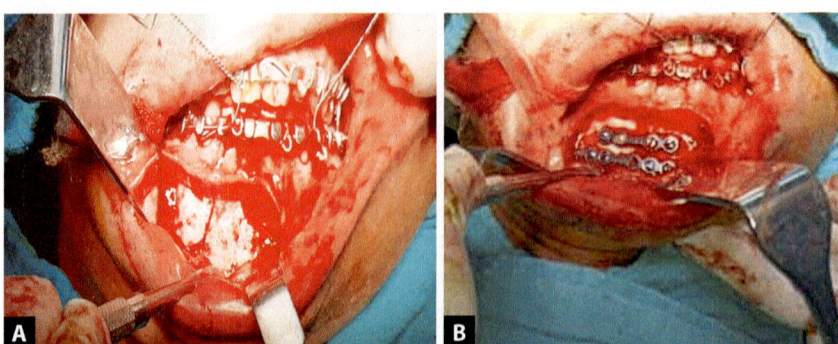

Figs. 14A and B: Two miniplates placed according to Champy's line of osteosynthesis.

The healing takes place without formation of intermediate callus between the fractured ends. These plates are based on the Swiss Arbeitsgemeinschaft für osteosynthese (AO) system and Association for the Study of Internal Fixation (ASIF) technique. All compression plates include at least two pear-shaped holes. The widest diameter of the hole lies nearest the fracture line. The screw is inserted in the narrow part of the hole and at the final moment of tightening its head comes to rest in the wider diameter countersunk area.

Because of the tendency for upper border to open when compression is applied across the fracture at the lower border it is necessary to apply a tension band (arch bar/monocortical plate with screws) at the level of upper border before tightening of the screw. Two types of compression plates are:

1. *DCP:* It requires tension band. This plate should be applied to the convex border of the mandible due to anatomic reasons. The screws incorporated in the plate are round/centric and does not cause inward movement of the screws.
2. *EDCP:* This does not require the use of tension band. It is designed with the most lateral holes angled in superior/medial direction to impart compression at superior border of mandible. The eccentric holes cause inward movement of the screw as well as the fractured fragments.

Noncompression plates allow a small gap to exist between the fractured bony ends which lead to small amount of primary callus formation.

Monocortical miniplates: These are form of load-sharing osteosynthesis.

Lag screws are most appropriate for sagittal or oblique fractures. Two or three lag screws are required to ensure stability.

Reconstruction plate is a type of internal surgical splint used for treatment of multiple segmental fractures. The fractured segments are held together with wires or miniplates and reconstruction plate is then contoured and screwed with two screws in each stable lateral segment. The segmental fragments are then secured to the plate.

Immobilization for an adequate time period is important to allow sufficient bone healing to occur. For example, a young adult who is receiving an early treatment for fracture of angle of mandible with tooth removed from the fracture line, an immobilization period of at least 3 weeks is required. This can be modified in various scenarios such as:
- Teeth retained in fracture line—add 1 week
- Fracture at symphysis—add 1 week (due to poor endosteal blood supply in this region)
- Age >40 years—add 1/2 weeks
- Children and adolescent—minus 1 week

Methods of immobilization:
- *Osteosynthesis without intermaxillary fixation*:
  - Compression plates—DCP and EDCP
  - Noncompression plates
  - Lag screws
- *Intermaxillary fixation:*
  - Bonded brackets
  - Dental wiring—direct/eyelet
  - Arch bar
  - Cap splint
- Intermaxillary fixation with osteosynthesis:
  - Transosseous wiring
  - Circumferential wiring
  - Bone clamp
  - Transfixation with Kirschner wire.

Osteosynthesis without IMF provides optimal rigidity across the fracture site eliminating the need of IMF. The patient can therefore continue normal day-to-day routine without compromising on dietary habits and oral hygiene maintenance.

Load-bearing versus Load-sharing Osteosynthesis

Load-bearing osteosynthesis: It is used in cases where mandible is incapable of handling the masticatory load by itself, e.g., atrophic mandible, comminuted fractures, and defect fractures. The reconstruction plate used bears all the functional force.

Load-sharing osteosynthesis: In this, both the implant and the bone share the functional load and works with the biomechanical principle of the mandible. This type of osteosynthesis includes miniplates along the ideal lines of osteosynthesis.

Special Areas of Mandible

- *Symphysis-parasymphysis* area fractures are defined as vertically unfavorable type fractures distracted by the mylohyoid muscle, thereby, closed reduction alone is difficult and acrylic lingual splint is required in addition to IMF. Open reduction with internal fixation is indicated which can be achieved by compression plates plus tension band arch bar or by lag-screws.
- *Fracture of body of mandible* is managed by either:
  - Eccentric dynamic compression plate through external incision along with tension band arch bar
  - Large reconstruction plate (in oblique/comminuted fracture)
  - Multiple lag-screw fixation plus tension band miniplates
- *Fracture of angle of mandible* can be managed by either of the following:
  - Inferior border compression plate with tension band plate
  - Tension band miniplates (noncompression)
  - Double miniplates
  - Lag-screws
- *Fracture of ascending ramus of mandible* is favorable and is managed by closed reduction with IMF for 3–4 weeks.
- *Condyle and condyle neck fractures* are mainly managed by closed reduction with exercise session every 2 weeks to avoid temporomandibular joint (TMJ) ankylosis. IMF is kept for 3–6 weeks followed by elastic band fixation.

The absolute and relative indications for open reduction of condylar fractures:
- *Absolute indications:*
  - Displacement into the middle cranial fossa
  - In cases where it is deemed impossible to obtain an adequate occlusion with closed reduction alone
  - Lateral extracapsular displacement of condyle
  - Invasion by a foreign body [gunshot wound]
- *Relative indications:*
  - Bilateral condylar fractures in an edentulous patient when splinting is impossible.
  - Unilateral or bilateral condylar fractures when splinting is not recommended for medical reasons or adequate postoperative therapy is impossible.
  - Bilateral condylar fractures associated with comminuted midfacial fractures.
  - Bilateral condylar fractures associated with significant pre injury malocclusion.

Studies have shown that closed reduction is associated with minimal pain and discomfort and does not limit functionality or pose any growth disturbances while open reduction is seen to be associated with facial nerve dysfunction depending upon the surgical approach chosen. However, patient can return to normal function early with open approach.

Teeth in the Line of Fracture

The absolute indications for *removal of tooth* from fracture line include:
- Infected fracture line
- Dislocation or subluxation of tooth from its socket
- Longitudinal fracture involving the root
- Presence of periapical infection

Relative indications for removal of tooth in fracture line:
- Functionless tooth which would eventually be removed electively
- Advanced caries or periodontal disease
- Teeth involved in untreated fracture presenting >3 days after the injury.

In *"pediatric age"*, mandible fractures are second most common site after the nasal bone. Most common site is the mandibular condyle, followed by angle and parasymphyseal region. Clinically, a kid presents with asymmetry on mouth opening/closing, malocclusion, trismus, swelling over TMJ, ecchymosis on floor of mouth and paresthesia of lower lip and chin. In age <3 years, crush injury of the spongy bone at the head of condyle is common (in contrast, adults have fracture at condylar neck) which may result in mandibular growth retardation and ankylosis of TMJ.

Management in pediatric age is mainly conservative. Greenstick and minimally displaced fractures are managed with soft diet, analgesia, and mouth opening/closing exercises while significantly displaced fracture requires close reduction followed by conservative treatment if reduction is stable. Displaced fractures can be reduced and fixation is maintained for 1-2 weeks with arch bars or acrylic splints, followed by several weeks of elastics to allow mobilization while maintaining occlusion. Open reduction and internal fixation is indicated only when closed reduction fails to achieve occlusion and is achieved by monocortical miniplates placed at inferior mandibular margins.

Geriatric Fractures

Certain biological and biomechanical differences occur in geriatric mandible when compared with the adult mandible:
- Decreased bone height, which leads to decreased buttressing effect.
- Alteration of blood supply pattern, i.e., decreased centrifugal (endosteal) blood flow. Therefore, the edentulous mandible is mainly dependent on centripetal (i.e., periosteal) blood supply.
- Reduced healing potential due to increasing age and/or associated systemic medical condition.
- Significant effect of muscular pull (digastric muscle).

Treatment includes closed reduction with the use of circummandibular wires fixated to pyriform rim and circumzygomatic wire with patient's existing dentures/gunning splint. Elderly patients usually require longer period of immobilization/IMF (6–8 weeks).

Open reduction with or without bone grafting can be done in cases where mandible is too atrophic for success with closed reduction, in case where there is nonavailability of splints/dentures, or when IMF is contraindicated.

External pin fixation has an added advantage that it avoids periosteal stripping. It can be used where open reduction is contraindicated. Large diameter screws (4 mm) are used for fixation with/without IMF.

Dislocation of mandibular condyle: It occurs after a blunt trauma to jaw with mouth opened. After ruling out subcondylar fracture by means of radiology, dislocated condyle should be reduced manually. Make the patient sit comfortably on the examination chair, stand in front and above the patient, grasp the mandible with the thumbs on the occlusal surface of teeth, while keeping the index and middle fingers below the lower border of the mandible, and apply sudden downward and backward movement bilaterally. Counter-traction is provided by an assistant who supports the head. This maneuver helps to cure the dislocation of the condyle. In some cases, local anesthesia can be injected around both jaws. While general anesthesia is given to pediatric patients and over anxious patients are sedated with intravenous midazolam.

■ PANFACIAL FRACTURES

These fractures are mainly seen after RTAs. Tracheostomy is required prior to reduction for general anesthesia. Intubation should not be attempted because of compromised and distorted upper airway. Facial bones are repositioned beginning at the cranium. Occlusion is achieved by IMF and remaining bones are repaired with open reduction and internal fixation. Suspension performed from stable points on the skull, depending upon the upper level of fractures which is usually orbital rim or forehead. Sometimes, external fixation devices, i.e., plaster head cap and metal outrigger especially in cases with gross anterosuperior instability are required.

■ CEREBROSPINAL FLUID LEAK

Cerebrospinal Fluid Otorrhea

Cerebrospinal fluid leak may manifest through ear as CSF otorrhea when ear drum is perforated (in longitudinal fracture of temporal bone) or may pass through eustachian tube to the nasopharynx in presence of intact ear drum (in transverse fracture of temporal bone). On examination, if drum is intact, there may be air fluid level as a meniscus or air bubbles but siegalization is contraindicated to prevent pneumocephalus. Patient is made to lean forward to look for rhinorrhea, which on white cloth reveals a *"ring sign" (target or halo sign)* with the CSF having a further diffusion point than blood. Other tests to diagnose CSF leak includes checking of beta-2 transferrin levels and checking the glucose content of the fluid.

In cases of perforated drum, careful suction and cleaning of external ear canal with sterile instruments under microscope is performed. Management includes keeping the ear dry and keeping a sterile cotton plug in the external ear canal, elevation of patient's head to 30° angle and bed rest, with the instructions to avoid straining, weight lifting, or bending over (to avoid increase in intracranial pressure). No topical ear drops are advised. Oral antibiotic prophylaxis and acetazolamide are advised. CSF otorrhea usually resolves spontaneously within 72 hours. Some authors advocate fluid restriction and diuretics. If CSF leak persists for several days, a lumbar drain may be added to conservative therapy. If leakage still persists or any complication of leakage occurs, neurosurgical opinion is sought for surgical intervention.

Cerebrospinal Fluid Rhinorrhea

Approximately 25% of fractures of sinuses are associated with CSF rhinorrhea and therefore should always be suspected even in presence of minor facial trauma. Mostly, it is due to anterior cranial fractures, through ethmoid roof or cribriform plate or CSF may pass through fractured posterior table of frontal sinus. Patient may present with intermittent or continuous watery or blood-stained rhinorrhea, provoked or increased by straining or change in posture. Mostly patient complains of continuous headache secondary to low pressure.

Management includes avoidance of straining and nose blowing, advising head elevation, bed rest with antibiotic prophylaxis, and acetazolamide. Surgical intervention for repair of dura is indicated after 7–10 days if CSF rhinorrhea does not resolve spontaneously.

■ TRAUMATIC OPTIC NEUROPATHY

It is one of the most common, forgotten, and overlooked cause of traumatic blindness especially in cases of substantial head trauma with loss of consciousness. The swinging flash light test for afferent pupil or *"Gunn pupillary sign"* is very important test, wherein the pupillary response is elicited. The pupil of the injured eye does not respond to direct light stimulus but does constrict with light stimulation of the contralateral retina. When the light stimulus is returned to the injured eye, the pupil dilates (normally pupil should constrict with this maneuver). This sign indicates failure to induce afferent signal for reflex bilateral pupillary constriction, localizing injury to optic nerve. Also lack of *"red color intensity"* is another sign elicited in conscious patients, in presence of some vision. Visual evoked responses (VERs) can confirm deficit in optic nerve transmission. High-resolution CT (axial cuts on a plane coaxial to optic nerve) is investigation of choice which may reveal fracture of optic canal.

Management includes mega dose dexamethasone [0.75 mg/kg body weight (BW) as initial dose followed by 0.33 mg/kg BW every 6 hourly for 24 hours, thereafter 1 mg/kg BW every 24 hours].

Surgical intervention is indicated in patients with absent light perception from the time of injury or in those who fail to show any improvement in vision within 12 hours of initiation of mega dose dexamethasone. Surgically, "optic nerve decompression" can be achieved by either transfrontal craniotomy, external ethmoidectomy, sublabial septal translocation technique, or by endoscopic sphenoethmoidal approach.

■ FURTHER READING

1. Alvi A, Doherty T, Lewer G. Facial fractures and concomitant injuries in trauma patients. Laryngoscope. 2003;113:102-6.
2. Foureca RJ, Barber HD, Powers MP, Frost DE. Oral and Maxillofacial Trauma, 4th edition. St. Louis: Saunders; 2012.
3. Hutchinon I, Lawler M, Skinner D. ABC of major trauma. Major maxillofacial injuries. BMJ. 1990;301:595-9.
4. Malik NA. Textbook of Oral and Maxillofacial Surgery, 2nd edition. New Delhi: Jaypee Brothers Medical Publishers (P) Ltd. 2011.

CHAPTER 8

Neck Trauma

*Venkata Surya Phani Bhushan Durvasula,
Jemy Jose, Parmod Kalsotra*

■ INTRODUCTION

Neck is a vital conduit between the torso and the head and due to its positioning in between, it is relatively unprotected and is vulnerable to both blunt and penetrating trauma. It is vital to have a clear concept of the anatomy of the neck, in order to manage the trauma to neck. *Six systems* with their vital structures course through the narrow neck, including vascular, respiratory, digestive, skeletal, neurologic, and endocrine systems. The vascular system includes great vessels of the neck: innominate, subclavian, axillary, carotid, jugular and vertebral vessels. The respiratory system is comprised of larynx, trachea that form a conduit to the lungs. The digestive system includes the oropharynx, hypopharynx and pharyngoesophageal sphincter that ends in esophagus. The neurologic system is limited to the spinal cord, brachial plexus, lower cranial nerves, and the cervical sympathetic chain. The thyroid and parathyroid comprise the endocrine system. The skeletal system includes the cervical spine.

Neck trauma may be due to either penetrating wounds or blunt injuries and the latter may be of low or high velocity **(Flowchart 1)**. "High velocity blunt trauma" is usually caused by injuries during road traffic accidents where the larynx is decelerated against blunt objects like the steering wheel or dashboard and is thus crushed between these and the rigid cervical spine. "Low velocity trauma" is due to a blow injury from a fist or foot or as a result of sport-related injuries by blow from a ball or a blunt object. Another important mode of blunt trauma is of the "clothesline" type caused by clothesline, chain or tree branch, and this carries a high risk of "laryngotracheal separation".

The "striking force vector" is from anterior to posterior in most blunt injuries while in "strangulation" injuries, the larynx is injured by lateral to medial compressive forces. Male larynx is prone to fractures because of acute thyroid alae angulation, larger size, and more brittleness. Pediatric laryngeal trauma tends to be less severe because the larynx is positioned very high in the neck and further its cartilages are very pliable and cricothyroid membrane is very narrow.

Flowchart 1: Management algorithm of different types of neck trauma.

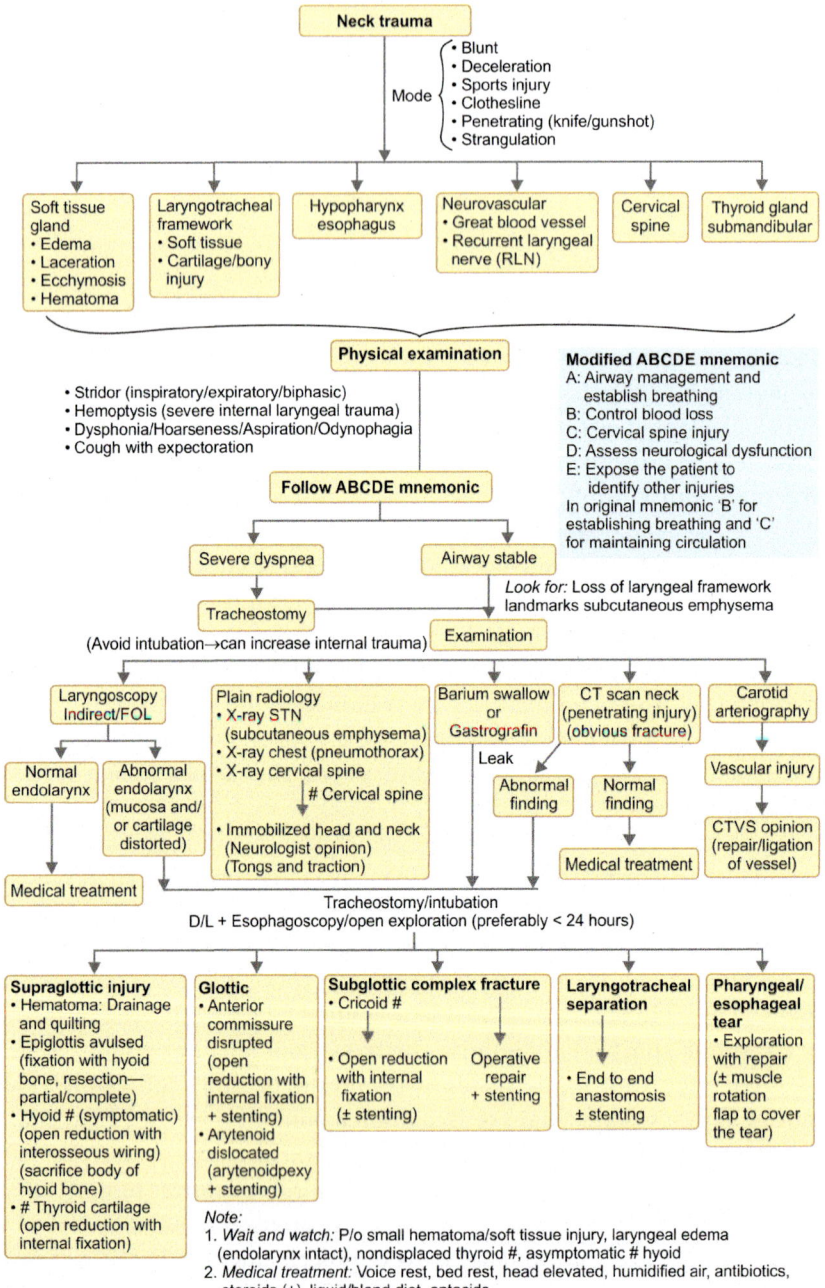

Penetrating neck trauma describes trauma to the neck by an injury that breached the platysma of the neck. It is usually caused by violent assault with knives, bullets, agricultural tools, etc.

Clinical presentation also varies depending upon the type of trauma, associated injuries to cervical spine or vascular injuries, compound fractures of laryngotracheal framework, respiratory distress, and shock.

Laryngotracheal injuries are usually life-threatening and may end up with permanent airway or voice changes. In clinical scenarios, acute cricoid cartilage injuries present with immediate airway obstruction because of subglottic hematoma that has limited space for expansion, while in thyroid cartilage injuries, delayed airway compromise may be expected from expanding hematoma and it is possible for hyoid bone injury to be completely overlooked.

■ ACUTE LARYNGOTRACHEAL TRAUMA

Simple contusions present as pain and hoarseness and tenderness of thyroid cartilage with mild edema or hematoma of endolarynx on flexible endoscopic examination provided patient has no airway distress. Dyspnea, dysphagia and slight aspiration may indicate cricoarytenoid dislocation which on inspection shows edema of arytenoid area and aryepiglottic fold, abnormal arytenoid position with a bowing and decreased mobility of vocal cord.

Hyoid bone fracture presents with pain and odynophagia with tender hyoid and a palpable crepitus, but bleeding into the preepiglottic and paraglottic space can cause swelling of the base of tongue with supraglottic edema and respiratory distress.

Vulnerability of the thyroid and cricoid cartilage to trauma is determined by the degree of their calcification which in turn is dependent on the age of patient. A blunt backward force pushing thyroid cartilage against the cervical spine usually splays the ala apart. The elastic thyroid cartilage usually springs back with no fracture or little damage and only disruption of anterior commissure will occur, with or without bleeding into the paraglottic space and posterior displacement of the epiglottis. The calcified thyroid cartilage on the other hand, will shatter like an eggshell with the loss of thyroid eminence. *Arytenoids* might be sandwiched between thyroid cartilage and cervical spine and can get dislocated. *Cricoid*, being the only complete ring in the respiratory tract behaves differently with tendency of resorption and ultimately stenosis, thereby reducing the airway lumen. Cricoid defects are the most difficult to repair.

Laryngeal membrane injuries: Penetrating injuries, on the other hand, tend to bounce off the relatively solid cartilages that form the skeleton of larynx but may cause more damage to the relatively thin thyrohyoid or cricothyroid membrane and thus manifest a different pattern of signs and symptoms and subsequent sequelae. Penetrating "thyrohyoid membrane" injury causes bleeding into the paraglottic space resulting in an airway obstruction but a relatively unaffected glottis, clinically presenting as localized painful wound with stridor, but with normal voice. Penetrating injury of the "cricothyroid membrane" causes air leak, presenting clinically as surgical emphysema. Bleeding into the subglottic space causes respiratory obstruction which gets compounded with severe coughing induced by blood trickling down the trachea.

Laryngotracheal separation can happen and is the most disastrous injury leading to death at the roadside. Sometimes, however, enough lumen may remain for the patient to breathe long enough to reach the hospital. Several tracheal rings may be damaged along with shearing of *cricotracheal membrane*. Symptoms include severe dyspnea, pain, aphonia or hoarseness and hemoptysis with severe airway distress, subcutaneous emphysema, tenderness, ecchymosis on examination with the head posturing forward to breathe.

Diagnosis

High index of suspicion for airway injuries is essential in all patients with injuries to the anterior part of the neck. The symptoms of laryngeal injury include cough and expectoration with laryngeal pain that increases on phonation or deglutition. Examination may reveal tenderness, swelling of neck and loss of laryngeal landmarks. Severity of symptoms can never be reliably correlated in patients with severity of injury in endolaryngeal trauma although dyspnea, hemoptysis, hoarseness, odynophagia and/or dysphagia are seen. Aphonia and apnea indicate possible compromised airway that warrants immediate tracheostomy. Emphysema of neck is a reliable indicator of perforation of either larynx or hypopharynx. Ecchymosis, laceration or strangulation marks may be noted on the skin, while external neck examination may reveal crepitus (subcutaneous emphysema), palpable fracture of thyroid cartilage and hyoid bone and loss of laryngeal landmarks. Type of stridor roughly indicates the level of injury (inspiratory stridor points to supraglottic, expiratory stridor indicates tracheal injury and biphasic stridor indicates the glottic level). Neurological deficit suggests cervical spine injury. Hypotension in a trauma patient must be assumed to be secondary to hypovolemia and not due to spinal shock.

■ WORKUP

One should always be mindful of associated neurovascular injuries and cervical spine injury. Active bleeding, expanding hematoma, bruits, loss of pulse—all indicate vascular injury that demands an urgent cardiovascular surgeon opinion.

"Plain radiographs of neck" are helpful in identifying and delineating air in the soft tissues, fractures of laryngeal framework and cervical spine injuries.

"X-ray chest" may detect mediastinal emphysema and/or pneumothorax. "Laryngogram", in absence of airway distress, outlines mucosal tears. A "computed tomography (CT) scan" (gold standard test) (2 mm cuts) in axial plane or spiral CT scan, is indicated in almost all patients to delineate the extent of injury after trauma and to localize the fracture site, especially in cases with suspected trauma. CT scan helps in identification of clinically inapparent cartilage fractures and to verify the laryngoscopic findings.

A CT scan is usually not recommended in patients with obvious fractures, large lacerations, penetrating trauma (who will require open exploration) and those patients with minimal trauma and normal clinical findings. Some authors, however, recommend routine CT scan in all patients with airway injuries that require operative management to allow better visualization of the subglottic area and anterior commissure preoperatively.

Carotid arteriography may be indicated in penetrating injuries to rule out vascular injuries. "Gastrografin-swallow or barium-swallow" (gastrografin being less irritant is preferred) is usually suggested to confirm suspected esophageal or pharyngeal tears.

Laryngoscopic examination is mandatory in all patients, usually indirect, or with flexible laryngoscopy or with direct endoscopic examination under general anesthesia.

Triple endoscopy (direct laryngoscopy, esophagoscopy and bronchoscopy) is considered the best method to assess the extent of damage, including edema with or without a hematoma, distortion of normal anatomy, mucosal tears of larynx and pharynx, bleeding, exposed cartilages and vocal fold weakness or displacement. It also allows better visualization of subglottic and tracheal area that may have been missed on the prior fiberoptic laryngoscopy with CT scan showing edema only.

Emergency Care

Follows the gold standard modified mnemonic "ABCDE":
- Airway assessment for stability and airway control
- Bleeding control with cardiac resuscitation
- Cervical spine stabilization
- Deficits in neurological function (Glasgow Coma Scale)
- Exposure of the full body beyond the neck to rule out other multiorgan injury that may need medical attention

Immediate airway management is the first line of treatment: Signs of impending airway obstruction are—stridor, dyspnea, shortness of breath, aphonia, accessory respiratory muscle use, air hunger. In these patients, perform immediate tracheostomy (urgent).

If intubation is planned, keep tracheostomy/cricothyroidotomy set ready. Intubation can be attempted in semiconscious or unconscious patients but because of distorted larynx (wherein oral intubation can increase the endolaryngeal damage, create false passage or precipitate loss of an already tenuous airway), tracheostomy is always preferred which may have to be performed in sitting or semisitting position in some patients. Some authors recommend low tracheostomy (4–5 tracheal ring) in cases of acute laryngeal trauma via "vertical incision" so that in case of laryngotracheal separation, the trachea may be better accessed if retracted inferiorly.

In inexperienced hands, cricothyroidotomy may be a safer and quicker option in emergency/casualty ward which should be converted to a standard tracheostomy within 24–48 hours.

In pediatric laryngeal trauma, bronchoscopy under inhaled anesthesia with spontaneous respiration, allows to assess the endolaryngeal damage and tracheostomy may be performed if required.

■ MEDICAL TREATMENT

Conservative approach is indicated in:
- Edema, small hematoma with intact mucosa
- Small glottic/subglottic laceration without exposed cartilage on endoscopic evaluation
- Single, undisplaced fracture of thyroid cartilage, hyoid bone fracture on endoscopic evaluation
- The conservative treatment includes:
  - Hospitalization for observation (minimum 24 hours) with "emergency tracheostomy set" kept bed side
  - Voice rest
  - Bed rest with head elevated (to prevent further swelling and reduce the edema)
  - Humidified air (to minimize crust formation and prevent progression of edema and throat irritation)
  - Steroid (useful in first few hours only)
  - Antibiotics (in presence of mucosal tear/laceration)
  - Nil orally (for hypopharyngeal tears), otherwise clear liquid diet with intravenous supplement
- Antacids to avoid reflux laryngitis especially in patients who underwent tracheostomy
- Nasogastric tube to be avoided because of risk of further injury, gastric acid reflux and mucosal ulceration in postcricoid region

Surgical Intervention

Open surgical reduction and repair is indicated in:
- Lacerations involving free margins of vocal cords
- Large mucosal laceration

- Palpable laryngeal fractures (single displaced fracture, more than two fractures) (note—for single undisplaced fracture conservative management is indicated)
- Increasing subcutaneous emphysema
- Exposed cartilage, hemorrhage
- Multiple/displaced cartilage fracture resulting in internal derangement
- Avulsed/dislocated arytenoids, anterior commissure disruption
- Vocal fold immobility
- Any neck trauma with airway obstruction
- Complete laryngotracheal separation

Current recommendation favors early intervention (with 24 hours) instead of old teaching of delayed surgical intervention (3–5 days) to allow resolution of edema. Because delayed surgical intervention has high incidence of infection (especially in supraglottic injuries), laryngeal dysfunction and laryngeal stenosis.

Initial step of surgical intervention is triple endoscopy, i.e., rigid direct laryngoscopy to evaluate the extent of endolaryngeal injury and palpate arytenoids for dislocation or immobility, rigid bronchoscopy to assess subglottis and trachea and esophagoscopy to look for any hypopharyngeal/esophageal tears.

Open Exploration

- Horizontal incision at level of cricothyroid membrane and gain exposure from hyoid bone to suprasternal notch.
- Assess visceral (hypopharynx/esophagus), neural and vascular structures.
  - Laryngofissure/midline thyrotomy for endolaryngeal exposure using oscillating saw or blade. Incision is made from cricothyroid membrane through the anterior commissure to the thyrohyoid membrane. Larynx can be entered from thyroid fracture if the fracture line runs 2–3 mm lateral to midline of thyroid cartilage.
  - Principle of minimal debridement is followed and muscle, cartilage, mucosal membrane with viable blood supply is preserved. Cover the exposed cartilage with mucosa which may get reabsorbed later on, forming a scaffold for firm fibrous tissue.
- Mucosal lacerations are approximated with fine absorbable sutures (5-0 or 6-0 sutures), with knots placed outside the lumen to prevent granulation tissue formation.
- Anterior margin of true cord is sutured to thyroid cartilage/external perichondrium to reconstruct the anterior commissure. During repair, maintain cartilage continuity in AP diameter especially at level of true vocal cords to achieve vocal cord length and tension (at the level of junction of inferior and middle one-third of thyroid cartilage). It is also

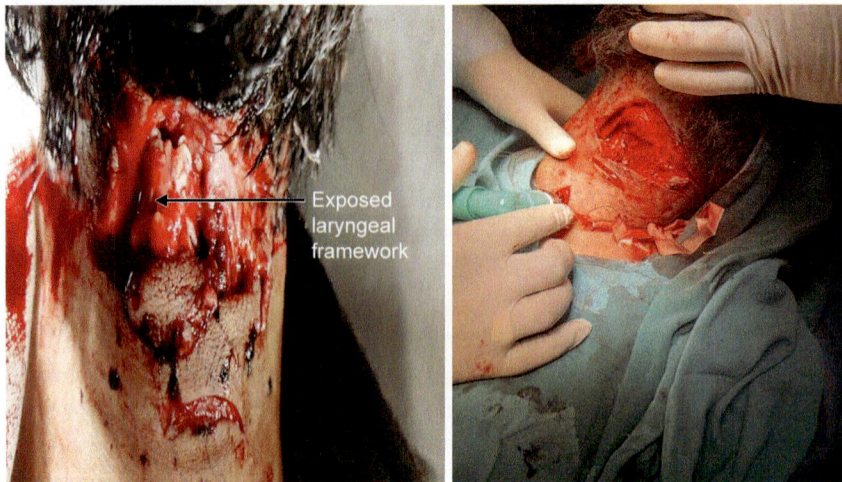

Fig. 1: Traumatic wounds on neck.

important to maintain cartilage continuity in craniocaudal position for proper alignment of vocal folds.
- In cases of large mucosal injury, pyriform sinus mucosal flap may be used to cover the cartilage or free buccal mucosal or dermal grafts may be used.
- Reduce and immobilize the fracture segments with wire, nonabsorbable sutures or mini plates. Titanium mini plates can be used for cartilage repair, which are secured with 4-6 mm screws (absorbable mini plates are also available). Suture or wire can also be used. In cases of multiple fractures: mesh or multiple mini plates are indicated. Even in undisplaced fracture some suggest mini plating in every case to avoid delayed displacement.

"Laryngeal stents" are indicated in cases of multiple cartilage fractures warranting stabilization, extensive lacerations involving anterior commissure or extensive soft tissue injury with limited plating option. Stents can be made of a finger cot packed with antibiotic-impregnated cotton gauze. Readymade stents (silicone, silastic or portex) can also be used which are fixed with two mattress sutures using heavy nonabsorbable suture (keeping superior end at the aryepiglottic fold and lower end above the tracheostomy site). Stent is kept in situ for 2-3 weeks. Stent is secured by suturing to a button on skin surface.

Closure of wound: Cover the laryngotracheal framework with anterior strap muscles to avoid skin tethering to it. Drain is kept for secretion and air **(Fig. 1)**.

Special Injuries

Hyoid bone fractures: This may need only symptomatic treatment. Open reduction and interosseous wiring of major fracture is performed very rarely.

Some authors prefer to sacrifice the body of fractured hyoid bone on either side of the fracture line.

Supraglottic injuries: These are more prone for infections and fibrosis. In cases of avulsed epiglottis, the epiglottis is fixed in position by anchoring it to the hyoid bone by two silk/PDS sutures. Alternatively, partial or complete epiglottic resection can be performed. Bleeding in the laryngeal spaces may need drainage of these spaces by opening them and then obliterating them with quilting sutures. Drains are not advised in these spaces and principle of minimal debridement is followed. In presence of significant bleeding in the larynx, midline thyrotomy is performed and control of hemorrhage with drainage of clot is achieved.

Glottic injuries: These occur because of fracture of thyroid cartilage at the level of attachment of true vocal cord.

Arytenoid cartilage if dislocated should be realigned at the earliest (within 48 hours) and should not be fixated or removed. Mucosal closure is achieved primarily or with an advancement flap of pyriform sinus mucosa. In cases of vocal fold immobility, one should follow wait and watch policy for spontaneous recovery. Anteriorly detached vocal cords may be sutured to the thyroid cartilage/external perichondrium thus achieving a reconstruction of the anterior commissure. Some authors recommend a "McNaught keel" (using 0.18 mm thick tantalum sheeting), placed in the laryngofissure with the external flanges sutured to the thyroid perichondrium with 3-0 chromic catgut, which can be removed after 4–6 weeks.

Cricoid cartilage fracture: It needs exposure with reduction and fixation along with laryngeal stenting. The fracture is usually anterior and it is extremely difficult to directly suture the mucoperichondrial tear because of poor access. Hence it is important to retain the cartilage as much as possible, with realignment of the cartilage fragments and place the laryngeal stent in situ (up to 3 months) especially in posterior fracture.

Laryngotracheal separation: It is dealt with tracheostomy, open reduction and suturing of cartilage. Damaged tracheal rings can be excised with a laryngeal drop thus mobilizing the larynx for an "end-to-end anastomosis" (cricotracheal anastomosis). All the sutures should be in place before tying, as it becomes very difficult to insert extra sutures once they are tied. Stenting should be avoided as it can cause infection and breakdown of anastomosis.

Penetrating neck trauma **(Fig. 2):** It describes trauma to the neck by an injury that breached the platysma of the neck. It is usually caused by violent assault with knives, bullets, agricultural tools, etc. For the assessment of

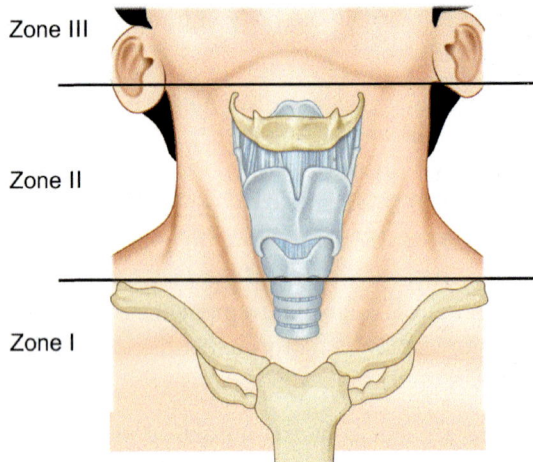

Fig. 2: Zones of neck for description of site of trauma.

penetrating neck trauma, the neck is anatomically classified into three zones anterior to the sternocleidomastoid muscle. Zone I extends between the level of the clavicles and sternal notch to the cricoid cartilage and includes the proximal carotid arteries, subclavian vessels, major vessels in the chest, lung and esophagus, trachea and the thoracic duct. Zone I injuries to right side are mainly explored via median sternotomy and on the left side are often approached by left anterior thoracotomy. Zone II extends between the cricoid cartilage and the angle of the mandible and comprises of the carotid arteries, jugular veins, larynx, and hypopharynx. Zone II is easily the most common area for penetrating injuries (60–75%) and has the easiest access for evaluation, surgical approach and assessment intraoperatively without the aid of preoperative diagnostic tests. Zone III extends from the angle of the mandibles to the base of the skull and includes the distal carotid arteries, jugular vein, and hypopharynx. Zone III requires craniotomy with or without a mandibulotomy for exploration and control of high carotid injury. Multiple cranial nerve involvement indicates high and grave vascular injury. In Zone I and III, in an otherwise stable patient with no airway obstruction or bleeding (external or internal or both), angiography and barium swallow should be performed to rule out other unidentified injuries.

In injuries of Zone II usually isolated venous and pharyngoesophageal injuries are missed clinically. In stable patients always monitor with repeated intraoral examination and look for expanding edema or hematoma in retropharyngeal or parapharyngeal spaces. Zone IV is classified by some authors to describe the transcervical penetrating wound cross the midline which tends to have more morbidity and mortality.

Management of Penetrating Neck Trauma

In the management, preliminary steps include securing of the airway after ruling out injury to cervical spine by intubation, cricothyroidotomy or tracheostomy. Tracheostomy is the preferred method in cases where intubation is not possible or prolonged. Maintenance of circulation with an intravenous line (large bore) is always advisable.

At this stage, the wound is assessed, for any hemorrhage or expanding hematoma (which responds to direct pressure instead of blind clamping through the wound). Avoid blind probing of penetrating neck wound as it may dislodge a clot and torrential bleeding can occur. Presence of pulse deficit, active bleeding, (external/internal or both), expanding hematoma, bruit, murmur, neurological deficit, hypotension, all indicate vascular injury (the most common cause of mortality in penetrating injury) and necessitate an urgent cardiothoracic and vascular surgeon (CTVS) opinion. Actively examine for a pneumothorax and manage with a chest tube insertion.

- In stable patients, X-ray STN (AP and lateral view) and X-ray chest may be indicated
- In the presence of spinal shock (hypotension without tachycardia) neurologist's opinion may be required
- High carotid injury may present with Horner's syndrome or multiple cranial nerve involvement
- Loss of facial skin along with bone loss after debridement will require plastic surgeon's intervention for grafting/flap rotation

Penetrating laryngeal injuries: Because of destructive nature of high velocity gun shots extent of tissue damage and tissue viability is difficult to assess at the time of presentation. Approaches vary and while some recommend delayed surgical repair, others recommend immediate intervention with wide area resection. In either approach, principles governing the tissue repair are same and all viable structures should be preserved, neurovascular damage assessed. In case of severe structural damage, endolaryngeal stenting (silicone or endotracheal tube) may be indicated as necessary. In severe cases, partial/total laryngectomy is often necessary.

Tracheal injury: Majority of the tracheal injuries are observed in the cervical trachea as the thoracic counterpart is protected by the sternum as it courses along the superior mediastinum. Signs and symptoms of a tracheal injury include crepitus, stridor, hemoptysis, and dyspnea. A vast majority of tracheal injuries are small, linear punctures, and defects up to 2–3 cm can be closed with debridement and primary repair with absorbable sutures. Large tracheal defects are rarely seen.

Larger injuries can be closed by mobilization of trachea using thyroid or suprahyoid release. Muscle flaps or musculofacial flaps or synthetic material has been used to close very large defects (>6 cm). Flexion of the neck can assist in closure very large defects. The neck is held in flexion by suturing the chin to the presternal skin for 7 days after surgery. The exact role of tracheotomy is unclear. Some authors have advocated using a distal tracheotomy for all proximal injuries, with the opinion that this is protective to the more proximal repair.

Broad spectrum antibiotics are always administered to prevent infection from mucosal tears and subcutaneous emphysema and to help avoid stenosis. Steroids are used for laryngeal edema. Feeding is achieved via nasogastric tube to prevent aspiration and to bypass dysphagia.

■ CERVICAL SPINE INJURY

Any blunt trauma to the neck may result in a cervical spine injury due to fracture or dislocation. This injury may lead to a life-threatening situation with neurogenic shock or it may cause quadriplegia. Patient complains of neck pain and neck swelling. On examination, there is tenderness with or without swelling over cervical vertebrae, paraplegia or quadriplegia and dyspnea.

Immediate cervical spine stabilization with an appropriate radiological investigation such as CT scan is usually confirmatory. Management includes immobilization of head and neck, i.e., packaging of the patient by means of cervical collar, long spinal board, etc., airway establishment as described earlier in the chapter by experienced ENT surgeon with an appropriate neurosurgical intervention for cervical spine and steroids for spinal cord injury.

While penetrating cervical injuries are usually devastating, presentation is profound neurologic deficit. The trajectory of the wound in addition to level of neurologic deficit suggests the level of spinal injury. Plain X-ray cervical spine reveals the bone injury, CT scan of cervical spine helps in assessment of geometry of the fracture. Early fixation within first three days by orthopedic/neurosurgeon is indicated.

■ INJURY OF MAJOR VESSELS IN NECK

Although blunt trauma rarely causes major vessel rupture, penetrating injuries especially bullet injuries are often associated with injuries to the vessels, and even if it is not obvious at the outset a very high index of suspicion is essential and every patient should be examined and investigated thoroughly for these injuries. If present, these vascular injuries, deserve immediate exploration in case of obvious injury. If no emergency exists, then a CT angiogram or an arteriogram should be performed to further delineate or rule out these injuries.

Clinically, patient presents with pain, swelling, tenderness and ecchymosis of skin or pharynx and airway distress. Progressing swelling is indicative of arterial or jugular vein injury unlike a static nonprogressive swelling seen in hematomas of blunt trauma. Workup consists of detailed physical examination, CT angiogram, endoscopy, esophagography and color Doppler ultrasound. Ultrasound or angiography can sometimes miss an isolated internal jugular vein (IJV) injury. Blunt trauma leading to soft tissue injury with hematoma which is static and patient is without dyspnea or shock can be managed conservatively. Carotid arterial injury or IJV injury needs urgent exploration of the neck with an aim of primary repair avoiding significant narrowing. Ligation of IJV is well-tolerated and is preferred to a repaired but compromised lumen. In isolated carotid artery injury, ligation should be avoided if possible and an opinion of a CTVS surgeon is essential. A CTVS surgeon should consider placing a shunt if restoration of blood flow is going to take longer than 20 minutes and follow-up with a postoperative imaging to rule out a cerebrovascular accident.

If primary repair of artery is not possible, CTVS surgeon can use saphenous vein or polytetrafluoroethylene (PTFE) graft, latter being more preferable especially in large defect and the repair is done using permanent monofilament suture. PTFE appears to be more resistant to infection than saphenous vein. Associated aerodigestive tract injury increases the risk of infection for which drains are required to control leakage from repair of aerodigestive tract injury.

■ INJURY TO PHARYNX AND ESOPHAGUS

The upper digestive tract injuries in the form of contusion, laceration or rupture in the wall may be caused due to blunt trauma or penetrating injuries. Although these may not be obvious initially, failure to recognize and treat them appropriately may lead to fatal complications. Clinical features include pain, crepitus, hematemesis, odynophagia, mild to moderate dysphagia, hemoptysis, edema or hematoma of the pharynx, subcutaneous emphysema. Tracheal deviation and a nonpulsatile hematoma may be seen. Patient may be initially asymptomatic but manifests later on with fever, odynophagia, neck abscess formation, mediastinitis and purulent discharge from the injury site. Soft tissue X-ray films (AP or lateral views) may reveal free air and/or retropharyngeal thickening is seen. CT scan usually delineates the accurate localization of injury site. Esophagography, endoscopy (direct laryngoscopy, hypopharyngoscopy and esophagoscopy) confirm the findings. Commonly flexible esophagoscopy is preferred over rigid esophagoscopy.

Surgical repair is essential for all blunt and penetrating trauma with an integrity compromising tear to the esophagus. Any laceration of the esophageal mucosa should be closed in several layers with only minimal debridement, and a drain should be placed. A nasogastric tube feeding with nil per orally is advised for 7–10 days and intravenous broad-spectrum antibiotics are essential. Primary repair offers a very high survival rate of

>90% but the survival rate falls to 64%, if the primary closure is delayed for >24 hours. This is because, with delayed diagnosis (>24 hours), the primary closure becomes difficult because of friable tissue. Even with early closure, the fistula formation rate is high (up to 57%). Some have advocated closure of wound over t-tube. Buttressing of the esophageal closure with strap muscles or pleura is also advocated. Proximal diversion of the esophagus, with a primary aim to drain the area and prevent abscess formation and secondary sepsis is also advocated after delayed esophageal closure.

INJURY TO SUBMANDIBULAR GLAND AND THYROID GLAND

In the submandibular gland injuries, the most important structure is facial artery owing to its propensity to significant bleeds and hematoma formation.

Trauma to thyroid is unlikely to produce any significant thyroid dysfunction, but a concern is bleeding because of its high vascularity. Management requires an exploration of the wound with direct sutures to control the bleeds which may necessitate a ligation of inferior thyroid artery. Larger injuries may need lobectomy. Trachea and esophagus inspection would be essential in these cases due to their proximity to trachea. An attempt is made to save some of thyroid gland and one or more of parathyroid glands, in cases which require extensive removal of the gland.

CAROTID BLOW-OUT

This is almost always seen in patients with complications after a major head and neck surgery. It usually presents weeks to months after the initial surgical treatment and some of these cases may present to the emergency with a major bleed.

Rupture of one of the major blood vessels of the neck is usually because of:
- Breakdown of skin wound with exposed great vessels when an improperly planned incision is made in irradiated skin (e.g., 3-point junction on the carotid artery).
- Superadded infection with exposed wound base especially in compromised patient.
- Presence of orocutaneous, pharyngocutaneous fistula or salivary leak infecting the wound.
- Blunt or penetrating trauma to the neck.
- Recurrent cancer in the neck that erodes the blood vessels, especially in terminal patients.

Radiation therapy commonly predisposes to a carotid blow-out, by affecting and weakening all the layers of the arterial walls including obliteration of vasa vasorum, adventitial fibrosis, sub endothelial vacuolization with edema, and fragmentation of the tunica media elastic fibers. Superadded infection may accelerate the gangrene of the arterial wall which predisposes to a rupture. During surgery, avoidance of stripping of the adventitia of the carotid sheath, preserving thyrocervical trunk that supplies vasa vasorum of carotid sheath and muscle graft used to cover the carotid (e.g., levator scapulae apron flap) may be protective against a subsequent blow.

Clinical Manifestations

Clinical presentation ranges from an asymptomatic exposure of a carotid artery to a frank hemorrhage which could present as one of three separate entities—threatened, impending or acute carotid blow-out.
1. *Threatened carotid blow-out* is when there is evidence on physical examination suggestive of inevitable hemorrhage with a radiological (angiographically) finding suggestive of tumor invasion of the carotid system and nonhemorrhagic pseudoaneurysm.
2. *Impending carotid blow-out* (sentinel hemorrhage), clinically small bleeds may present as an episode of transcervical or transoral bleeding and these herald the onset of a possible full blow-out that may occur within next 48 hours. These small bleeds are usually from a pseudoaneurysm which has either resolved spontaneously or after packing or pressure. This prodromal bleeding may also be observed through a surgical wound or fistula and will eventually lead to a blow-out, especially if quick action is not taken.
3. *Acute carotid blow-out* presents active bleeding. A clinical entity called the recurrent carotid blow-out syndrome (recurrent bleeding because of progressive disease or treatment failure) and internal jugular vein hemorrhage has also been reported.

Management

Principles of management of carotid blow-out include:
- Control of airway with cuffed tracheostomy tube
- Control of bleeding with local pressure
- Fluid resuscitation
- Multiple units of cross-matched blood arranged
- Manipulation of neck wound beyond the application of pressure for control of hemorrhage should be avoided. Once the patient is stabilized (cardiac and respiratory), further diagnostic and therapeutic maneuvers are considered.

Surgical Options

If there is an apparently healthy carotid artery that is exposed in an infected, fistulas or otherwise irradiated neck wound with no history of prior bleed, plan for carotid coverage with vascularized tissue flap. In presence of unhealthy (devascularized or aneurysmal) carotid, i.e., threatened carotid artery blow-out, treatment is directed toward dealing with artery. Contrast enhanced CT scan will be useful in terms of delineating a tumor or air-interface with carotid artery, outlining the site and degree of exposure. CT angiography is extremely useful and if available, helps to study of bilateral carotid artery with their contributions to the cerebral circulation, tumor blush, site of bleed and/or aneurysmal dilatation. Venous phase is also studied for any internal jugular vein (IJV) bleed.

Use of coils to achieve the occlusion in case of external carotid artery or IJV bleed has been reported. In case of internal carotid or common carotid artery (site of bleed), a temporary balloon occlusion test is performed and monitoring of the patient for neurologic sequelae and arterial back pressure is done. This may help plan permanent occlusion of artery in cases where patient is able to tolerate the occlusion. If patient tolerance is not achievable, then the temporary shunting of the bleed site is performed until definitive surgical extra-anatomic vascular bypass and subsequent permanent occlusion can be achieved.

Presence of interventional radiology is helpful and it is preferable to transfer such patients to a better center if time is available and the patient remains stable. Otherwise, operative intervention for carotid artery ligation should be undertaken based on principles explained above. No attempt is made to repair it or tie it in the middle of any infected area to avoid recurrence of blow-out. Vascularized myocutaneous flap (pectoralis major or latissimus dorsi flap) may be used to cover the wound after appropriately debriding the wound. Any fistula, if present, is externalized.

Morbidity and mortality of carotid blow-out is very high. At least one-third of these patients die, out of those who survive, half will have hemiplegia.

■ FURTHER READING

1. Flint PW, Haughey BH, Lund VJ, Robbins KT, Thomas JR, et al. Cumming's Otolaryngology Head and Neck Surgery, 7th edition. New York: Elsevier; 2020.
2. Mohmoodie M, Sanai B, Moazeni-Birtgani M. Penetrating neck trauma review of 192 cares. Arch Trauma Res. 2012;1:14-8.
3. Van Waes OJ, Chevek KL, Navsaria PH, van Riet PA, Nicol AJ, Vermeulen J. Management of Penetrating Neck Injuries. Br J Surg. 2012;99(Suppl 1):149-54.
4. Vishwanatha B, Sagayaraj A, Huddar SG, Kumar P, Datta RK. Penetrating neck injuries. Indian J Otorhinolaryngol Head Neck Surg. 2007 Sep;59(3):221-4.
5. Watkinson JC, Clarke RW. Scott-Brown's Otorhinolaryngology Head and Neck Surgery, 8th edition. New York: CRC Press; 2018.

CHAPTER 9

Deep Neck Space Infections

Parmod Kalsotra, Venkata Surya Phani Bhushan Durvasula, Jemy Jose

■ INTRODUCTION

The morbidity and mortality in any head and neck infection depends upon many parameters, including virulence, pathogenicity, and antibiotic sensitivity of the invading organism and the host factors (age, general health, and immunologic capability of the host). The deep neck infections may end up with life-threatening complications, despite antibiotic therapy because of different reasons such as complex anatomy, deep location within the neck causing difficult access and its proximity to important neurovascular structures. Different spaces also communicate with each other and to other portions of the body such as mediastinum and coccyx and can be a potential nidus that may allow the spread of infection to other areas of the body. A deep understanding of anatomy of the fascial planes and potential spaces of the neck is essential for the surgical management of these infections. The cervical fascia consists of fibrous connective tissue that ensheaths the organs, muscles, nerves, and vessels of the neck, binding them into functional units and thereby forming planes and potential compartments. The "tube within tube" concept helps one to visualize the three layers of the deep cervical fascia namely the—(1) superficial, (2) middle, and (3) deep layer **(Fig. 1)**.

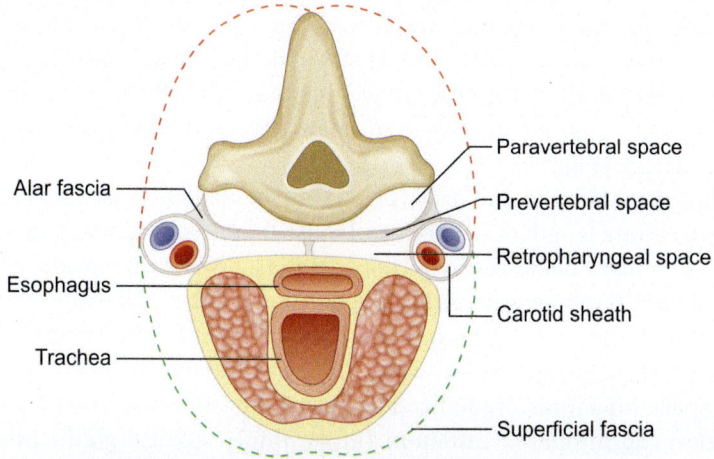

Fig. 1: The various deep neck spaces (transverse section).

■ SUPERFICIAL LAYER OF DEEP CERVICAL FASCIA

Superficial layer of deep cervical fascia (DCF) is a clear continuous sheet of fibrous tissue surrounding the neck and enclosing two glands, two muscles, and two spaces (the rule of two) and attaches to the ligamentum nuchae and vertebral spines posteriorly. Two glands are; a submandibular on each side, two muscles on each side are the trapezius and sternocleidomastoid and the two spaces are the suprasternal space of burns and posterior triangle.

■ MIDDLE LAYER OF THE DEEP CERVICAL FASCIA

Middle layer of the deep cervical fascia or *pretracheal fascia* has muscular and visceral division. Muscular division envelops the anterior strap muscles the sternohyoid, sternothyroid, thyrohyoid, omohyoid, and the adventitia of the great vessels. The visceral division of middle layer of deep cervical fascia extends around the constrictor muscles of the pharynx and esophagus to create the buccopharyngeal fascia posteriorly and anterior wall of retropharyngeal space. The middle layer of DCF is attached superiorly to the base of skull superiorly and extends with the fibrous pericardium via the carotid sheath, inferiorly, and envelops the larynx, trachea, and thyroid gland.

The *deep layer* surrounds the muscles around vertebral column and includes sympathetic trunk. All the three layers contribute to the carotid sheath as it courses through the neck. The deep layer of DCF consists of two divisions—(1) the alar and (2) the prevertebral layer. The alar layer is sandwiched between the prevertebral layer behind and the visceral (middle) layer at front, forming the posterior wall of retropharyngeal space and anterior wall of prevertebral or danger space. The retropharyngeal space extends from skull base to T1 or T2 level. The prevertebral layer forms the posterior wall of prevertebral space and anterior wall of paravertebral space, extending from skull base to coccyx. It is important to recognize that spread of an infection follows planes of least resistance and there is a continuum of these potential spaces and all the layers of deep cervical fascia that allows rapid spread of an abscess. A knowledge of these potential spaces helps guide a careful surgeon in a diseased, edematous, inflamed, and abnormally enlarged neck **(Fig. 2)**.

Clinically, the spaces of neck **(Fig. 3)** are divided into space that extends along the entire length of the neck and those that lie anterior and are limited to either above or below the hyoid bone **(Box 1)**. Because of these fasciae and musculofascial planes anteriorly, infections tend to be held within the neck, gravitate to the mediastinum, and cause asphyxiation and dysphagia from the resulting pressure, pain and swelling. The areas that tend to be the sources of deep space infections of the head and neck are—tonsillar and pharyngeal infection, odontogenic infection (anaerobic), salivary gland infection (staphylococcal), iatrogenic trauma (esophagoscopy, bronchoscopy, and removal of suspension wires from oral cavity), oral surgical procedures and

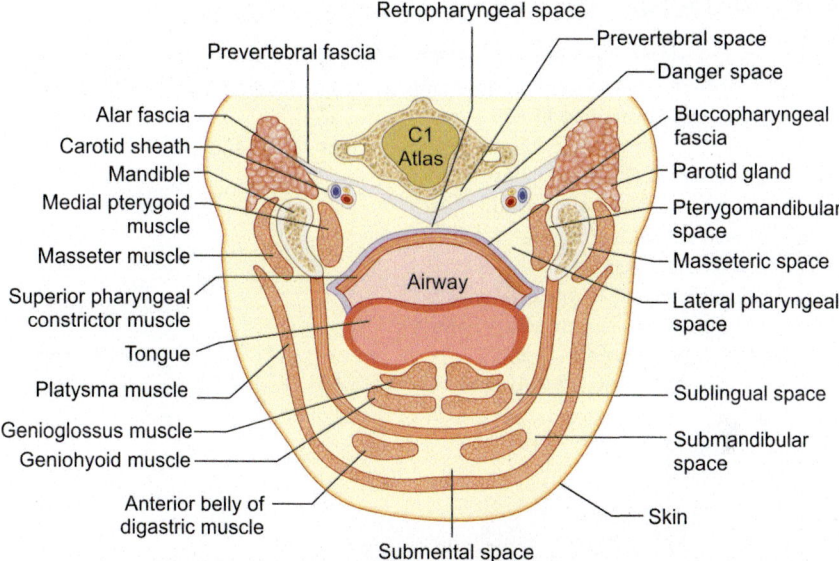

Fig. 2: The fascial spaces seen as a transverse section cut at an oblique angle.

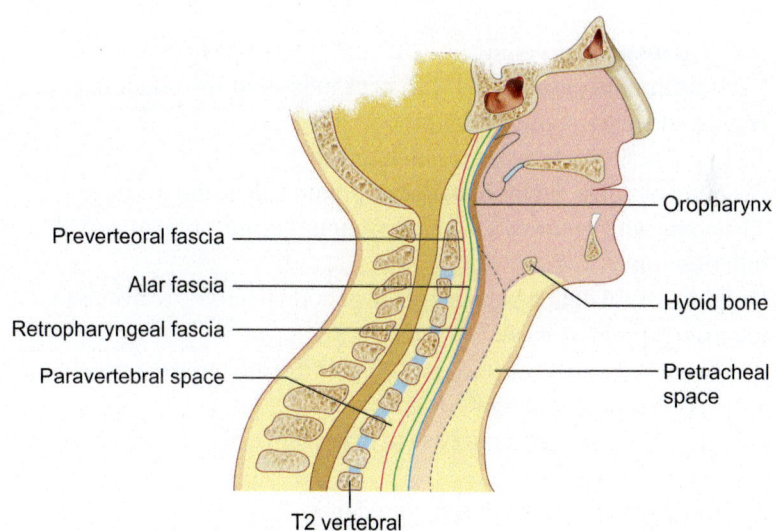

Fig. 3: The fascial planes of neck on saggital section

oral/oropharynx trauma, foreign body aspiration/ingestion, cervical nodal infection, and intravenous drug use. Rare causes include thyroiditis, branchial cleft anomalies, thyroglossal duct cyst, and mastoiditis with petrous apicitis. In majority of patients (20–50%), source of infection may not be identifiable.

■ SYMPTOMS AND SIGNS

They depend upon the mass effect of the inflamed tissue on surrounding structures and direct extension to the other critical spaces.

BOX 1: Clinically potential neck spaces.

- Spaces involving the entire length of the neck
  - Retropharyngeal space (posterior visceral, retrovisceral, or retroesophageal space) (base of skull to T1–T2)
  - Danger space (prevertebral space) (skull base to diaphragm)
  - Paravertebral space (skull base to coccyx)
  - Visceral vascular space (carotid sheath)
- Spaces above the hyoid bone
  - Submandibular space
    - Superior space (sublingual space)
    - Inferior space (submaxillary space)
      - *Medial*: Submental space
      - *Lateral*: Submaxillary proper
  - Parapharyngeal space (lateral pharyngeal and pharyngomaxillary)
  - Masticator space
  - Parotid space
  - Peritonsillar space
- Spaces below the hyoid bone (anterior only)
  - Anterior visceral (pretracheal space)

A "sick" patient presents clinically with any of following features:
- Neck asymmetry, associated with neck masses or lymphadenopathy.
- High grade fever, sometimes in septic shock.
- Tachypnea, sitting forward to catch the air.
- Drooling of saliva, odynophagia, hot potato voice, and dysphagia.
- Torticollis with restricted neck movement because of paraspinal muscle inflammation.
- Variable neural deficit because of lower cranial nerve involvement and/or metastatic brain abscess.
- Presence of trismus is an indicator of spread of infection to parapharyngeal space, pterygoid, or masseteric space.
- Odontogenic infection mainly seen in presence of decayed, loose, tender, or broken tooth.
- Always examine floor of mouth for edema.
- Examine Stensen's and Wharton's duct opening for purulent discharge and palpate for any obstructing stone.
- Examine oropharynx for lateral or posterior wall bulge or deviation of uvula.
- Examination of eye for any ophthalmoplegia or absent pupillary light reflex.
- Flexible fiberoptic evaluation of upper airways is must in all patients of deep neck infections.
- Pulse oximetry is must in all patients.

INVESTIGATIONS

The investigation includes the following:
- Complete blood count to rule out neutropenia, clotting profile, blood biochemistry, and blood culture in case of septic patient.
- X-ray of soft tissue neck (STN) (lateral view) will reveal soft tissue swelling in prevertebral region or pretracheal area, presence of any radiopaque foreign body, air fluid levels, subcutaneous air, and vertebral body involvement like Pott's spine.
- X-ray mandible (especially panorex view) for complicated odontogenic infections.
- X-ray chest for features suggestive of mediastinitis and aspiration pneumonitis.
- Contrast-enhanced computed tomography (CECT) scan is the "gold standard" in evaluation of deep-neck infection, for its extent, location, boundaries, and involvement of surrounding neurovascular structures.
- *Ultrasound (USG):*
  - It is very useful in pediatric patients.
  - It is useful for follow-up to look for status of residual or recurrent abscess.
  - *Limitations:* In presence of significant neck edema and in presence of retro or parapharyngeal abscess, ultrasound has limitation in differentiating phlegmon stage from abscess.
- Magnetic resonance imaging (MRI) and angiography have limited role as compared to CECT scan and is not available at every center. MRI is only indicated when suspecting spread of infection to intracranial cavity, parotid and prevertebral space, also in strong suspicion of suppurative thrombi of internal jugular vein (IJV), sigmoid sinus, or cavernous sinus.

MANAGEMENT (FLOWCHART 1)

The management includes the following:
- Oxygenated face stents with cool mist humidity.
- Epinephrine nebulization.
- Maintenance of airway, which may require intubation or tracheostomy. Intubation is quite difficult because of trismus, oropharyngeal edema, tracheal deviation, and because of additional risk of abscess rupture leading to aspiration. Tracheostomy or cricothyroidotomy is preferable.
- Intravenous fluids to correct dehydration secondary to trismus, odynophagia, and dysphagia.
- Check for electrolyte imbalance and maintain acid-base balance.
- Intravenous steroids (controversial)
- Intravenous broad-spectrum antibiotics to cover both gram-positive, gram-negative, and aerobic and anaerobic bacteria. Intravenous antibiotics (clindamycin, ampicillin/sulbactam, cefuroxime, etc.) are

Deep Neck Space Infections

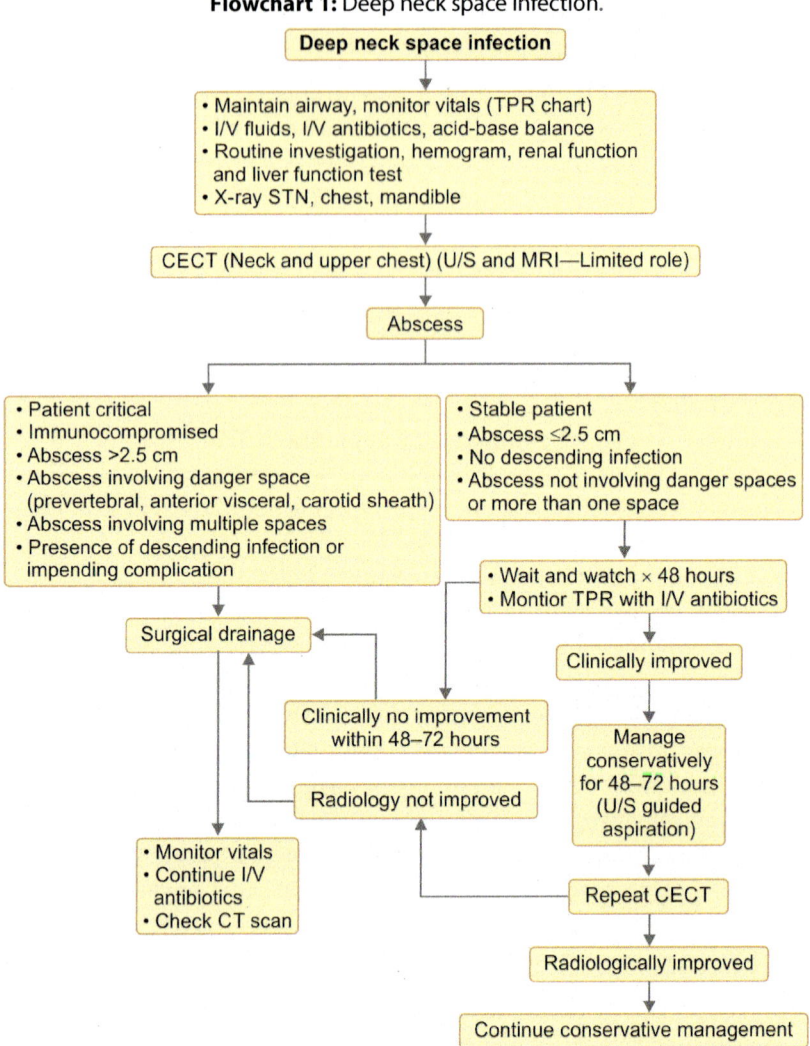

Flowchart 1: Deep neck space infection.

(CECT: contrast-enhanced computed tomography; MRI: magnetic resonance imaging; STN: soft tissue neck; TPR: temperature, pulse, respiration)

continued until the patient is clinically improving and has been afebrile for at least 48 hours. The patient is then put on oral antibiotics. Antibiotic regimen can be altered as per the blood culture or pus culture report and after taking microbiologist opinion.

- Control of concomitant medical problems like diabetes.

CONSERVATIVE/MEDICAL THERAPY

- Some authors recommend conservative approach (wait and watch) for deep neck space abscess based on CECT findings. If the patient is clinically stable, abscess is <2.5 cm, absence of descending infection, absence of involvement of >2 spaces and absence of involvement of danger spaces (prevertebral, anterior visceral, and carotid sheath). Recommendation is broad-spectrum empiric intravenous antibiotics for 48–72 hours, with nil per orally and close vital monitoring including total leukocyte count (TLC) and differential leukocyte count (DLC).

SURGICAL MANAGEMENT

Surgical Treatment Principles

- Mainstay is incision and drainage because intravenous antibiotics have poor penetration in pus-filled spaces due to poor vascularity. The incisions for external drainage of various deep neck space abscesses are depicted in **Figure 4**.
- Involved tooth should be extracted (ideal time is at the time of I and D) but take preoperative consent for tooth extraction too.
- Open all primary and secondary spaces and keep drain or irrigation catheters.

Indications for Surgical Intervention

- Frank abscess/air fluid level in neck or infection proven to be due to gas producing organisms
- Compromised airway
- Failure to medical therapy within 48–72 hours
- *Impending complications:* Immediate surgical intervention in deep neck space infection is indicated in the presence of sepsis, respiratory distress or hemorrhage from the pharynx or ear. Repeated hemorrhage of small

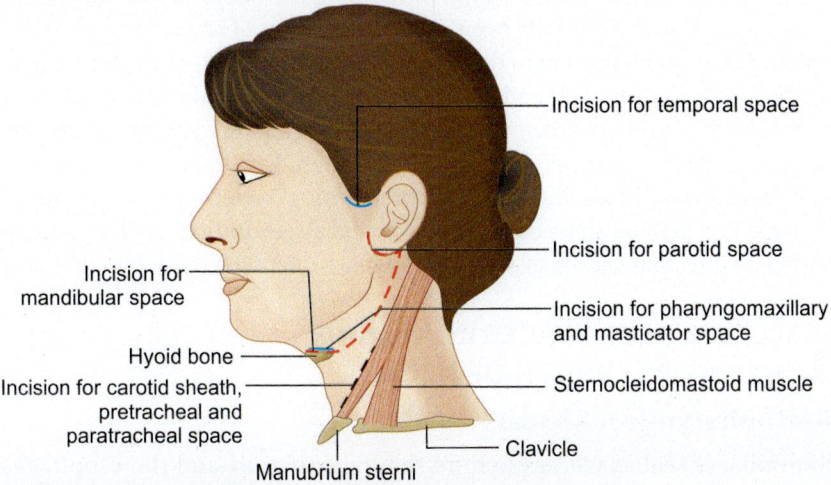

Fig. 4: Incisions for deep neck space infections.

amounts of blood into the pharynx or ear indicates vessel erosion. Erosion of the walls of the jugular vein may be accompanied by thrombus formation and its embolization may result in repeated chills with spiking temperature.

Transoral drainage is indicated in selective cases and includes:
- Quinsy
- Odontogenic infection with alveolar abscess
- Buccal space (via per-oral incision parallel to branches of the facial nerve through buccinator muscle)
- Masticator space (via retromolar trigone)
- Retropharyngeal space abscess.

Transcervical Drainage

General surgical rules are similarly followed including proper drainage of abscess cavities along with antibiotic coverage based on culture and sensitivity studies. When surgery is indicated, drainage of both primary site, and secondarily involved areas should be performed. Neck space infections cause immense swelling and distortion of landmarks, and this should be kept in mind and reliance on fixed surgical landmarks (like cricoid cartilage angle of mandible) will allow safe drainage. Surgical approach to external drainage is based on identification of the carotid sheath which is followed to the abscess, opening the potential spaces along the path. Retract the submandibular gland anteriorly and blunt finger dissection is carried out superior and medial to posterior belly of digastric muscle along the medial surface of mandible to open parapharyngeal space. Retract strap muscle medially and carotid sheath laterally, at a level inferior to carotid bulb and enter the prevertebral and retropharyngeal space. Blunt finger dissection can be carried superiorly or inferiorly depending on radiological extent of abscess. Access to deep neck compartments even requires excision of secondary inflamed/enlarged lymph nodes. Try to do minimal debridement as, because of edema and inflammation, vessels and nerves are at high risk. Cultures for aerobic and anaerobic bacteria are taken whenever possible, and the abscess is irrigated thoroughly with saline before insertion of drains. The drains are left in place and carefully advanced and removed when timing is appropriate as suggested by local and general signs of inflammation, soakage and sepsis. The primary source of infection should also be treated like a offending tooth by extraction.

INFECTION OF SPACES INVOLVING THE ENTIRE LENGTH OF NECK

Retropharyngeal Abscess

Retropharyngeal space lies behind the hypopharynx and the esophagus, extends superiorly from the base of skull and inferiorly up to the superior mediastinum to the level of T1–T2 where middle and deep layers of cervical fascia fuse. Retropharyngeal abscess occurs most frequently in infants and young children with three cardinal features, i.e., dysphagia, drooling of saliva, and sore throat. Infection springs from nasal chambers, posterior nasal sinuses, adenoids, and nasopharynx to involve the retropharyngeal lymph nodes. In adults, tuberculosis is an important causative factor. Other causes include foreign bodies piercing the posterior esophageal wall, endoscopic complication, esophageal rupture, vertebral fractures, syphilis, upper respiratory tract infection, and dental infections. Infection in ear, nose, and throat spreads via lymphatics to retropharyngeal lymph nodes, which are found in greatest number in children under the age of four and hence, account for relatively greater incidence of retropharyngeal abscess in this age group. Symptoms of this abscess in children differ from those in adults. Most common organisms are Group A *Streptococcus*, *Staphylococcus aureus*, and aerobic and anaerobic pharyngeal microorganisms. In children, most common features are abrupt onset of high-grade fever, odynophagia with drooling of saliva, dysphagia, neck pain with torticollis, and interference with breathing. Child maintains his neck in extended position and holds his head slightly forward known as *sniffing position*. X-ray soft tissue neck (lateral view during inspiration with fully extended neck) reveals air, air fluid level or foreign body in the retropharyngeal soft tissues or widening of prevertebral area. Normally the retropharyngeal tissue on lateral plain X-ray is equal to width of the body of C2 in small children. Normal soft tissue shadow should be <½ of the width of the adjacent vertebral body [(<7 mm over C2 in children and adults (retropharyngeal space) or <14 mm in children and 22 mm in adults over C6 (retrotracheal space)]. Contrast-enhanced computed tomography scan may be indicated in doubtful cases. The classical appearance of retropharyngeal abscess is a unilateral (posterolateral) swelling of the posterior pharyngeal wall, which may push the palate forward, because of midline fascia dividing the retropharyngeal space and restricting the abscess to one side along with cervical lymphadenopathy. In adults, the most common symptoms are pain, dysphagia, dyspnea, noisy breathing, snoring, nasal obstruction, anorexia, regurgitation, and swelling of glands of the neck. Extension of infection into the mediastinum is characterized by chest pain, severe dyspnea, persistent fever, and X-ray evidence of widening of the mediastinum **(Table 1)**.

- *Differential diagnosis* of retropharyngeal abscess includes cervical osteomyelitis, meningitis, Pott's disease, and calcified tendonitis of the longus colli muscle.
- *Surgical management* is done mainly by external approach, while the peroral approach is indicated in selected patients **(Fig. 5)**.
  - *Transoral/peroral approach:* This is indicated in an early retropharyngeal abscess with no respiratory obstruction. Head is kept in extreme

TABLE 1: Comparative chart of retropharyngeal abscess, parapharyngeal abscess, and peritonsillitis.

Clinical features	Retropharyngeal abscess	Parapharyngeal abscess	Peritonsillitis
Age	<4 years	Older children, adolescents, and adults	Adolescents and adults
Site of origin	Pharyngitis, dental infection, and trauma	Tonsillitis, otitis media, mastoiditis, and parotitis and dental infection	Tonsillitis
On examination	• Unilateral posterolateral pharyngeal wall bulging • Hyperextension of neck • Drooling of saliva • Respiratory difficulty (±)	*Anterior compartment:* • Parotid area swelling • Trismus • Tonsil/tonsil fossa pushed medially • Uvula pushed to same side *Posterior compartment:* • Septicemia • Pain • Trismus (±)	• Unilateral tonsil swelling • Uvular displacement toward opposite side • Trismus (±) • Muffled voice
May complicate to	Spread to parapharyngeal space, posterior mediastinum	• Carotid blow-out • Airway obstruction • Metastatic abscess • Lung aspiration • Mediastinal extension • Septic shock	Spread to parapharyngeal space
Treatment	Antibiotics, I and D and secure airway	• Airway management • Antibiotics—I and D	Antibiotics—I and D

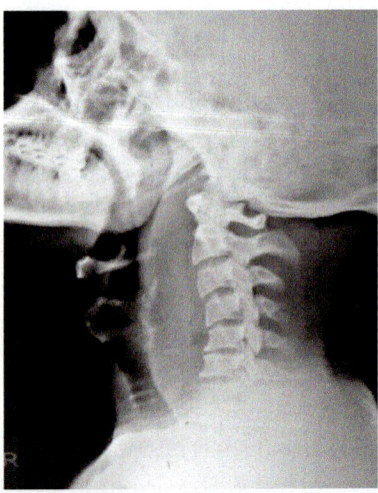

Fig. 5: X-ray lateral neck showing retropharyngeal abscess.

"Rose's" position, mouth gag is utilized, and incision and drainage is done. Tracheostomy is indicated in presence of airway obstruction.
- *External approach:* This is indicated in large retropharyngeal, paravertebral, prevertebral and carotid sheath abscess, where *anterior external approach* is employed. A transverse incision is made along the anterior border of sternomastoid muscle at a desired level between the hyoid bone and the sternum. Alternatively, the *Dean approach*, a lateral oblique incision anterior to the sternocleidomastoid muscle is a better option with excellent exposure. The sternocleidomastoid muscle and carotid sheath are retracted laterally, and the thyroid gland and superior thyroid pedicle is retracted medially and the middle thyroid vein, the superior thyroid artery and the omohyoid muscle may be sectioned for better exposure. The abscess may resemble a distended bag and lies between the carotid sheath and the paravertebral muscles behind the inferior constrictor muscle. The abscess is then opened and drained. If it extends inferiorly into the neck and upper mediastinum, finger dissection can be carried into mediastinum along the esophagus and a drain is left in place. Another external approach is *posterior approach*, incision is made behind the sternomastoid muscle avoiding the carotid sheath and the abscess is entered from the fascia behind the sternomastoid muscle. If the abscess has spread past the level of T4 posteriorly or the tracheal bifurcation anteriorly, as documented on CT scan, drainage by external thoracotomy may be contemplated.

■ INFECTION OF SPACES ABOVE THE HYOID BONE

Submandibular Space

Involvement of this space occurs mainly in dental or periodontal infections, submandibular gland infection or suppuration of submandibular lymph nodes, leading to Ludwig's angina **(Fig. 6)**. Streptococci and staphylococci are the most common organisms but Vincent's organism and common spirochetal commensals of the mouth may be primary or secondary invaders. Ludwig's angina (described by Ludwig in 1836) is the infection involving this space. It is usually caused by the infection of the lower second and third molars that begins in their subgingival pocket but spreads into submandibular space along the lingual aspect of the mandible, as their roots extends below the attachment of mylohyoid muscle, the so-called *mylohyoid line*. The lingual aspect of mandible, being thinner facilitates the spread along the sub lingual and then submandibular space that usually presents as a patient in acute pain and difficulty in breathing with characteristic finding—extremely swollen and inflamed tissues of the floor of mouth that show a brawny induration initially in the submandibular compartment

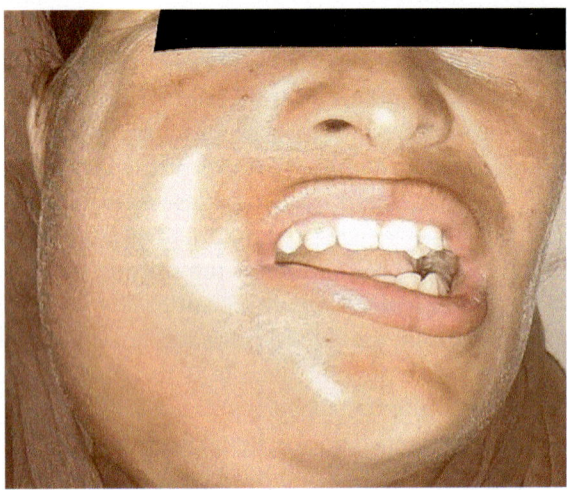

Fig. 6: Submandibular space abscess.

(but can spread quickly to the infrahyoid compartments leading to mediastinitis and upper airway obstruction) with upward and backward displacement of the tongue that has been pushed by these swollen tissues toward the palatal vault, trismus, hoarseness, and dyspnea. This highly virulent infection is a cellulitis and not a true abscess. Wide surgical drainage is indicated and airway is managed with tracheostomy. On drainage, a straw-colored weeping exudate rather than the true abscess fluid is released. Trismus and hypopharyngeal mucosal edema contraindicate preliminary intubation. Transverse incision is made in submental space and is carried down to the deep fascia of the mylohyoid muscle. Mylohyoid muscle is divided perpendicular to the course of its fibers and a drain is kept. If the infection localizes to the floor of mouth above the mylohyoid line, intraoral drainage is sometimes possible **(Figs. 7 and 8)**.

Parapharyngeal Space

This space is most commonly involved in children because the portals of infection here are most often from the pharynx, tonsils and adenoids, teeth (usually from masseteric space), parotid glands, and the lymph nodes that drain the nose and pharynx. Also, uncommon cause is Bezold's abscess (mastoiditis leading to abscess in inner aspect of mastoid tip). *Staphylococcus aureus*, *Streptococcus* sp. and anaerobic bacteria are the most common causative organisms. The styloid process divides *parapharyngeal space* into two compartments. The *anterior compartment* infection results in high grade fever and chills, rapidly growing unilateral tender neck swelling obliterating the angle of mandible, and trismus mainly because of medial pterygoid muscle irritation. Most of patients are acutely ill, have odynophagia,

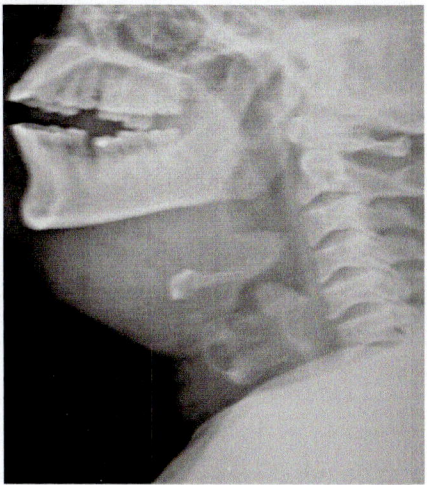

Fig. 7: X-ray lateral neck in Lugwig's angina.

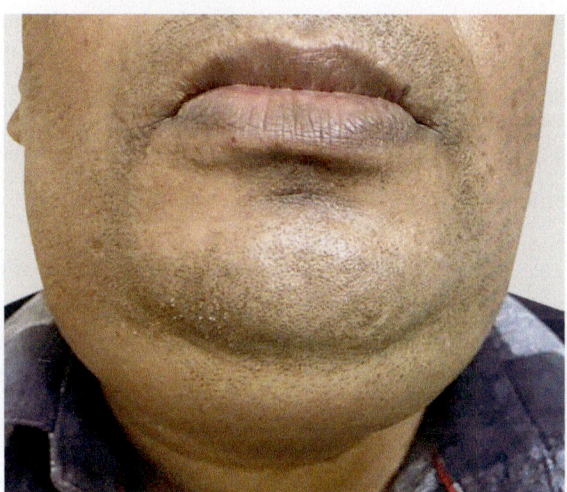

Fig. 8: Lugwig's angina.

dysphagia, and mild dyspnea, along with medial displacement of normal looking inflamed tonsil and lateral pharyngeal wall. Torticollis toward the side of abscess, caused by reflex neck muscle spasm, is also seen (similar to that seen in acute cervical lymphadenitis). *The classical triad is—a normal looking but prolapsed tonsil due to its medial displacement with trismus and swelling of the parotid area.*

Infection of the "posterior compartment" causes signs and symptoms of septicemia without pain or trismus. Swelling may be overlooked because it lies deep behind the palatopharyngeal arch. Flexible laryngoscopy reveals swollen lateral pharyngeal wall with ipsilateral obliteration of the pyriform fossa. Later on, patient may also show features of toxicity and altered sensorium. Plum color of the swollen oral mucosa indicates submucosal hemorrhage suggesting arterial erosion. Externally, there is swelling in the neck with ill-defined margins, absence of fluctuation but with pitting edema of neck, mostly seen in patients with diabetes, nephritis, tuberculosis or acquired immunodeficiency syndrome (AIDS). Ear hemorrhage is a grave prognostic sign of vascular involvement. Dissection of the abscess through the junction of the cartilaginous and bony external auditory canal may present as purulent otorrhea. Hemorrhage due to the erosion of internal carotid artery may occur and may require immediate surgical intervention.

Treatment

Management of parapharyngeal abscess depends on the size of abscess and general condition of the patient. There are several studies quoting that a small abscess <25 mm size can be managed conservatively with IV antibiotics, especially in pediatric age groups, provided the general condition of the patient remains stable and patient can be monitored daily. The role of serial CECT scans in such cases becomes important and can help objectively assess the increase in size of such abscesses thus facilitating appropriate management. It should also be borne in mind that such cases can occasionally deteriorate quickly due to sepsis and early drainage remains invaluable in such cases.

Surgical drainage is best performed after localization of the infection unless hemorrhage or respiratory obstruction necessitates earlier intervention. Tracheostomy may be required prophylactically because airway obstruction due to laryngeal edema may develop abruptly. In case of arterial erosion, carotid artery may be ligated.

The proper time for surgical drainage depends on the stage of infection which can be monitored effectively by CECT scan. Rarely, the abscess ruptures spontaneously and drains externally. It should be drained surgically, even when no complication has occurred. However, no drainage attempt should be made during the stage of phlegmon formation (cellulitis), when antibiotics alone are sufficient (clindamycin, chloramphenicol, metronidazole, cefoxitin, or imipenem and a combination of penicillin plus a β-lactamase inhibitor are more appropriate antibiotics). Surgical drainage by submaxillary approach can be accomplished by a modification of the Mosher-T shaped incision. Make a horizontal incision at the level of hyoid bone, follow the carotid sheath and insert the finger below the submandibular gland, dissect bluntly with finger along the posterior border of digastric muscle, deep to mastoid tip toward the styloid process. The tip of greater cornu of hyoid bone serves as a fixed inferior surgical landmark.

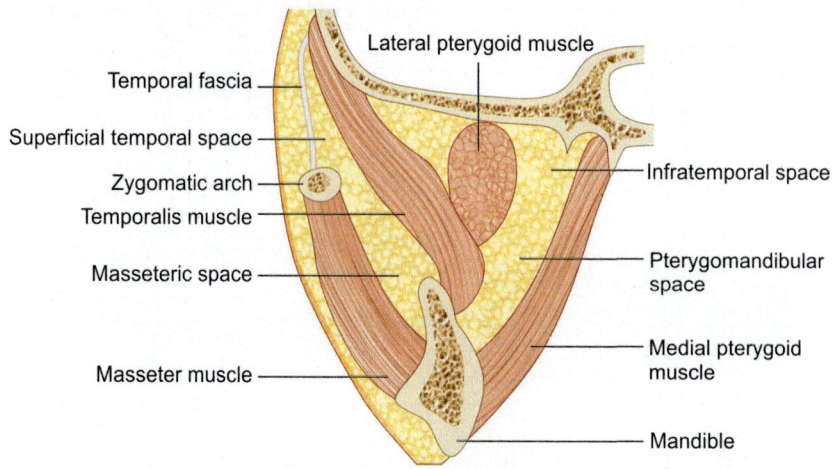

Fig. 9: Masticator space.

Masticator Space or Masseteric Space

Masseteric space **(Fig. 9)** abscess is a subperiosteal abscess and cellulitis of the mandible and soft tissue and may involve the fascial sling containing the muscles of mastication (i.e., masseter, pterygoid, and the temporalis muscle). It presents as a brawny induration over the area of the angle and body of the mandible externally, with marked trismus. Incision and drainage is achieved via intraoral approach or by external incision made below the horizontal ramus of mandible posterior to facial artery, carrying it down till the periosteum and then blunt dissection is carried on each side of the mandible.

Parotid Space

The parotid space formed by the superficial layer of deep cervical fascia, is not a true anatomic space, many fascial septa run vertically through it. A parotid space abscess is actually an infection of the gland with loculated microabscesses. The most common pathogen is *Staphylococcus*. The patient presents with erythematous skin and a swollen parotid gland with high grade fever and tenderness but with absence of trismus or swelling of lateral pharyngeal wall. Stenson's duct usually reveals a purulent flow on massage. Surgical drainage is necessary when antibiotics are unsuccessful and achieved via "Furstenberg" incision, where multiple incisions are made through the fascia parallel to the branches of facial nerve and opening of spaces with a blunt clamp **(Fig. 10)**.

Peritonsillar Space

This space is between superior constrictor muscle and tonsil capsule. Peritonsillar or paratonsillar abscess (quinsy) is the most common deep

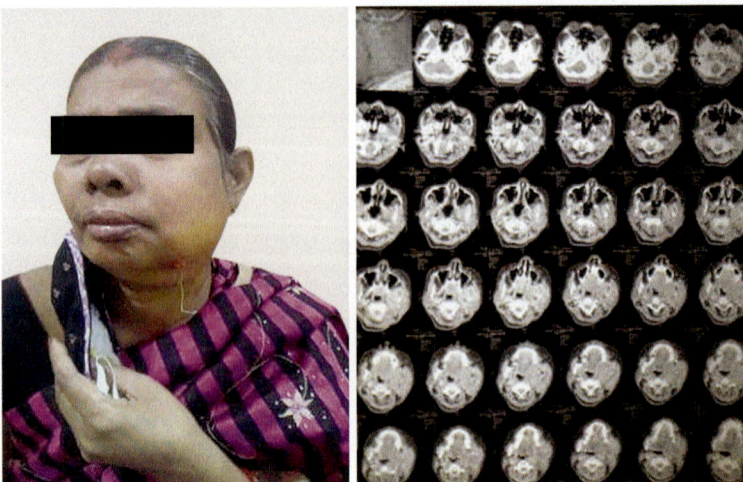

Fig. 10: Deep neck space infection involving left submandibular, masticator, and parotid spaces.

head and neck infection. It generally occurs in adolescents and adults as a complication of repeated episodes of bacterial tonsillitis or as a secondary complication of viral infection. Infection begins in intratonsillar fossa and extends around the tonsil. Suppuration is into the space between tonsillar capsule and superior constrictor, the most common location being the upper pole. In contrast, the "tonsillar abscess" is uncommon and is because of retention of pus within a follicle. Quinsy is usually unilateral and rarely bilateral. The patient may be apprehensive and pale, with the temperature and pulse rate increasing, often preceded by a rigor. There is difficulty in swallowing and speaking (hot potato voice) with pain radiating to ipsilateral ear. Trismus is because of pterygoid muscle spasm. Breath has a foul odor along with salivary dribble. Tonsil is swollen, inflamed and medially deviated, but the soft palate even if edematous, does not bulge. The uvula is edematous and pushed toward the opposite side and the affected tonsil is usually hidden by the surrounding swelling. Ipsilateral cervical lymph nodes are enlarged and tender. Bilateral abscess is rare and difficult to diagnose because the classic signs like congestion on the affected side of the palate and edema of the uvula, with a shift to the opposite side are absent.

Most common cause for hospitalization is dehydration. Abscess is drained using quinsy forceps intraorally through the most fluctuant area (by making stab incision or using 16G or 18G needle for aspiration) or just lateral to the point of junction of an imaginary line drawn through the base of uvula and a vertical line through the anterior tonsillar pillar. Some advocate emergency tonsillectomy but bleeding may be more troublesome in the acutely infected tonsils (especially opposite side) **(Fig. 11)**.

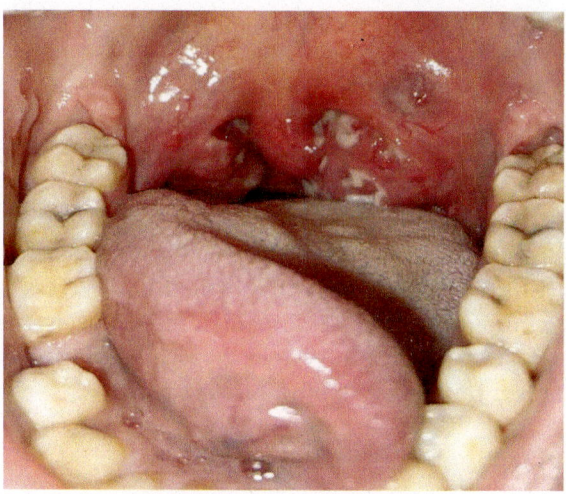

Fig. 11: Peritonsillar abscess.

■ INFECTION OF SPACES BELOW THE HYOID BONE
Anterior Visceral Space
Infection of this space occurs through the perforation of the anterior esophageal wall by trauma, foreign bodies, and endoscopic instruments. Infection can easily extend into the mediastinum. Clinically, patient complains of severe dyspnea, dysphagia, and occasionally hoarseness and nasal regurgitation. Abscess is drained via a transverse incision made along anterior border of sternomastoid muscle. Carotid sheath is retracted laterally along with sternomastoid muscle. Abscess is drained and drain is kept.

Complications of Deep Space Abscess
Complications of deep space abscess include:
- *Osteomyelitis* due to local spread of infection to bones such as spine, mandible, and skull base.
- *Grisel syndrome:* Inflammatory torticollis causing cervical vertebral subluxation.
- *Mediastinitis* (severe dyspnea, chest pain, and persistent fever with widened mediastinum on X-ray chest).
- Acute renal failure.
- Disseminated intravascular coagulation (DIC)
- Airway compromise because of tracheal compression or secondary laryngeal edema.
- Aspiration, especially due to rupture of retropharyngeal or parapharyngeal abscess or while intubation, the abscess may rupture open and drain into the airway.

- Septicemia and septic shock.
- Metastatic abscess to liver, brain, lung and joints.
- Direct intracranial extension (meningitis and cavernous and lateral sinus thrombosis).
- Erosion of arteries like carotid blow-out (may present as external auditory canal bleed).
- Dysphagia.
- *Neurological involvement:* Vagus involvement can lead to hoarseness; 12th nerve involvement can cause ipsilateral tongue paralysis and Horner's syndrome because of sympathetic chain involvement.
- *Toxic shock syndrome:* Multisystem involvement occur secondary to growth of toxin-producing *Staphylococcus aureus*.

Diagnostic criteria for toxic shock syndrome:
- Systolic BP <90 mm Hg
- Temperature >39°C
- Rash with desquamation focused on palms and soles
- Involvement of three or more organ systems (mentioned underneath)
  - *Musculoskeletal system:* Myalgia and increase in creatine phosphokinase levels
  - *Mucous membranes:* Frank hyperemia
  - *Gastrointestinal system:* Vomiting/diarrhea
  - *Renal system:* Renal insufficiency
  - *Hepatic system:* Hepatitis
  - *Hematology:* Low platelet count (<150,000 platelets/µL)
  - *Nervous system:* Disorientation without focal neurological signs

Treatment involves aggressive intravenous fluid hydration and intravenous broad-spectrum antibiotics. Emergency surgical consultation for any wound debridement.

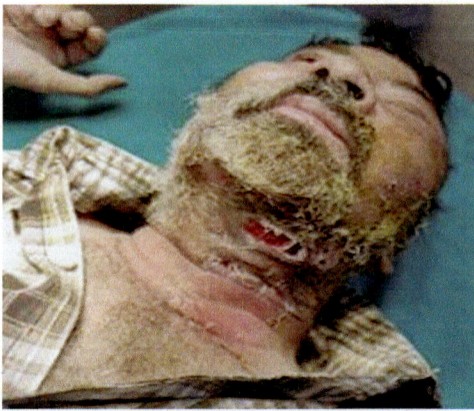

Fig. 12: Lemierre's syndrome.

Lemierre's syndrome is a rare complication of bacterial tonsillitis that extends into the lateral pharyngeal spaces of the neck thus causing internal IJV thrombophlebitis and septicemia resulting in septic emboli and metastatic abscesses **(Fig. 12)**. This needs immediate drainage of the abscess and evacuation of these thrombi and long-term IV antibiotics for at least 3-6 weeks.

■ OTHER IMPORTANT CERVICAL INFECTIONS
Necrotizing Fasciitis

It is a fulminant soft tissue infection of the skin, subcutaneous tissue and deep fascia with relative sparing of muscle and spreads along fascial planes. These infections do not have clear local boundaries or palpable margins and thereby result in delayed diagnosis and subsequent management. Necrotizing fasciitis (also known as hospital gangrene, Meleney's gangrene, hemolytic streptococcal gangrene, and synergistic necrotizing cellulitis) is caused by aerobic and anaerobic microorganisms resulting in massive tissue destruction and toxic shock syndrome.

In most cases, the route of entry of pathogen is via trauma or surgery. Initially, there is cellulitis, followed by progressive tissue necrosis and normal floral invasion. The combined effect results in decreased oxygen tension, local ischemia and proliferation of anaerobic organisms. Localized gangrene is evident within 4-5 days and after 8-10 days, necrotic tissue separates from underlying ischemic but viable tissue. Bacterial metabolic gaseous end-products results in subcutaneous emphysema **(Fig. 13)**.

The causative organisms are clostridial and nonclostridial such as *Escherichia coli, Klebsiella, Peptostreptococcus, Bacteroides melaninogenicus,* and *Fusobacterium*. The most common cause of cervical necrotizing fasciitis is dental infection (lower molars). Other sites of origin of infection are tonsils, pharynx, salivary glands, and cervical lymph adenitis. Predisposing factors are diabetes, malnutrition, obesity, corticosteroid therapy, and immune-deficiency but can also be seen in normal healthy patients.

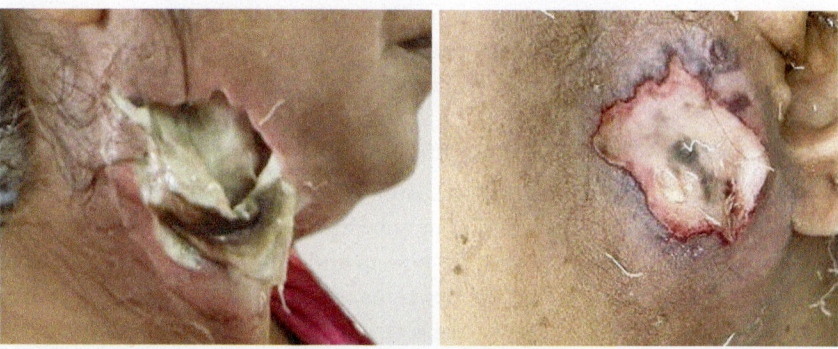

Fig. 13: Necrotizing fasciitis.

Histology reveals obliterative endarteritis and thrombosis of the subcutaneous vessels. Necrosis of superficial fascia, foci of polymorphonuclear and mononuclear cell infiltration and microbial colonization of the skin and fascia are other changes. Myonecrosis is not seen which is otherwise a typical finding in clostridial infection (*Clostridium perfringens*).

Clinically, the picture is of an acutely febrile patient with tender, erythematous and edematous overlying skin with occasional bulla formation and crepitations of underlying soft tissue (**Figure 13**). The pain is severe and out of proportion to other clinical findings. Occasional presentation is because of streptococcal toxic shock syndrome. Additionally, patient may also present with other sequelae such as pneumonitis, pleural effusion, mediastinitis, pericarditis, and pericardial effusion and DIC leading to septic shock.

Necrotizing fasciitis is always suspected whenever odontogenic infection spreads rapidly to lower neck or anterior chest with abnormal accumulation of gas in tissue and an orange-peel appearance of the involved skin and progressive soft tissue involvement despite broad-spectrum antibiotic coverage, showing no clinical response. Contrast-enhanced computed tomography is the investigation of choice. Common CT findings include diffuse thickening of skin and subcutaneous tissues, with reticular enhancement of the subcutaneous fat of face and neck signifying cellulitis, thickening and/or enhancement of cervical fascia due to fasciitis and cervical muscles due to myositis with gas and fluid in multiple neck spaces and possibly mediastinum.

Management

The management includes:
- Maintaining the vitals (BP support with vasopressin), intravenous fluid, intravenous antibiotics (start with empiric broad spectrum antibiotics, e.g., third generation cephalosporin combined with clindamycin or metronidazole). Heavy doses of pencillin are effective.
- Early but wide local surgical debridement of cervical fascia compartment (debridement of all necrotic tissue). Surgical finding is extensive soft tissue necrosis with fat liquefaction. Excision to the point of bleeding is the clinical guide for debridement. Use of hyperbaric oxygen is reported in the literature but is not available at every treating center. Mortality is high, 6–76% with mediastinitis being most common cause of death.

Acute Suppurative Thyroiditis

It is a rare but potentially life-threatening infection. Clinically, patient presents with tender firm swelling in anterior aspect of neck with local rise of temperature, fever, erythema, dysphagia and dysphonia/hoarseness. The swelling, moves with deglutition, develops over days to a few weeks with or without fever. Neck movements are restricted especially the extension and chin is depressed during deglutition. Fluctuation may appear later on, in the swelling. Suppurative thyroiditis may occur as a part of cellulitis in the neck or because of infection of a cyst in a multinodular goiter.

Causative microorganisms are *Staphylococcus aureus, Streptococcus pyogenes, Staphylococcus epidermidis,* and *Streptococcus pneumoniae*. Serum T3 and T4 are elevated because of release of hormones from the inflamed gland. Ultrasound is helpful to detect the local abscess formation, involvement of contiguous structures, to differentiate from other causes of anterior neck pain, and ultrasound-guided needle aspiration of abscess. Computed tomography scan or MRI scan are of limited value. Thyroid scan will not visualize the thyroid with diffuse inflammation, although "patchy uptake" or a cold area may be reported with localized thyroid abscess or less severe involvement. Diagnosis can be facilitated by needle aspiration of the neck mass and Gram staining of the aspirated material.

Management includes intravenous broad-spectrum antibiotics, analgesics, intravenous fluids and β-blockers if the raised T3/T4 causes tachycardia after taking opinion of physician. If antibiotic treatment fails, surgery as incision with drainage can be necessary. Drainage can be repeated if the abscess persists. In cases of extensive necrosis or pretracheal space, persistence of infection, lobectomy can be considered. Necrotic tissue should be debrided and wound allowed to heal by secondary intention.

On follow-up, transient or prolonged hypothyroidism may occur in some patients and may require L-thyroxine replacement. Local complications, most commonly seen are vocal cord paralysis, abscess extension (into anterior mediastinum, trachea, and esophagus), pericarditis, pneumonitis, septic shock, and Lemierre's syndrome (IJV thrombophlebitis).

Cervicofacial Actinomycosis

Actinomycosis (by *Actinomyces israelii*) tends to spread along connective tissue planes, with little tendency to ulcerate or lymphatic spread. Poor orodental hygiene, dental caries, and minor trauma are common predisposing factors. Clinically, patient presents with painful or painless indurated swelling with fixed overlying skin, a few weeks after dental extraction or oral trauma, usually at the angle of the jaw (lumpy jaw), which suppurates with multiple draining sinuses or fistulae where from "sulfur granules" are discharged. Trismus may be seen. Direct extension of disease causes osteomyelitis and periostitis of mandible, orbital or paranasal sinus involvement and central nervous system (CNS) spread.

Treatment is high dose of penicillin because of poor penetration into the actinomycotic mass which is continued 2–3 weeks beyond subsidence of all clinical signs of disease. Surgical excision may be indicated if large area is involved.

Cat Scratch Disease

Bartonella henselae causes cat scratch disease with swollen tender cervical lymph nodes, ultimately forming an abscess. Management is mainly nonsurgical, followed by incision and drainage (I and D).

Descending Necrotizing Mediastinitis

This is a rare but most dreaded and probably the most lethal form of mediastinitis, occurring as a complication of oropharyngeal infection with quoted mortality rate, as high as 40% even in the antibiotic era. Majority of cases of descending necrotizing mediastinitis (DNM) develop from odontogenic infection, typically lower second or third molar abscess, which spreads from the submandibular space to the parapharyngeal space and then into the mediastinum via retrovisceral, pretracheal or perivascular space. Other causes include peritonsillar abscess, retropharyngeal abscess, cervical trauma, epiglottitis, parotitis, cervical lymphadenitis, intravenous drug abuse, etc.

Causative microorganisms are typically highly virulent mixed aerobes and anaerobes often acting synergistically. Rapid spread of infection is facilitated by tissue necrosis, gravity, and negative intrathoracic pressure. The diagnosis of DNM is clinically different because of vagueness of early symptoms. One should consider DNM diagnosis if:

- Clinical condition does not improve or worsen despite adequate medical treatment and/or surgical drainage, e.g., quinsy drainage.
- Increasing neck swelling, surgical emphysema, rash, and chest or back pain.
- Additional feature of respiratory insufficiency along with septicemia.
- Rising inflammatory markers such as TLC, C-reactive protein, liver function tests (LFT), and renal function tests (RFT).
- *Management includes:*
  - Admission of all suspected cases of DNM
  - Baseline TLC, DLC, LFT, RFT, and C-reactive protein
  - Pus culture and blood culture
  - Intravenous fluids and electrolyte balance
  - Intravenous broad-spectrum antibiotics
  - Plain X-ray chest, soft tissue neck may reveal widening of retropharyngeal space (with or without air fluid level), anterior displacement of tracheal air-column, mediastinal emphysema, and widening of superior mediastinal shadow.
  - Contrast-enhanced CT scan (skull base to diaphragm) may reveal soft tissue infiltration with loss of normal fat planes or collection of fluid density with or without presence of gas bubbles.

Computed tomography evidence of disease below carina has been recommended as an indication for thoracotomy in addition to cervicotomy.
- Blood transfusion for concomitant anemia or serum protein depletion.
- O_2 inhalation because cyanosis is often present in mediastinitis.
- Surgical drainage of cervical and mediastinal collection, debridement of necrotic tissue and wide mediastinopleural drainage.

"Cervical mediastinotomy" is an approach described for drainage of mediastinitis above the level of sixth thoracic vertebra. Incision is made parallel to the lower, medial border of sternomastoid muscle (some prefer horizontal incision). Sternomastoid is retracted and fascia lateral to sternothyroid muscle is divided to expose the carotid sheath and thyroid gland. Lateral and inferior thyroid vein are ligated and divided. By lateral displacement of great vessels and medial displacement of the thyroid gland, trachea, and esophagus are exposed. Inferior thyroid artery may be ligated and divided and carotid sheath and pretracheal space may be inspected. If the infection is in anterior mediastinum, "anterior mediastinotomy" is indicated wherein pretracheal space is opened and blunt finger dissection is carried to the level of tracheal bifurcation. In case of posterior mediastinal abscess, dissection is carried behind the esophagus and retrovisceral space is opened and pus is aspirated and drain is kept at the bottom of cavity. If pus is encountered on dependent pockets on either side of the midline, it should be drained through separate incision on the corresponding sides of the neck because a drain crossing the midline can get pinched between the spine and the esophagus causing obstruction to the drainage of abscess. This approach is inefficient in the diffuse and necrotizing form with unencapsulated collections.

Cardiothoracic and vascular surgeons (CTVS) opinion is always sought for DNM. CTVS intervention includes "subxiphoid" approach for extensive cases of anterior mediastinitis or "posterior mediastinotomy" in posterior mediastinitis. Standard "posterolateral thoracotomy" may be indicated in some patients which provides good exposure of the pleural cavity, the pericardium and all compartments of the mediastinum; allowing radical surgical debridement, complete excision of tissue necrosis, drainage of the pericardial and pleural cavities. "Clamshell approach" is reported in literature which includes bilateral anterior thoracotomy and a transverse sternotomy.

■ FURTHER READING
1. Brook I. Microbiology and management of peritonsillar, retropharyngeal, and parapharyngeal abscesses. 2004;62(12):1545-50.

2. Daneil E, Meltzer, Shatzkes DR. Masticator space: imaging anatomy for diagnosis. Otolaryngol Clin North Am. 2012;45(6):1233-51.
3. Larawin V, Naipao J, Dubey SP. Head and neck space infections. Otolaryngol Head Neck Sur. 2006;135(6):889-93.
4. Singh B, Paparella M, da Costa SS. Paparella's Otolaryngology Head and Neck Surgery, 1st edition. New Delhi: Jaypee Brothers Medical Publishers (P) Ltd; 2019.
5. Singh M, Kambalinath DH, Gupta KC. Management of odontogenic space infection with microbiology study. J Maxillof Oral Surg. 2014;13(2):133-9.
6. Vieina F, Allen SM, Stocks RM, Thompson JW. Deep neck infection. Otolaryngol Clin North Am. 2008,41(3):459-83.

CHAPTER 10

Pediatric Stridor

Sahil Kalsotra, Gopika Kalsotra, Ghanshyam Saini

■ INTRODUCTION

Stridor is a physical sign of turbulent airflow through a partial obstruction in the airway, characterized by an audible noise (harsh, high-pitched sound). Presentation of a kid with stridor merits immediate investigation and intervention, otherwise the pathological lesion causing airway narrowing can cause death. The loudness of stridor does not necessarily correlate with the severity of obstruction and hence important to take other symptoms into account.

Infant larynx and trachea are anatomically different from adult one:
- Infant larynx is approximately one-third of an adult larynx
- Infant's vocal cords are 6–8 mm long and vocal process of arytenoids make up approximately 50% of the glottis (in adults, the vocal process makes up approximately 25% of the glottis).
- In infants, epiglottis tilts more posteriorly and hyoid overlies the thyroid notch due to short thyrohyoid membrane. The cricoid is at level of C4 rather than C7 as in adults.
- Subglottis is the narrowest segment of the pediatric airway (5-7 mm being normal diameter, <4 mm diameter is indicative of subglottic stenosis). In adults, the narrowest portion is glottis.
- Mucosa is lax in pediatric age especially subglottis, therefore, minimal swelling of the airway produces significant narrowing of the subglottic airway. In fact, in the subglottis 1 mm of circumferential oedema leads to over 60% narrowing and 1 mm of glottic edema leads to 35% obstruction of airway.
- Tongue size is relatively larger in infants, this makes the obstruction more acute in presence of micrognathia, and also practical aspect wise makes airway securing more difficult.

■ TYPES OF STRIDOR

Types of stridor (**Fig. 1**) depends upon the location and severity of the obstruction:
- Airway obstruction at the level of nasopharynx or oropharynx produces "low-pitched" sound known as "stertor" or "snoring" (oropharyngeal mass lesion produces classical *gurgle* sound).

- *Inspiratory stridor:* This occurs due to airflow obstruction above or at the level of the vocal cord, is typically "high pitched" and is because of collapse of structures with negative inspiratory pressure.
- *Biphasic stridor:* It has both inspiratory and expiratory component and is localized to subglottic and extrathoracic trachea, with an "intermediate pitch". It means breathing requires tremendous effort to move air through critically narrowed airway lumen and often heralds respiratory collapse. Biphasic stridor is a "medical emergency" and often requires intubation or tracheotomy since both inspiration and expiration are very limited.
- *Expiratory stridor:* It is usually produced by airflow limitations in distal tracheobronchial tree (intrathoracic trachea and bronchi) and characterized by more prolonged, sonorous, lesser harsh than stridor sound with a musical quality (often known as wheeze).

■ EVALUATION

It is organized as per the Holinger's (1997) mnemonic SPECS-R **(Box 1)**.

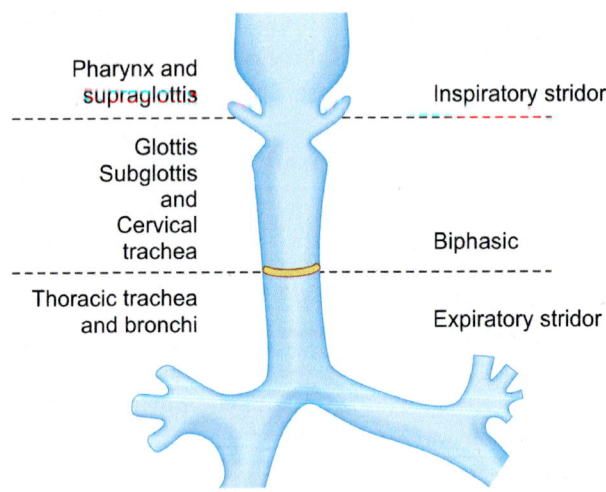

Fig. 1: Types of stridor.

BOX 1: Stridor: SPECS-R.

S: Severity
P: Progression
E: Eating or feeding problem (aspiration, failure to thrive)
C: Cyanotic episode
S: Sleep disorder
R: Radiographic anomalies

HISTORY TAKING

- If time permits, a detailed, careful history is taken including birth history, time of onset (congenital or acquired), severity, progression, associated fever (infective pathology).
- Any abnormality of cry should be recognized. Presence of hoarseness suggests a laryngeal pathology such as laryngeal papillomatosis, vocal cord palsy
- Relationship of stridor to feeding and possibility of aspiration (laryngeal paralysis), reflux may indicate gastrointestinal pathology
- *Fluctuation of stridor:* In vocal cord paralysis, stridor is more in awake kid as compared to when child is asleep. Similarly, in "laryngomalacia", child has more pronounced stridor when excited, crying or in supine position. The stridor decreases when child is resting and in prone position.
- *Mode of onset:* Sudden (foreign body, edema), gradual and progressive (laryngomalacia, subglottic hemorrhage, juvenile papilloma)
- Always have a high degree of suspicion of an "aspirated foreign body". Severe apnea and aphonia may not be the features of a laryngeal impacted foreign body only but also of an upper esophageal foreign body (cricopharyngeal foreign body).
- *Presence of cough:* It is usually seen in tracheomalacia, tracheoesophageal fistula and rarely, in infantile asthma.
- Look for any congenital craniofacial anomalies
- "Drooling of saliva" may be a presenting feature of acute epiglottitis.

PHYSICAL EXAMINATION

- While keeping the child comfortably in the parent's arm, assess the severity of respiratory distress and need for emergency airway management.
- Respiratory rate and level of consciousness are the most important indicators of severity. Tachypnea is often the first sign of respiratory distress. Flaring of the nasal alae and use of accessory neck or chest muscles (increased work of breathing with suprasternal, subcostal, and intercostal retraction) indicate significant airway obstruction.
- Increasing cyanosis and air hunger (especially in supraglottic infection or foreign body), causes the patient to "sit with neck hyperextended" (always let the child maintain that posture).
- Relatively quiet, shallow breathing indicates late respiratory failure/exhaustion
- *"Mental status examination":* Confusion or lethargy indicates impending respiratory arrest. Presence of "cyanosis" is a late and inconsistent sign of respiratory failure.
- On "palpation" look for fever, presence of any swelling, crepitations (in subcutaneous emphysema). Also look for any "birth marks" (seen in

subglottic hemangioma). Palpate laryngotracheal framework for any deviation from midline, any palpable fracture, presence of any transmitted pulsations or thrills.
- *Auscultation* is done over lung fields, along the neck, mouth, and nose to define the respiratory phase (inspiratory, expiratory, biphasic) and the intensity and pitch and quality of stridor. Type of stridor tells the level of obstruction.
- Hoarse cry/voice suggests laryngeal cause at vocal cords and normal cry indicates laryngomalacia or subglottic stenosis.
- Look for change in "respiratory cycle". Normally, it is composed of a shorter inspiratory and longer expiratory phase. Any change of inspiratory or expiratory phase and presence of stridor during that phase is noted.
- The child may be placed in various positions to look for any change in stridor. In laryngomalacia, macroglossia, micrognathia and innominate artery compression, stridor decreases in prone position.
- Check the nasal patency with a "cold spatula" or a wisp of cotton wool.
- If respiratory failure is not imminent, internal examination is done which includes nasal, oral cavity and oropharyngeal airway examination to rule out any possible inflammatory lesions, neoplasm, adenotonsillar hypertrophy, etc. Indirect laryngoscopy is possible in older cooperative children.

Flexible fiberoptic airway endoscopy in the awake child is the most preferred way to assess the upper airway. Topical anesthesia 2% xylocaine with decongestant (oxymetazoline 0.05% nasal drops) is applied and semisitting position is preferred (always keep resuscitation tray available). Both nares are evaluated followed by nasopharyngeal patency and velopharyngeal function. Also inspect the oropharynx, hypopharyngeal and laryngeal airway dynamics.

■ RADIOLOGY

If airway distress is noted secure airway before radiological investigations, however, in a more stable patient with no distress, radiological investigations can be extremely useful and diagnostic.
- X-ray soft tissue of neck lateral view (especially during inspiration because during expiration mobile pharyngeal tissue may buckle or bulge, appearing as retropharyngeal abscess or mass) helps to identify adenotonsillar hypertrophy, epiglottitis, deep neck space infection [while AP view of soft tissue neck (STN) shows tracheal deviation and narrowing of subglottis].
- Inspiratory and expiratory chest X-ray may help in evaluation of radiolucent airway foreign bodies. X-ray chest may also diagnose pneumonia, areas of hyperaeration or atelectasis.
- Fluoroscopy can be performed to ascertain respiratory effort and segmental ventilation. It is useful in identifying dynamic obstruction such as laryngomalacia, tracheomalacia, vocal fold palsy, etc.

- Barium swallow for evaluation of suspected vascular rings and tracheoesophageal fistulae.
- CT scan with contrast is helpful in evaluation of suspect choanal stenosis/atresia, mediastinal masses and aberrant vessels compressing the trachea.

■ MANAGEMENT

The priority in pediatric stridor, remains assessment of patients and evaluate for distress and if necessary, the re-establishment of an adequate airway and correction of the underlying pathology and avoiding the tracheostomy, if possible. The management includes:

1. Look for respiratory distress and respiratory failure signs.

   Signs of impending respiratory failure include:
   - Biphasic stridor
   - Retraction (suprasternal, subcostal and intercostal)
   - Neck hyperextension
   - Severe tachypnea
   - Oxygen desaturation (least reliable sign)
   - Gravely ill and listless/lethargic child

2. Assist ventilation by positioning the patient with the head extended and the lower jaw thrust forward
3. Secretions are cleared with suction
4. Place the ventilation mark with a self-inflating bag over the nose and mouth and apply positive pressure ventilation with 100% oxygen to stabilize the patient before attempting definitive airway management.
5. If positioning and positive airway pressure are not adequate, endotracheal intubation is contemplated. Endotracheal intubation is nowadays preferred over tracheostomy because of inherent problems and complications of pediatric tracheostomy (such as esophageal perforation, uncontrolled bleeding, inadequate gas exchange). Airway maintenance should be done, preferably in operation theater, with a team of anesthetist, pediatrician and ENT surgeon with the availability of resuscitation equipment, tracheostomy set, endoscopes and suction machines. The intubation can be performed by any member of team including otolaryngologist, anesthetist, or any person who is adequately trained to do so. Using a straight blade laryngoscope, the airway is carefully visualized and after pushing the large infant tongue aside, the laryngoscope is secured in vallecula to expose the inlet of larynx which is then intubated under visualization. This needs practice and this is good to establish teams that are dedicated and work in such scenarios and this improves outcomes. The importance of teamwork cannot be overemphasized, sometimes otolaryngologists are better at intubating

some distressed patients especially with congenital malformations owing to their prior knowledge of deformed airway. A ventilating bronchoscope with mounted endotelescope may also be used as a backup in a rare case, when intubation is not possible to pass the bronchoscope under vision into larynx then hold the bronchoscope in airway with jet ventilation, while arrangements are made for other modes of securing airway. Intubation should be performed gently to avoid damage to already inflamed subglottic mucosa. If an oral tube is used initially, it should be replaced with a nasal tube, which is more secure in cases of prolonged intubation.

6. In children >2 years, the approximate size of endotracheal tube (mm) (internal diameter) can be estimated by dividing the age (in years) by 4 and then adding 4 mm (uncuffed) or 3.5 mm (cuffed). It is recommended that a tube one size smaller than the one required for the normal child is selected for the inflamed larynx. In emergency, a tube is chosen which is approximately the width of 5th (pinkie) fingernail **(Table 1)**.

   Extubation is possible within 48–72 hours with acute epiglottitis but in laryngotracheobronchitis, tube may be kept in for 1 week also.

7. Tracheobronchial secretions should be sucked out. If secretions are very tenacious, or there is a suspected foreign body, bronchoscopy should be performed.

8. Tracheostomy may be indicated in presence of unexpected pathologies (subglottic stenosis, impacted foreign bodies, advanced acute epiglottitis, etc.) or failed intubation. Tracheostomy set with pediatric range of tracheostomy tubes should be readily available.

TABLE 1: A guide to the size selection of pediatric tracheostomy tube, endotracheal tubes, and bronchoscopes.

Age	Tracheal transverse diameter (mm)	Bronchoscope size (Storz)	Endotracheal tube (Portex) (inner diameter mm)	Tracheostomy tube (Portex) (ID mm)	Chevalier Jackson tracheostomy tube
Preterm to neonate	5	2.5	2.5–3.0	3.0	14
Neonate to 6 months	5–6	3.0	3.5	3.5	16
6–18 months	6–7	3.5	4.0	4.0	18
18 months to 3 years	7–8	4.0	4.5	4.5	20
3–6 years	8–9	4.5	5.0	5.0	22
6–9 years	9–10	5.0	6.0	5.0	24
9–12 years	10–13	6.0	7.0	6.0	26
12–14 years	≥13	6.0	8.0	7.0	28

9. Cricothyroidotomy is not recommended in infants and young children because of narrow cricothyroid membrane and other complications such as stenosis (some authors recommend "needle cricothyroidotomy" with large-bore intravenous catheter).
10. Once the airway has been secured, the patient can be further assessed and managed accordingly, which includes airway endoscopy laryngotracheobronchoscopy (LTB) and surgical intervention such as laser.

Concurrent basic medical support measures include:
- Antipyretics for fever control (cold sponging is not recommended in obstructed airway patients)
- Maintaining temperature, pulse, and respiration (TPR) chart
- Intravenous fluid, fluid-electrolyte balance maintenance
- Humidifier to loosen the secretions and improve patient comfort
- Oxygen therapy to manage hypoxemia (monitor with pulse oximeter)
- Intravenous antibiotics
- Corticosteroids, both by intravenous route or by nebulizer
- If available, apnea and bradycardia monitors, pulmonary function test and arterial blood gas evaluation can be helpful.

AIRWAY BRONCHOSCOPY (LARYNGOTRACHEOBRONCHOSCOPY)

Anesthesia: Induction as dictated by overall situation of the patient. Intravenous induction (suxamethonium) is preferred in older children, otherwise in infants, precarious airway or poor venous access patients, gas induction is indicated. Premedication with atropine helps to reduce secretions and prior xylocaine spray helps to avoid laryngeal spasm. The child can be intubated and ventilated to a level of anesthesia to allow the passage of endoscope without gagging while maintaining spontaneous respiration and the laryngoscope can be manipulated with the tube-in. Otherwise, after induction, patient may not be intubated and endoscope directly introduced and airway is controlled via ventilating endoscope. Other options available are—jet ventilation, laryngeal mask or via tracheostomy tube anesthesia. Halothane and oxygen maintain a level of anesthesia that allows thorough examination.

Laryngoscopy: With any anesthesia technique, laryngoscopy with microscope [(microlaryngeal surgery (MLS)] is used to examine the larynx and a ventilating bronchoscope with telescopes to examine tracheobronchial tree. Laryngeal examination begins with the endotracheal tube in-situ, by gently inserting the laryngoscope from right corner of mouth and pushing the tongue to the left, while taking care to protect the teeth and lips. Tip of laryngoscope is pushed forward against the base of tongue to open the pharyngeal lumen and visualize the epiglottis. Supraglottis, glottis and laryngopharynx are examined. Laryngeal examination with the endotracheal tube removed provides a superior view, using a probe to move the arytenoids independently (cricoarytenoid joint movements). Also, the posterior laryngeal cleft can be probed and the cords can be gently moved to assess subglottis.

Bronchoscopy: An appropriate size of bronchoscope as per the age of child is used. In a suspected narrow airway, a bronchoscope of size smaller than the size recommended for the age should be used. In significant stenosis, an ultrafine telescope passed through laryngoscope helps in evaluation. Bronchoscope is inserted using anesthetist's laryngoscope (Mackintosh laryngoscope). After careful insertion of this laryngoscope, by keeping the laryngoscope in vallecula to lift the larynx forward, bevel of the bronchoscope is passed through the rima glottidis of the vocal cords. Both the main bronchi, the carina, the trachea, and the subglottis are systematically examined. Tracheomalacia should also be looked for. A practical point to emphasize in bronchoscopy is that—it is important that the surgeon performing the procedure is aware of oxygen desaturation as the pulse oximeter is about 20–30 seconds behind the actual physiological desaturation in the body and hence keeping an eye in the saturation levels on monitor or following anesthetist advice without delay is very helpful.

At the end, "dynamic assessment of the larynx" on recovery from anesthesia is made by withdrawing the bronchoscope to just posterior to the tip of the epiglottis. This helps in diagnosing vocal cord palsy and laryngomalacia.

Therapeutic microlaryngoscopy and bronchoscopy: It includes:
- Laser laryngeal surgery (CO_2 or KTP laser) for various intralaryngeal lesions such as laryngeal papillomatosis, laryngeal cysts, subglottic hemangioma, tracheal or subglottic stenosis, anterior laryngeal web, etc.
- MLS procedure for various lesions where laser is not available
- Therapeutic bronchoscopy includes foreign body removal, tenacious secretion removal and KTP laser via bronchoscope.

■ COMMON CAUSES OF PEDIATRIC STRIDOR (TABLE 2)

The differential diagnosis of common causes of stridor is described in **Table 3**.

Acute Epiglottitis (Supraglottitis)

Acute epiglottitis (supraglottitis) is relatively uncommon, but potentially lethal, caused by *Haemophilus influenzae* type B. *Staphylococcus aureus* represents large proportion of pediatric patients in vaccinated children. The child is quiet, looks pale and terrified because of systemic infection and bacteremia causing shock giving rise to pallor. The child assumes an

TABLE 2: Important causes of stridor.

Congenital	- Web, cyst - Subglottic stenosis - Laryngomalacia, tracheomalacia - Vocal cord paralysis - Vascular anomaly - Micrognathia, macroglossia - Subglottic hemangioma - Cleft larynx, tracheoesophageal (TE) fistulas

Acquired	- *Apyrexial*
	  – Foreign body
	  – Injury
	  – Scald
	  – Papillomas
	  – Laryngismus stridulus
	- *Pyrexial*
	  – Acute epiglottitis, tracheitis
	  – Acute laryngotracheobronchitis (LTB)
	  – Diphtheria, retropharyngeal abscess
	- *Allergy*
	  – Angioedema
	- Neoplasm
	- Vocal cord paralysis
	- Laryngeal/tracheal stenosis

upright sitting posture with the chin up and mouth open, bracing him or herself on the hands (the "tripod" position), with drooling of saliva because of odynophagia and looks very "toxic". There is severe throat pain, high grade fever, muffled voice, irritability, and respiratory distress that are rapidly progressive. Inspiratory stridor is a late finding and indicates progressive airway obstruction. (The mnemonic to remember the clinical presentation is AIR RAID—**Box 2**.)

Clinical Features of Acute Epiglottitis

- 3–5 years age
- Supraglottic area involvement
- Rapid onset
- High grade fever
- Toxic look
- Cough is usually absent
- Drooling of saliva
- Stridor is usually a late finding, and represents that airway may be almost completely blocked.

TABLE 3: Differential diagnosis of common causes of stridor.

Diagnosis	Epiglottitis	Laryngotracheal bronchitis	Bacterial tracheitis	Retropharyngeal abscess	Airway foreign body
Cause	Hemophilus influenza-B	Viral: Parainfluenza type 1	S. aureus	S. aureus	—
Age	3–5 years	<3 years	6 months to 8 years	1–5 years	Any age
Onset	Rapid (<6 hours)	Slow (approx. 48 hours)	Rapid	Slow	Rapid
Fever	High	Variable—none	Usually high	Usually high	Afebrile
Voice	Muffled voice (cough usually absent)	Hoarse/Barky cough	Hoarse/Barky cough	Hoarse	Hoarseness ± Paroxysm of cough
Drooling	Marked with severe dysphagia	No drooling, no dysphagia	Drooling and dysphagia	Drooling and dysphagia	Occasional drooling and dysphagia
Stridor	Inspiratory	Biphasic	Expiratory	Inspiratory	Inspiratory
Posture	Quiet-terrified, in sitting, leaning forward	Lying on back, struggling	No characteristic posture	Sitting, stiff neck	Variable
Toxic appearance	Toxic (pale or grey)	No toxicity, pink (cyanosis in late stages)	Yes	Variable (flushed)	No
Radiology	Thumb sign	Steeple sign	Steeple sign ±	Retropharyngeal space widened markedly	Opaque foreign body visible
Management	Humidification, IV antibiotics, artificial airway	Humidification, steroids, antibiotics	IV antibiotics, Bronchoscopy suction, ICU	Antibiotics, airway I and D	Airway endoscopy and removal

BOX 2: AIR RAID.

- **A** Airway closed
- **I** Increased pulse
- **R** Restlessness
- **R** Retractions
- **A** Anxiety increased
- **I** Inspiratory stridor
- **D** Drooling

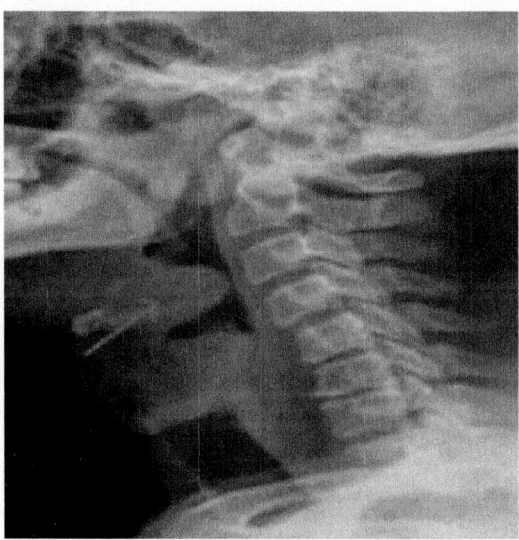

Fig. 2: Thumb sign on X-ray soft tissue neck (STN) in case of acute epiglottitis.

The role of radiology (X-ray: STN lateral view) is controversial because of risk of causing delay and adds to respiratory distress because of handling and positioning of an already terrified child. "Thumb sign" as mentioned in literature because of swollen acutely inflamed epiglottis is seen **(Fig. 2)**. Also, the examination of oral cavity, throat by tongue depressor is contraindicated because of fear of increasing and spreading of swelling in the preepiglottic space or inducing vasovagal reflex.

Management
- High index of clinical suspicion
- Oxygen inhalation
- Keep OT ready. In OT, larynx is visualized and intubation is done if required
- Blood culture and swab from epiglottis for culture
- Intravenous line for fluid replacement and antibiotics
- Antibiotics against causative microorganisms. Ampicillin/Sulbactam (200 mg/kg body weight/day ampicillin component), Ceftriaxone (100 mg/kg body weight/day), Cefotaxime (100 mg/kg body weight/day)
- Shift to pediatric ICU
- Immobilize the child with strong restraints or paralyze the child so that airway is not compromised
- Intubation may be required for 2–4 days till edema settles.

Bacterial Tracheitis

It is also known as bacterial laryngotracheobronchitis, membranous laryngotracheobronchitis or pseudomembranous croup. It is rare, but potentially life-threatening disease, caused by *Staphylococcus aureus, Streptococcus pyogenes, Haemophilus influenzae*, etc., with the involvement of subglottis and trachea with marked edema, mucosal ulceration and pseudomembrane formation. Clinical features are—acute illness, respiratory distress, biphasic stridor, barky cough and hoarseness, high grade fever, toxic appearance and may mimic acute epiglottitis (odynophagia and drooling of saliva are absent). X-ray STN may show a "steeple sign" similar to viral croup. Management includes intubation and ventilatory support. Airway endoscopy is both diagnostic and therapeutic by suction of copious secretion and pseudomembrane. Intravenous antibiotics (cefotaxime or ceftriaxone), humidified oxygen, intravenous fluids and if needed, repeated bronchoscopy (to handle unusually tenacious secretions) are important tools of management protocol.

Croup (Laryngotracheobronchitis, Viral Croup)

This is most common form of infectious airway tract obstruction in children (approximately 90% of all cases, recurrent in 5% of children). Parainfluenza virus 1 and 2, Influenza, RSV, *Mycoplasma pneumoniae* are common causative agents, involving children of 3 months to 3 years, mainly in late autumn and winters. Clinically, a "nontoxic" child presents with history of prodromal upper airway infection with low grade fever followed by acute onset of inspiratory stridor. Hoarseness and barky cough are the cardinal findings. Changing of symptomatology to biphasic stridor, retractions, tachypnea, anxiety or restlessness, oxygen desaturation (on pulse oximetry), altered sensorium indicates severe respiratory distress.

X-ray (AP view and lateral view) of STN reveals "steeple" sign (wine bottle sign), i.e., narrowing in the subglottis and ballooning of the hypopharynx **(Fig. 3)**.

Management

- Humidified air (portable humidifier, steamer or mist tents)
- *Corticosteroids (controversial):* Dexamethasone 0.6–1.0 mg/kg single intramuscular or intravenous dose followed by prednisolone 2.0 mg/kg/day or dexamethasone 1.0 mg/kg/day in divided doses. Nebulized steroid (budesonide) can also be used.
- Intravenous fluid, supplementary humidified oxygen
- Nebulized racemic epinephrine

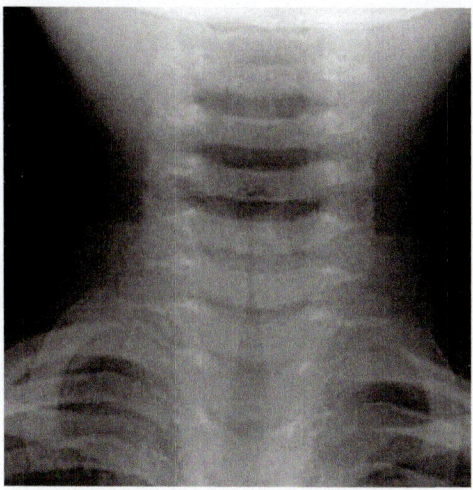

Fig. 3: Steeple sign seen on X-ray in case of laryngotracheobronchitis.

- Antibiotics to avoid secondary bacterial infection
- Endotracheal intubation (orotracheal or nasotracheal) with a tube 0.5 mm smaller than the one estimated for the child, is indicated in presence of severe respiratory distress signs as already explained in the text.
- Antivirals have no role because maximum cases are caused by parainfluenza virus.

Laryngomalacia

It is the most common congenital abnormality of larynx. It is caused by flaccidity or incoordination of the supralaryngeal structures, including the cartilages and the soft tissue. In 60% of cases, stridor starts by first week of life and persists thereafter, is worse with crying and feeding, during excitement or activity, or in supine position with head and neck flexed. Stridor may improve when child is kept in "prone" position or when head and neck is extended. Cyanosis, dysphagia, and aspiration are not seen and the presence of any of these features indicate suspicion of other cause of congenital stridor. On direct laryngoscopy, epiglottis is abnormal: tall, narrow or folded on itself (omega/W shaped), lax, flaccid; with aryepiglottic folds which tend to get sucked in during each inspiration and get blown up and out on expiration and prominent arytenoids. It is often a self-limiting condition that gets better with age and only 10–12% patients presenting to ENT OPD may need surgical intervention. Stridor is the most common presentation in these patients in whom most of the complaints are usually managed with adequate control of laryngopharyngeal reflux and very rarely these patients present with acute respiratory distress.

Management

Usually, most complaints are managed with adequate control of laryngopharyngeal reflux. Usually H2 blocker, famotidine 0.5 mg/kg BID orally or a proton pump inhibitor such as lansoprazole 7.5 mg BID orally will help control reflux. Thus, very rarely these patients present with acute respiratory distress. Even the emergency presentations of distress settle with adequate conservative measures and laryngopharyngeal reflux control but surgery may be needed only in cases that fail to respond to conservative measures: Surgical intervention is indicated in cases with failure to thrive as indicated by lack of weight gain, obstructive sleep apnea, severe chest deformity (Pectus excavatum), cyanotic attacks, desaturation noted during observation, pulmonary hypertension and cor pulmonale. Surgical intervention includes supraglottoplasty (aryepiglottoplasty) that can be performed either with CO_2 laser or cold steel technique using laryngeal microscissors or microdebrider. It involves excision of prolapsing supraglottic tissue over lying aryepiglottic folds, cuneiform cartilage, and lateral aspect of epiglottis. Care should be taken to protect interarytenoid mucosa to avoid stenosis.

"Epiglottopexy" is indicated in severe omega shaped epiglottis wherein mucosa from lingual surface of epiglottis and corresponding base of tongue is removed with CO_2 laser and then epiglottis sutured to the base of tongue.

Tracheostomy is usually not needed unless complicating comorbidities are present, as supraglottoplasty and maintenance of airway to tide over acute situations is usually sufficient.

Recurrent Croup

A set of infants and toddlers, between 6 months and 3 years or after, present with recurrent bouts of croup especially during spring and fall seasons. They have history of more than two episodes of croup a year that necessitate the emergency visits, although these are not severe enough to cause a respiratory airway emergency and can be managed by conservative measures.

These patients tend to be seen by pediatricians or emergency staff. However, these patients need an ENT opinion and a thorough investigation with MRI neck delineating soft tissue anatomy of upper airway and also diagnostic laryngobronchoscopy, as apart from simple conditions such as gastroesophageal reflux and asthma, potential airway pathologies like subglottic stenosis, subglottic hemangioma, laryngotracheal cleft, tracheoesophageal fistula may also be identified by an alert ENT physician.

Choanal Atresia

Infant being an obligate nasal breather, will present with neonatal airway obstruction in presence of bilateral choanal atresia. The airway obstruction is relieved by crying (as oral airway is normal) and the neonate can have cyanosis and respiratory collapse. Feeding difficulty may lead to failure to thrive. A unilateral choanal atresia may remain undiagnosed, presenting with unilateral nasal discharge.

Physical examination reveals no misting of a mirror placed at the nostrils, inability to pass a nasal catheter or flexible scope and suctioning of thick mucoid secretions from the nasal passages.

X-ray lateral soft tissue with contrast in nose will reveal atresia while axial CT scan helps in defining the thickness and character (bony/cartilaginous) of the atretic plate.

Management includes maintenance of airway (oral airway, tracheostomy) and definitive surgical repair (transpalatal, transnasal or transseptal route) of the atresia. Also look for associated anomalies if present (*CHARGE* association: Coloboma, heart anomalies, choanal atresia, growth retardation, genital hypoplasia, and ear anomalies).

Respiratory Papillomatosis or Laryngeal Papillomatosis

This is a condition caused by Human Papilloma viruses usually types 6 and 11. This infection may result in multiple papillomata in a child and the most common site of papilloma is glottis but the supraglottis, subglottis and trachea may also be affected. The method of transmission is due to exposure to the virus in the birth canal. It can present in neonates or infants and toddlers with the stridor and worsening respiratory distress leading to airway emergency. Diagnosis is usually by endoscopic visualization of papilloma and may necessitate an emergency procedure to clear the papillomata. Cold-steel techniques or laser may be utilized and adjuvant therapies such as quadrivalent human papilloma virus vaccine, intralesional cidofovir, interferons and cetuximab have been used in infants and toddlers with good outcomes. It may regress spontaneously or may worsen and run a protracted course, thus necessitating periodic surgeries whether planned or emergency procedures.

Retropharyngeal Abscess

Please refer chapter on "Neck Space Infection".

Airway Foreign Body

Please refer chapter on "Foreign Bodies".

The clinical features and management of the common causes of stridor in children are summarized in **Flowchart 1**.

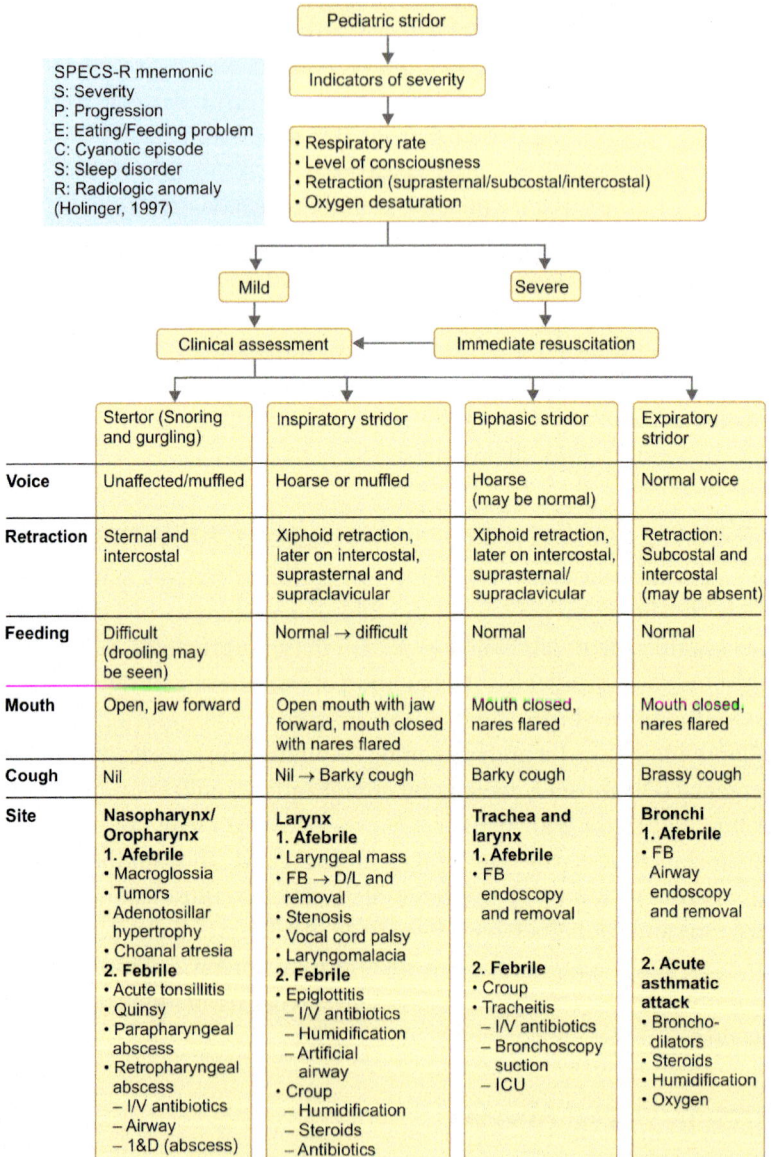

Flowchart 1: Clinical features and management of the common causes of pediatric stridor.

FURTHER READING

1. Holinger LD. Etiology of in neonate, infant and child. Ann Otol Rhinol Laryngol. 1980;89(5 Pt 1):397-400.
2. Ida JB, Thompson DM. Pediatric stridor. Otolaryngol Clin North Am. 2014;47(5):795-819.
3. Roybal JL, Liechty KW, Hedrick HL, Bebbington MW, Johnson MP, Coleman BG, et al. Predicting the severity of congenital high airway obstruction syndrome. J Pediatr Surg. 2010;45(8):1633-9.

CHAPTER 11

Sudden Sensorineural Hearing Loss

Sachin Gupta, Venkata Surya Phani Bhushan Durvasula, Arvind Kairo

■ INTRODUCTION

Idiopathic sudden sensorineural hearing loss (SSHL) is a medical otological emergency condition with a reported incidence of 5-20 per 100,000 population per year. This condition has been defined as 30 dB or more of sensorineural hearing loss (SNHL) over at least three contiguous audiometric frequencies occurring within 3 days or less. If hearing loss progression is slow, i.e., it takes >3 days, then the term is known as rapidly progressive instead of idiopathic SSHL.

Most widely accepted etiologic theories are the vaso-occlusive and viral (cytomegalovirus, mumps, rubella, etc.). Other reported causes include brain stem abnormalities, possible vitamin deficiency, autoimmune inner ear injury, and inner ear membrane rupture **(Table 1)**. The diagnosis of

TABLE 1: Important causes of sudden sensorineural hearing loss (SSHL).

Infectious	Meningitis (viral/bacterial/fungal), labyrinthitis (viral/bacterial), and acquired immunodeficiency syndrome (AIDS)
Traumatic	Perilymph fistula, otologic surgery, temporal bone fracture, and inner ear concussion
Vascular	Anomalous carotid artery and cardiopulmonary bypass
Hematological	Anemia, embolism, coagulation disorder, sickle cell disease, and leukemia
Neurologic	Multiple sclerosis, Friedreich's ataxia, and Vogt–Koyanagi–Harada syndrome
Metabolic	Thyrotoxic hypokalemia, diabetes mellitus, and renal failure/dialysis
Neoplastic	Vestibular schwannoma, myeloma, and metastasis to petrous apex
Autoimmune disease/vasculitis	Wegener's granulomatosis, temporal arteritis, Cogan's syndrome, and primary immune inner ear disease
Miscellaneous	Sarcoidosis, scleroderma, dental surgery, ulcerative colitis, and snake bite
Ototoxicity	
Endolymphatic hydrops	
Central deafness	
Idiopathic	

idiopathic SSHL is by exclusion akin to Bell's palsy. Some of these cases may however have implicated causes in 10-15% of patients and do not constitute idiopathic SNHL.

Most common symptom reported is the *"blocked ear"* for which patient tends to consult general physician or self-medicate with decongestants, antihistaminics or antibiotics before eventually asking for ear, nose, and throat (ENT) opinion. This accounts for the delayed diagnosis.

Patient evaluation includes asking for known and potentially treatable causes of SSHL such as ototoxicity and diabetes. Routine otoscopy should be performed in every patient followed by tuning fork tests. Lateralization of Weber test even in presence of obvious occlusive wax plug should make one suspect of SSHL. Other commonly reported symptoms are variable degree of hearing loss, tinnitus (ipsilateral or central), and/or vertigo. Fistula test should be performed to look for perilymph fistula (gentle positive pressure in the ear canal may cause subjective dizziness or objective nystagmus). Audiometry at the earliest is mandatory for documentation and severity of hearing loss. Hearing loss may be mild (<40 dB), moderate (40-90 dB), or profound (>90 dB) which has prognostic significance. Spontaneous recovery is commonly seen in mild hearing loss cases while those presenting with profound hearing loss seldom recover. Caloric test or electronystagmography (ENG) is not very useful in routine cases except for aminoglycoside ototoxicity. Role of routine magnetic resonance imaging (MRI) with gadolinium enhancement is controversial, although it is an ideal way to detect a retrocochlear lesion like vestibular schwannoma in these cases.

■ MANAGEMENT

In case of idiopathic SSHL (majority of cases), the treatment is controversial. Many treatment protocols have been proposed, but no single treatment is found to be more effective than other **(Table 2)**. The American Academy of Otolaryngology—Head and Neck Surgery in its guidelines for treatment of idiopathic SSHL has suggested that oral steroids, intratympanic steroids and hyperbaric oxygen therapy as recommended options. Approximately two-thirds of the patients recover spontaneously, especially with mild hearing loss (<40 dB), upward sloping audiogram, and no history of vertigo. Profound hearing loss (>90 dB), especially with downward sloping audiogram and vertigo, rarely recover spontaneously. Moderate hearing loss patients (40-90 dB) have an adequate time window of opportunity (2-4 weeks) for treatment, especially with systemic steroids.

■ PROGNOSTIC INDICATORS OF IDIOPATHIC SENSORINEURAL HEARING LOSS

- *Severity of loss:* More severe the loss, poorer are the chances of recovery
- *Age:* Children and adults >50 years have poor prognosis

TABLE 2: Treatment options for sudden sensorineural hearing loss (SSHL).

Vasodilators	Pentoxifylline/oxpentifylline, papaverine, buphenine, thymoxamine, prostacyclin, nicotinic acid, and carbogen inhalation
Immunologic agents	Corticosteroids and prostaglandins
Diuretics	Lasix and hydrochlorothiazide-triamterene
Calcium antagonists	Nifedipine
Defibrinogenation therapy	Batroxobin
Volume expanders/hemodilution agents	Low-molecular-weight dextran and hydroxyethyl starch
Antiviral	Acyclovir and valacyclovir
Miscellaneous	Bedrest, acupuncture, iron and multivitamins, and procaine
Hyperbaric oxygenation	
Anticoagulants	

- *Presence of vertigo:* Poor prognostic indicator
- *Presence of tinnitus:* Good prognostic indicator
- *Audiogram shape:* Upsloping and mid frequency loss have better recovery than flat and down sloping audiogram
- *Erythrocyte sedimentation rate (ESR):* Patients with normal ESR have better prognosis.

■ TREATMENT

It is generally accepted that early onset of treatment within first 7 days increases the chances of recovery in cases with idiopathic SSHL. *"Systemic steroids"* have been the hallmark of therapy for SSHL. The mechanism of action is still unknown but probably steroids help in inflammatory and immune mediated conditions. 1 mg/kg body weight of prednisone per day for at least 10 days, tapered later on, is most widely prescribed regimen. If patient has partial recovery by the end of 10 days, full dose is extended for another 10 days. Maximum benefit is seen in cases of moderate hearing loss. Recently, many centers have reported use of "transtympanic dexamethasone" injection in profound SSHL. 0.3 cc dexamethasone (24 mg/mL) is injected into middle ear space with 27 G needle over the area of round window. Steroid is allowed to perfuse the middle ear for 30 minutes by keeping the injected ear in upward position. The procedure is repeated twice weekly for 2 weeks (i.e., four sessions). The main indication is those cases where "oral steroids" are contraindicated. Combination of systemic steroids and intratympanic steroids for treatment has also been advocated and may provide an additional benefit. But all the sittings should be ideally completed in first 4 weeks to be deemed effective.

Low salt diet and diuretic, usually prescribed for Meniere's disease, is also helpful and inexpensive. Low salt diet (2 g sodium/day) along with avoidance of salty food is advised. Potassium sparing diuretic (hydrochlorothiazide with triamterene) is usually prescribed.

Vasodilators and volume expanders: In past (early 70s and 80s), vasodilators (intravenous papaverine and pentoxifylline) and volume expanders (low-molecular-weight dextran—Rheomacrodex—molecular weight of 40,000 as 10% solution, either in 5% dextrose or saline) were very popular when SSHL was considered due to hyperviscosity or hypercoagulability state. Volume expanders are contraindicated in patients with cardiac failure and bleeding disorders.

Stellate ganglion block: This induces increase in blood flow, but usefulness is limited to SSHL presenting within 2 weeks of onset. Limitation is the requirement of high skill for the procedure.

Carbogen inhalation (95% oxygen and 5% carbon dioxide mixture) has been found to be useful in improving the rate of spontaneous recovery by increasing perilymphatic oxygen. The dose is carbogen inhalation for 10 minutes, six times daily for 3 days (other reported regimen of carbogen inhalation is for 30 minutes, 8 times per day at intervals of 1 hour). The limitations include—hospitalization, proper monitoring, and close coordination with anesthetic team.

Systemic *"antivirals"* (acyclovir, valacyclovir, ganciclovir, or famciclovir) have been advocated by many authors, considering SSHL secondary to viral cochleitis, but their role is still controversial.

In case of nonimprovement of hearing loss, appropriate hearing aid may be advised and patient should be kept under follow-up for possible delayed symptoms and contralateral ear disease.

The importance of generating awareness among general practitioner for SSHL cannot be ignored and message should be conveyed in order to facilitate rapid diagnosis and subsequent management.

■ OUTCOMES

It is generally accepted that one-third principle works here with one-third improving while one-third remain same and another one-third get worse, further no one treatment is proven to be better than the other, except possibly management with steroids.

■ ASYMMETRIC SENSORINEURAL HEARING LOSS

It is often a finding in outpatients on audiograms and is important as it may signify an underlying vestibular schwannoma and is the most common symptom associated with it. However, the degree of asymmetry between patients varies greatly; hence, it becomes important to identify the subset of patients who need further investigations like gadolinium-enhanced MRI scan to rule out the presence a retrocochlear lesion.

It has not been possible to define asymmetrical SNHL adequately to make it 100% sensitive for identifying retrocochlear pathology. According to current available literature an interaural asymmetry of >20 dB hearing loss at two contiguous frequencies or >15 dB hearing loss at any two frequencies between 2,000 Hz and 8,000 Hz is considered significant asymmetry.

■ FURTHER READING

1. Conlin AE, Parnes LS. Treatment of sudden sensorineural hearing loss: I. A systematic review. Ach Otolaryngol Head Neck Surg. 2007;133:573-81.
2. Darino J, Jaochim HZ, Eliacher I, Podoshin L, Ben-David Y, Fradis M. Tinnitus as a prognostic factor in sudden deafness. Am J Otolaryngol. 1984;5:394-6.
3. Hughes GB, Freedman MA, Habcrkamp TJ, Guay ME. Sudden sensorineural hearing loss. Otolaryngol Clin North Am. 1996;29:393-405.
4. Watkinson JC, Clarke RW. Scott-Brown's Otolaryngology Head and Neck Surgery, 8th edition. Florida, United States: CRC Press; 2018.

CHAPTER 12

Caustic Ingestion

Shallu Jamwal, Shyam Gupta, Parmod Kalsotra

■ INTRODUCTION

Caustic ingestion results in significant morbidity and mortality and continues to be a common and controversial problem faced by otolaryngologists. Presentation of caustic ingestion displays a bimodal distribution with a peak occurring in children (accidental) and the second one in adulthood (suicidal, intentional). Caustic agents constitute both alkaline agents and acids, the former being more common than latter.

Alkalis tend to cause more damage that continues to happen as long as there is contact with the mucosa of the aerodigestive tract and this causes liquefactive necrosis resulting in rapid and deep burns that can be transmural. The damage continues as long as the alkali is in contact with soft tissue. Acids on the other hand, tend to produce coagulative necrosis and get converted into the acid proteins in the process. The coagulum prevents further damage thus reducing chances of full thickness injuries.

■ ALKALINE BURNS

Common alkaline agents include lyes (sodium hydroxide, potassium hydroxide), miniature or disc batteries, hair relaxers, ammonia and clinitest tablets. Solids (crystalline form) are usually spit out by a child before large amounts are ingested. Therefore, liquid alkalis carry much greater risk of severe esophageal and gastric burns. Also, solids usually do not reach the stomach owing to gastroesophageal sphincter spasm while liquids can cause transmural necrosis of esophagus and stomach. Bleaches cause mild to moderate gastrointestinal irritation with symptoms such as nausea, vomiting and diarrhea. Mucosal ulceration usually does not occur with bleaches except with concentrated ammonia solutions. Esophageal injury and stricture formation after ingestion of household bleach is very rarely seen.

Symptoms and Signs

- Burning sensation in the mouth and chest (esophagus)
- Dysphagia and increased salivation leading to drooling of saliva and vomiting which may be blood stained.

- Stridor due to laryngeal swelling secondary to aspiration.
- Mouth or pharynx may have white patches or inflamed ulcerated mucosa. In the presence of two or more symptoms (vomiting, drooling or stridor) there is a 50% chance of an associated esophageal burn.
- Hoarseness, stridor, accessory respiratory muscle movement indicates injury to laryngeal mucosa secondary to aspiration.
- Fever, chest pain, abdominal pain, and shock is suggestive of esophageal or gastric perforation, mediastinitis and shock.
- Severe complications include hemolysis, renal failure, peritonitis, mediastinitis and ultimately death.
- Sinister symptoms and signs include tachycardia, shortness of breath, odynophagia, hoarseness, severe dysphagia, severe chest pain and abdominal pain.
- Clinically, 25–70% of oropharyngeal burns do not have associated esophageal burns. The reverse is also true and 15% of esophageal burns have a normal oral cavity and oropharyngeal findings.

There is no reliable relationship among the signs–symptoms, physical examination, and degree of injury except for dysphagia, retrosternal pain or abdominal pain which indicates severe injury.

Management (Flowchart 1)

Initial management of the caustic ingestion patient follows a standard emergency protocol as under:
- Securing an airway
- Cardiovascular support
- Intravenous line to be commenced and blood samples sent for complete blood count and electrolytes [including arterial blood gas (ABG) analysis, if indicated]
- Urine analysis is also done
- Keeping the patient on *"nil orally"*
- Determine the type and amount of caustic agent ingested and whether the patient has aspiration, emesis or respiratory distress by asking relevant questions from patient or attendants.
- Note vital signs and perform complete physical examination and look for any skin burns due to agent spilled onto the clothing.
- Any obvious skin or oral cavity burns should be washed with a copious amount of water.
- Flexible fiberoptic laryngoscopy is most helpful in determining the presence of upper airway injury.
- X-ray chest routinely and abdominal radiography, if indicated.
- Water or milk (a neutral buffer) can be administered (15 mL/kg BW) to dilute or neutralize the agents unless immediate surgery is planned.

Flowchart 1: Management algorithm for the different types of caustic ingestion.

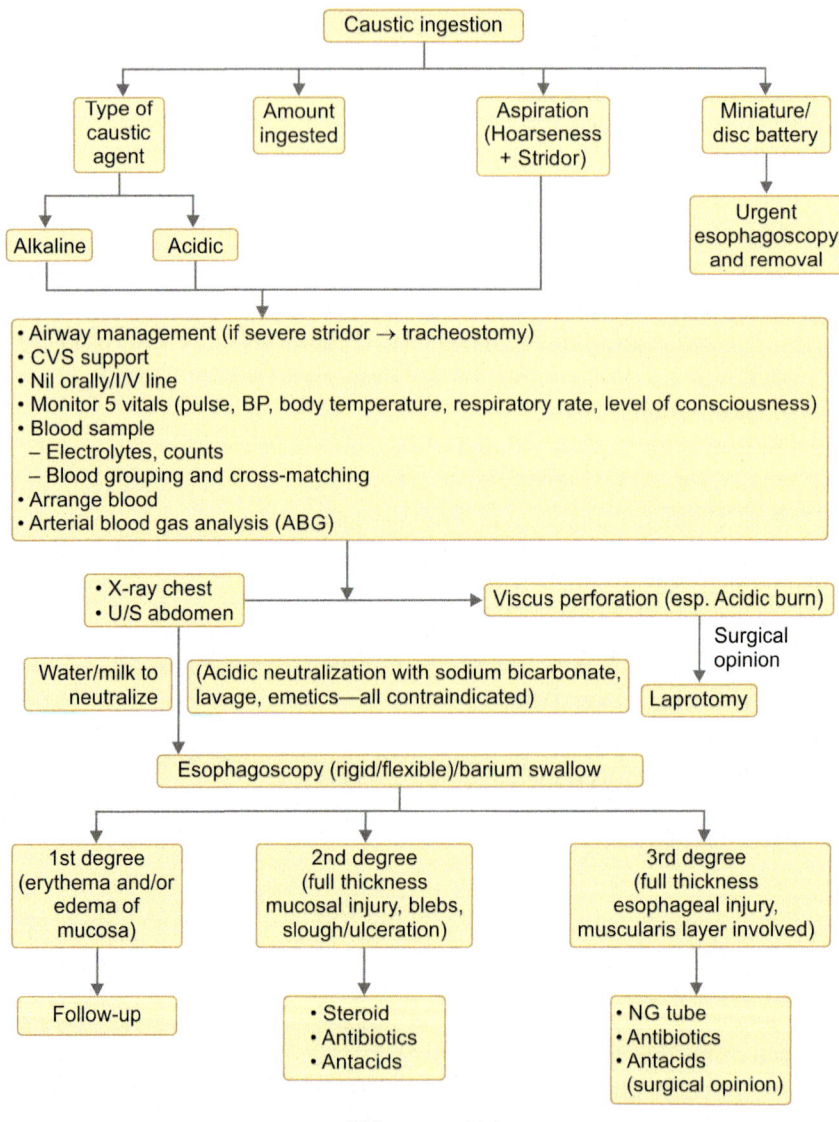

(NG: nasogastric)

- Induction of vomiting, gastric lavage, emetics (ipecac) are contraindicated because vomiting will cause repeated exposure of esophageal mucosa to the offending agent, and gastric lavage being a blind procedure, can cause iatrogenic esophageal perforation.
- Also contraindicated is the use of neutralizing agents (vinegar for lye and sodium bicarbonate for acids) because of risk of exothermic chemical reactions. Same is the risk with usage of acids (citrus juice) for alkaline ingestion, which can increase the internal trauma.

- Role of blind nasogastric tube insertion is controversial and usually not recommended.
- Hoarseness and stridor indicate possible damage to pharynx, larynx or trachea. Such patients may require tracheostomy.
- Acute chest or abdominal pain indicates a possible viscus perforation usually seen in an adult who has ingested large amount of a strong acid or base in a suicidal bid and may require emergency laparotomy with possible esophagogastrectomy.
- *Button batteries* (dead or working) are dangerous as electrical energy from these reacts with saliva to produce hydrolysis with caustic injury within 2 hours of ingestion. Sometimes leakage from these batteries can cause perforation within hours. Delayed diagnosis often results in grade 2-3 esophageal burns, perforation, tracheoesophageal fistula, bilateral vocal cord palsy and may prove fatal. Plain X-ray reveals *"double halo sign"* which distinguishes it from coin ingestion and demands a *very urgent endoscopy and removal*. However, if the battery passes into the stomach, it can be allowed to transit with the patient kept under a general surgeon's observation. Stools should be checked daily and inability to detect in stools within 4 days, would prompt a repeat X-ray. As long as the battery continues to progress through the gastrointestinal tract (GIT), no intervention is required but constant checkup from a general surgeon is mandatory.
- *Bleach ingestion* rarely causes significant esophageal injury and many of these patients can be sent home directly from the emergency room depending on the clinical status.
- Attempted suicide patients require urgent psychiatric consultation and preventive precautions.
- After taking care of the emergency, subsequent evaluation, and management of injury of upper aerodigestive tract especially esophagus is initiated. Definitive evaluation of esophagus should be performed, 12-48 hours after the injury. Before 12 hours, injury is usually not fully manifested and one may underestimate the damage. Delayed examination in presence of increased structural weakness of esophagus carries high risk of iatrogenic injury. Therefore, the ideal time recommended in literature is between 24 and 48 hours.
- Esophagoscopy is critical to assess the esophageal involvement and helps to identify the patients with 2nd degree esophageal burns who will benefit from oral steroids.

Role of Endoscopy

Ideally, every known or suspected case of ingested strong acid or base (except bleach) should undergo esophagoscopy under general anesthesia by an experienced endoscopist unless there are contraindications for esophagoscopy such as impending airway obstruction, evidence of esophageal perforation such as mediastinitis or shock.

Much is written in literature regarding "pros and cons" of rigid versus flexible endoscopy. Rigid esophagoscopy has always been preferred by ENT surgeons and carries no extra risk of perforation in experienced hands. Esophagoscopy is performed cautiously and should not be passed distal to a visualized full thickness burn. If it is encountered, a nasogastric tube or esophageal stent is passed. Flexible gastroduodenoscopy should always follow rigid esophagoscopy in case of any suspicion of gastric injury and carries the additional advantage of its ability to assess the gastric and duodenal mucosa.

If esophagoscopy is not possible, contrast barium-swallow may sometimes help delineate the extent of esophageal injury. Delayed passage of contrast or edematous esophageal mucosal folds and linear ulcerations suggest a mild injury, with severe injury revealing either a rigid, poorly distensible narrowed esophagus, a dilated atonic esophagus or an esophagus showing increased irritability and uncoordinated peristaltic activity. An esophagogram is sometimes helpful in evaluation of esophagus in the presence of a circumferential burn that may prevent passing of a rigid esophagoscope. Some authors recommend barium swallow as initial assessment if >48 hours have passed.

Thus, esophageal endoscopy is the cornerstone in assessment of caustic injuries and helps to stage the extent of injury and is usually performed between 12 and 48 hours and not advised between 5 and 15 days due to friability of tissue during healing. Flexible esophagoscopy may be preferred over rigid as it is less traumatic and ability to evaluate gastric and duodenal mucosa is better. Occasionally, in the presence of esophageal injury, tracheoscopy may be necessary to assess the damage of the posterior tracheal wall.

Further management depends upon degree of burns **(Table 1)**. If esophagoscopy reveals no burn or only minor "first degree burn" (erythema

TABLE 1: Degree of esophageal burns based on endoscopic appearance.

Degree	Endoscopic appearance
1st degree (superficial injury)	• Nonulcerative esophagitis • Mild erythema, oedema of mucosa
2nd degree (transmucosal)	• Whitish exudate/slough • Erythema • Underlying ulceration may extend into the muscularis
3rd degree (transmural)	• Dusky or blackened transmural tissue • Deep ulcerations extending into the periesophageal tissue • Lumen may be obliterated

and/or edema of the mucosa), patient is advised only topical antibiotic ointment and local oral hygiene for oral burns. When oral ulcer heals satisfactorily and allows eating, patient can be discharged and kept on follow-up in OPD. Patients with "second degree burns" (second degree: full thickness injury to the mucosa, including bleb formation) are given steroids (prednisone 1 mg per kg/day to maximum 60 mg/day in twice daily dosage for 2 weeks and then tapered over another 4 weeks) in order to decrease collagen deposition with subsequent fibrosis during healing. Use of lathyrogenic agents (which reduce collagen cross-binding) to decrease esophageal structures, i.e., beta-aminopropionitrile, acetylcysteine, penicillamine has been reported in the literature but their role is yet not established. Antibiotics (ampicillin, cephalosporins or clindamycin) for a period of 10–14 days along with liquid antacids and H2 blockers are given for 2–4 weeks. Intravenous fluids with correction of electrolyte-imbalance are advised, followed by oral clear liquid diet and subsequently soft diet when swallowing is possible. Repeat barium esophagogram is performed at 3 weeks of caustic ingestion. On detection of esophageal stricture, esophageal dilatation procedure is commenced.

For "circumferential 2nd degree and all 3rd degree burns" (3° burns: full thickness esophageal injury, with perforation into or through the muscular layer), a nasogastric tube (Ryle's tube) is left in place for 6 weeks. Antibiotics along with antacids and H2 blockers and prokinetic agents (cisapride) are used. Steroids are contraindicated in these severe injuries. Mechanical stenting of esophagus to avoid stricture formation has been reported but long-term outcome is still controversial.

CT Scan

A computed tomography (CT) scan likely offers a more detailed evaluation than early endoscopy about the transmural damage of esophageal and gastric walls, and the extent of necrosis. It is more valuable than endoscopy in assessing threatened and established stomach perforation, and a CT graded system has been proposed to predict esophageal stricture **(Box 1)**. With the advantage of not being invasive, CT has a promising role in the early evaluation of caustic injury damage.

BOX 1: CT scan grading system for caustic lesion.

- *Grade 1:* No definite swelling of esophageal wall
- *Grade 2:* Edematous wall thickening without periesophageal soft tissue involvement
- *Grade 3:* Edematous wall thickening with periesophageal soft tissue infiltration plus well demarcated tissue interface
- *Grade 4:* Edematous wall thickening with periesophageal soft tissue infiltration plus blurring of tissue interface or localized fluid collection around the esophagus or descending aorta

Some authors recommend early surgical resection of damaged esophagus/stomach with reconstruction (especially grade three). Severely burnt patients are kept in hospital for long time due to risk of massive hemorrhage as a result of esophagogastric necrosis.

If stricture becomes evident, serial dilators are commenced which may be carried out either in anterograde method (e.g., mercury filled Maloney Bougies) or by Tucker retrograde method via gastrostomy.

Role of Thoracic and/or Gastric Surgeon

Their opinion is sought in cases of:
- Severe esophageal necrosis with risk of esophageal perforation and major blood vessel rupture
- Progressive and/or complete esophageal stricture (long segmental) and atony, which are long-term complications.

The surgeon can opt for total esophagectomy with replacement with either gastric pull up, isoperistaltic ileum with cecum or transverse or left colon interposition or jejunal free flap.

Also, surgical intervention is required for correction of hiatus hernia due to shortening of esophagus secondary to stricture formation.

Important point to be kept in mind during follow-up is higher risk of developing squamous cell carcinoma of esophagus due to caustic ingestion induced esophageal injury and that the late onset dysphagia may be due to stricture, tumor or both.

ACID BURNS

Hydrochloric, sulfuric and nitric acids are most common agents ingested. Acids are less likely to cause severe esophageal burns but more commonly involve the gastroduodenal region which on healing produce gastric outlet obstruction. Clinically, patient presents with burning sensation in the mouth, chest and abdomen with dysphagia and hematemesis. Oral examination may reveal inflamed mucosa with whitish slough covered ulcerated areas. On palpation of abdomen, acute abdominal signs may be elicited.

Initial management includes checking vitals, intravenous fluids, and supportive care. Neutralization of acid with sodium bicarbonate, lavage and emetics are contraindicated. Prophylactic antibiotics and steroids are not indicated. Cutaneous burns are treated in the conventional way. Patient is closely monitored for signs of gastric perforation when laparotomy is required.

During follow-up, upper gastrointestinal contrast (barium) radiography is performed 3–6 weeks post ingestion of acid to look for gastric outlet obstruction where general surgeon's consultation and intervention is indicated.

Sequelae: Esophageal strictures are common after caustic injury that happen between 6–8 weeks and pose a significant cause of morbidity. Sequential dilatation and use of stents are used to manage these strictures that are known to be precancerous for formation of squamous cell carcinoma.

■ FURTHER READING

1. Ananthkrishnan N, Kalayalrasan R, Kate V. Injury of oesophagus and stomach. In: Mishra PK (Ed). Textbook of Surgical Gastroenterology, 1st edition. New Delhi: Jaypee Brothers Medical Publishers (P) Ltd.; 2016.
2. Chirica M, Kelly MD, Sibioni S, Aiolfi A, Riva CG, Asti E, et al. Oesophageal emergencies: WSES guidelines. World J Emerg Surg. 2019;14:26.
3. Zorgar SA, Kochher R, Nagi B, Mehta S, Mehta SK. Ingestion of strong corrosive alkalis spectrum of injury to upper GI tract and natural history. Am J Gastroenterol. 1992;87:337-41.

CHAPTER 13

Complicated Otitis Media

Parmod Kalsotra, Sachin Gupta, Kapil Sikka

■ INTRODUCTION

Spread of infection to outside the confines of middle ear cleft causes variety of clinical symptomatology and presents usually in emergency as complicated otitis media. In preantibiotic era, acute otitis media was mainly responsible for complications but nowadays chronic otitis media is the greater mode of presentation.

■ SPREAD OF INFECTION

Different Possible Routes of Spread of Infection

- *Direct extension via bone:* By either of three processes.
    - Demineralization of bone due to hyperemia secondary to acute infection
    - Resorption of bone by cholesteatoma
    - Due to osteitis
- *Thrombophlebitis:* Infected clot spread within small veins/within its Haversian vascular system.
- *Iatrogenic route:* Postsurgical such as stapedectomy and fenestration of lateral semicircular canal.
- Natural anatomical pathway, e.g., round window, oval window, internal auditory meatus, cochlea, vestibular aqueduct, and persistent suture lines.
- *Nonanatomical bony defects:* Post-traumatic, erosion due to neoplasm.
- Along periarteriolar spaces of Virchow–Robin into brain tissue.

Overall, acute infection spreads mainly by thrombophlebitis or preformed anatomical pathways while chronic otitis media spreads by direct erosion of bony border.

Predisposing Factors

- *Patient's/host factors:* Age, immune status, and chronic debilitating conditions.
- *Bacterial infections:* Presence of antibiotic resistance, virulent species such as *Streptococcus pneumoniae* type III and *Haemophilus influenzae* type B
- Presence of anaerobes.

COMPLICATIONS (FIG. 1)

- *Intratemporal complications:*
  - Facial palsy
  - Labyrinthitis
  - Petrositis
  - Mastoiditis
- *Intracranial (extratemporal) complications:*
  - Extratemporal abscess
  - Subdural abscess/empyema
  - Lateral (sigmoid) sinus thrombophlebitis
  - Meningitis
  - Brain abscess
  - Otitic hydrocephalus
  - Subclavian vein thrombosis
  - Internal carotid artery aneurysm.

Intratemporal Complications

Petrositis

Generally, 80% of mastoid bones are pneumatized and approximately 30% have petrous apex pneumatization.

Two groups of cells are described connecting middle ear with petrous apex.
1. Posterosuperior chain extending from attic and antrum, around the semicircular canal and into the apex.

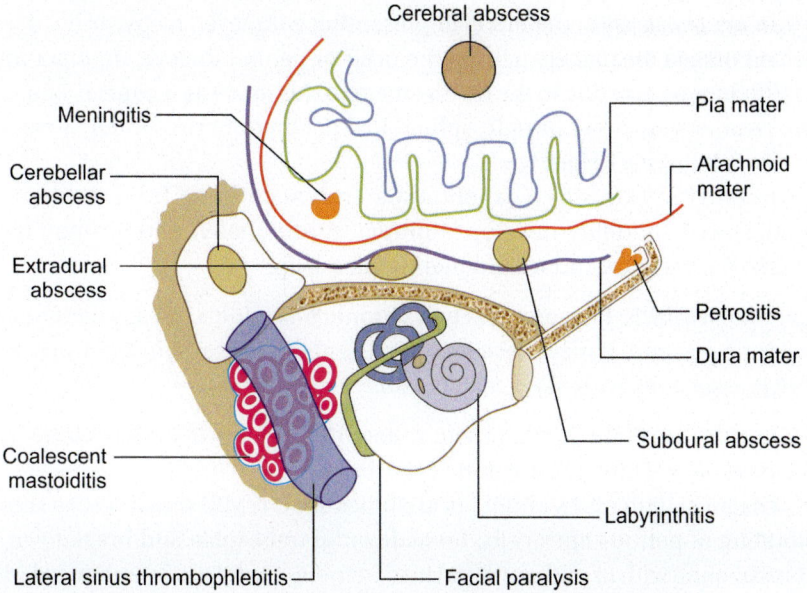

Fig. 1: Complications of chronic suppurative otitis media (CSOM).

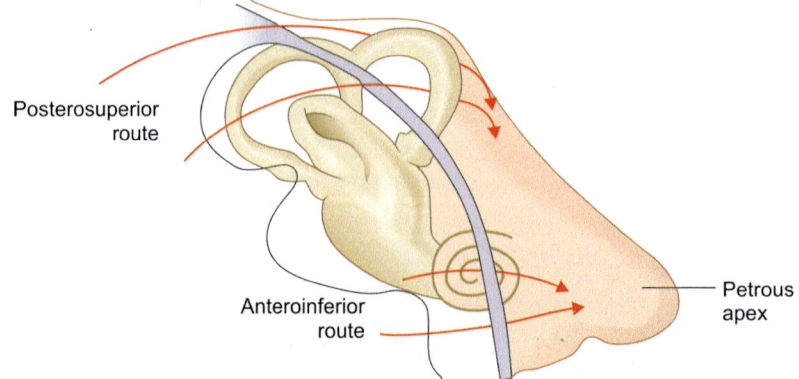

Fig. 2: Routes of spread from middle ear to petrous apex.

2. Anteroinferior chain from hypotympanum and peritubal, around the cochlea into the apex **(Fig. 2)**. Infection of petrous apex occurs much less commonly than mastoiditis. As the free drainage of pus from the petrous apex is limited by bony labyrinth naturally, it can potentially cause more complications.

Clinically petrositis is mainly due to trigeminal (Vth CN) and abducent (VIth CN) nerve irritation which are separated from petrous apex only by dura mater. Typical clinical triad of middle ear infection, paralysis of ipsilateral external rectus muscle (VI CN irritation) and pain in ipsilateral orbit or behind the eye (Vth CN irritation) (Giuseppe Gradenigo 1904) is known as Gradenigo syndrome.

In *acute petrositis*, patient is ill presenting with fever, tachycardia, deep-seated otalgia, headache, pain in the orbit or behind the eye, diplopia (due to VIth nerve palsy due to the involvement of this nerve as it courses beneath the Gruber's ligament or petrosphenoidal ligament in the Dorello's canal), and vomiting (neck rigidity ±).

In *masked petrositis*, (patient apparently recovering from acute otitis media) will suddenly develop diplopia. Additionally, patient may have headache, anorexia and will frequently fall asleep.

Chronic petrositis: It is rarely seen as chronic mastoiditis, mostly confined to sclerotic mastoid. It may present as persistent discharge from a petrous tract and is associated with deep-seated pain.

Management: Plain X-ray towne's view (35° fronto occipital view) and Stenvers view. These are not done these days.

Diagnosis is made by radiological studies like CT/MRI scan. CT scan shows clouding of petrous apex cells, breakdown of trabeculae and breakdown of cortical bone with or without dural involvement. Gadolinium-enhanced MRI scan shows lesion as isointense on T1-weighted images and hyperintense on T2-weighted images. MRI reveals any associated inflammatory change, meningeal involvement or any abscess.

When osteomyelitis is suspected, bone scans are very useful, both in diagnosis, and monitoring progression of disease. Looking for asymmetry between right and left petrous bone is important to avoid misdiagnosing marrow as petrositis.

In acute petrositis, start intravenous antibiotics (broad-spectrum) and review after 24 hours, if signs and symptoms remain static or improve, continue intravenous antibiotics for next 24 hours. By 48 hours, maximum patients improve clinically, i.e., fall in temperature and decrease in earache and/or discharge (Vth and VIth nerve signs may persist for longer time due to nerve sheath edema, even up to 3 months).

If there is no response or inadequate response to antibiotics after 24 hours of adequate antibiotics, surgery is indicated. Perform a simple (cortical) mastoidectomy and open up posterosuperior group of cells from all around the semicircular canal and curette any fistulous track. It may be necessary to convert the cortical mastoidectomy into a radical mastoidectomy, in order to facilitate adequate drainage.

In case of *masked petrositis,* patients commonly present with diplopia after apparent control of acute otitis media (AOM). Surgical procedure is same, i.e., cortical mastoidectomy with antibiotics.

In *chronic petrositis,* the patient presents as persistent Gradenigo syndrome or there is persistent discharge from petrous track despite cortical mastoidectomy for acute or masked mastoiditis.

General principle of petrous apex syndrome: Acute petrositis generally extends via perilabyrinthine group of cells (posterosuperior tract). Chronic petrositis usually involves the track beneath or in front of cochlea.

Posterosuperior tract is explored first via **(Fig. 3)**:
- *Frenckner's approach:* Through the arch of superior semicircular canal
- Above the horizontal and behind superior vertical superior semicircular canal (SSC)
- *Dearmin and Farrior's infralabyrinthine approach:* Beneath the posterior canal and behind vertical part of facial nerve.

Anterior track is explored via **(Fig. 3)**:
- *Farrior's subcochlear hypotympanic approach:* In this approach we explore the hypotympanum between carotid artery and jugular bulb. Eustachian tube area also explored between cochlea and carotid artery.
- *Almoor's approach:* Petrous apex is approached through an area bounded by cochlea, carotid and tegmen tympani.
- *Ramadier-Lempert approach:* The anterior track is explored between carotid artery and cochlea. Tegmen is removed. Tensor tympani and

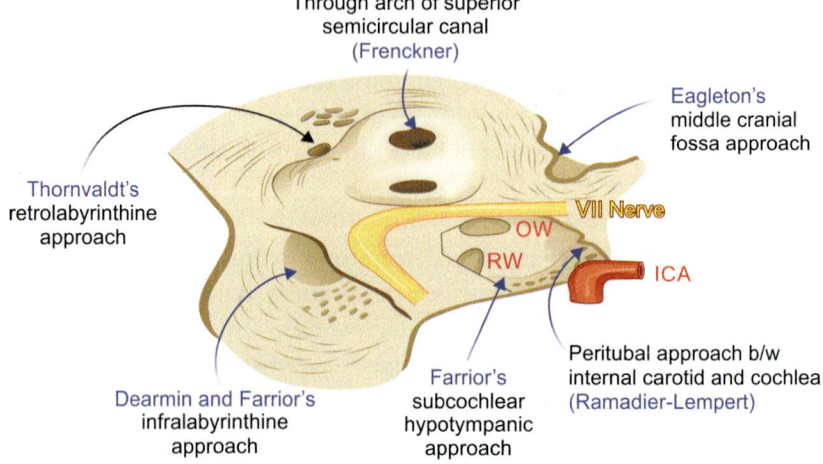

Fig. 3: Petrous apex—various surgical approaches.

wedge of bone between carotid and cochlea and middle fossa is also removed.

Other approaches include:
- *Thornvaldt's approach:* This approach is also along the supralabyrinthine tracts. As the dissection proceeds, it merges with that of Eagleton's approach.
- *Eagleton's approach:* This is the superior approach to the petrous apex that involves removal of the tegmen to the base of the zygoma together with removal of part of the squamous temporal bone. The dura of the middle cranial fossa can now be elevated to expose the petrous apex.

Despite adequate surgical management, patients with petrositis need long-term antibiotics guided by culture and sensitivity for 6–12 weeks or longer and these treatments are often guided by inflammatory markers such as erythrocyte sedimentation rate (ESR), C-reactive protein (CRP), serial computed tomography (CT) scans, and nuclear scans looking for inflammation along the temporal bone.

Facial Paralysis

This can be seen as a complication of both acute and chronic otitis media.

In acute otitis media, it occurs only in those patients who have congenital dehiscence of fallopian canal (8–10%). The cause is mainly neuropraxia due to infection/inflammation acting on perineurium of otherwise intact facial nerve.

Differential diagnosis: Ramsay Hunt syndrome (look for the presence of blisters on tympanic membrane).

Treatment:
- Systemic antibiotics

- Myringotomy ± cortical mastoidectomy (facial nerve decompression is not indicated).

In chronic otitis media, facial nerve is exposed and subjected to inflammatory reaction/pressure/bone eroding cholesteatoma. Onset is usually slowly progressive with ear discharge.

Patient presenting with above infection needs proper evaluation including otoendoscopic/microscopic examination of ear (especially look for posterior superior quadrant and attic) and HRCT temporal bone.

Send granulation tissue for histopathological examination (HPE) examination.

Management: Urgent exploration of middle ear is indicated and if necessary, radical mastoidectomy is done.
- Facial nerve is exposed in horizontal and vertical segment.
- Gently peel off cholesteatoma matrix from facial nerve.
- Attached granulation tissue should be left untouched to avoid further neural injury.
- Facial nerve decompression by decapping the fallopian canal bone on either side of the diseased segment to allow space for edema of the nerve.
- Gentle packing with gelfoam in the cavity to avoid pressure on the nerve.

Labyrinthitis

In acute otitis media, routes of spread for labyrinthine infection are:
- *Round window:* Pus cells can enter scala tympani by diapedesis from inflamed labyrinthine blood vessels.
- Preformed labyrinthine fistula, e.g., poststapedectomy.
- Inflammation induced fibrillary precipitate in both endolymphatic and perilymphatic spaces, ultimately destroying the membranous labyrinth.
- The disease process may culminate at any stage. If end result is reversible, the clinical entity is termed as serous labyrinthitis and if cochlea and vestibule are destroyed, the clinical entity is termed as suppurative labyrinthitis.

In chronic otitis media: Four stages of labyrinth involvement are seen.
1. *Paralabyrinthitis (circumscribed):* Bony erosion leads to thinning of the bony labyrinthine wall to produce a fistula, followed by vestibular irritation (Para labyrinthitis). Most common, seen in 10% cases of CSOM (perilabyrinthitis—problems caused by a fistula into an active labyrinth in an ear of postoperative mastoidectomy).
2. Inwards spread of infection leads to *serous labyrinthitis* which is diffuse intralabyrinthine inflammation without pus. No permanent loss of vestibular and cochlear function.

3. *Suppurative labyrinthitis*: Pus formation resulting in permanent loss of hearing and vestibular function.
4. Rarely, sequestration of labyrinth—due to necrosis of whole otic capsule.

Clinical features: Patient of acute or chronic otitis media presents to ear, nose, and throat (ENT) emergency with violent, prostrating vertigo, and vomiting.

Patient avoids any head movements, lies still, on the side with infected labyrinth upward.

On examination: Spontaneous irritative jerk nystagmus beating toward infected ear is the initial finding. Later on, it changes its direction toward healthy ear because of paralytic nystagmus.

Due to this, patient lies on healthy ear side because an effort to look at bedside visitor involves turning the eyes toward the damaged labyrinth and in this direction of gaze; the degree of nystagmus is least.

Masked bone conduction test indicates retained inner ear function in serous labyrinthitis and loss of cochlear function means irreversible suppurative state.

Patient warrants microscopic/endoscopic examination of ear.

Management:
- Complete bed rest.
- Avoid head movements.
- Intravenous fluids for hydration.
- Labyrinthine sedative—prochlorperazine.
- Look for signs and symptoms of meningitis.
  AOM: Myringotomy ± cortical mastoidectomy if intravenous antibiotics fail
  COM: Exploration of mastoid
- Premature surgical treatment can promote dissemination of infection so wait till signs and symptoms of acute vertigo settles down we should wait for 7–10 days with conservative medication.
- Initially, dead labyrinth was drained intraoperatively nowadays, it is not advised.

Labyrinthine fistula: It is seen in 10% of all COM with mastoiditis. Most common site is dome of lateral semicircular canal (LSCC) followed by promontory. Typically, CSOM patient presents with a brief period of vertigo/unsteadiness.

Cold air caloric test is indicated for testing vestibular function test.

Fistula test: Air pressure in external canal is increased with finger on tragus or pneumatic otoscope/Siegel speculum.

Classical clinical finding of fistula test in presence of LSSC fistula in most common site (dome of LSSC) is mentioned underneath:

- Increased pressure in external canal causes conjugate deviation of eyes away from the examination side.
  - If pressure maintained, jerk nystagmus beating toward involved/tested side.
  - On release of pressure, eye return to midline.
- Continuous pressure on the meatus.
  - Repeated eye deviation to healthy side with return to primary gaze position.
- During the test feeling of dizziness complained.
  - Deviation of eye toward normal ear (as discussed) is commonly seen.

Note:
- If fistula is anterior to ampulla, conjugate deviation of eye is toward the side of fistula is seen.
- If vestibule is eroded, fistula test reveals rotatory horizontal deviation toward the diseased ear.
- In presence of fistula in superior SCC, fistula test shows rotatory movement toward the normal ear.
- In presence of fistula in posterior SCC, vertical deviation of eyes is seen.

False negative fistula test:
- Inadequate sealing of the speculum in the meatus
- Cholesteatoma sealing the fistula
- Dead labyrinth

[*Note*: False positive fistula test—in presence of intact tympanic membrane is seen in congenital syphilis (Hennebert's sign) and in Meniere's disease.]

Management: In case of chronic otitis media with vertigo, always suspect labyrinthine involvement and plan for surgical exploration. High-resolution computed tomography may be helpful.

Intraoperative: Always peel off the matrix from LSSC very carefully, away from the areas where fistula is suspected. Remove the matrix from other sites first (under high power magnification) slight change of color at the junction of matrix and adjoining bone—suggests possibility of fistula.

In modified radical mastoidectomy (MRM)/radical mastoidectomy (open cavity) matrix can be safely left-over fistula.

Bony fistula will close by new bone formation later on.
- If matrix is removed completely, seal fistula by connective tissue such as temporalis fascia and perichondrium.
- In case of intact canal wall tympanoplasty (closed cavity) if matrix is left over fistula this will require second exploration after 6–12 months to let the epithelial pearl formation which can be easily removed.

Cochlear Complication

Transmission of toxic substances/enzymes due to active inflammation-through the dependent round window membrane into the basal turn of the cochlea can cause initially temporary and later on, permanent high frequency sensorineural hearing loss (SNHL).

Risk of hearing loss is more in acute otitis media than chronic otitis media as round window membrane is thicker in COM. Also, pus is under pressure in acute otitis media.

Mastoiditis

Two types of mastoiditis are typically seen as per the primary middle ear cleft pathology.
1. *Acute mastoiditis*—symptomatic, or masked mastoiditis by antibiotics.
2. *Chronic mastoiditis*—as a part of continuation of disease process of chronic otitis media, leading to formation of granulation tissue in the mastoid bone.

Acute mastoiditis: In case of a very active acute otitis media, pus collected in middle ear cleft is under pressure and if drainage is inadequate, it induces pressure necrosis of bony trabeculae, coalescence of air cells and empyema formation (in pneumatized mastoid), ultimately cortex gets penetrated, resulting in subperiosteal abscess (**Fig. 4**). The process takes about 10 days to three weeks depending upon severity of infection, virulence of microorganisms and antibiotics resistance. If drainage is adequate, pus production and drainage continue resulting into *mastoid reservoir*.

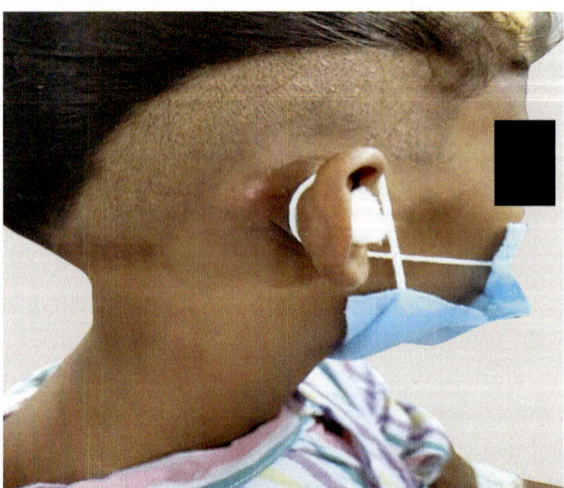

Fig. 4: Acute mastoiditis.

Failed antibiotics in acute mastoiditis (in pneumatized mastoid), due to short course of antibiotics results in *masked mastoiditis*. Acute signs and symptoms get masked but coalescence process continues, resulting in extensive destruction of bony trabeculae, granulation tissue, and destruction of bony tegmen/sinus plate with dura/sinus covered with granulations.

- *Black cholesteatosis:* A condition seen in children, where in air cells are filled with black fluid rich in cholesterin crystals.
- *Clinical signs and symptoms:* In preantibiotic era, classical acute mastoiditis presented with retroauricular edema, with pinna pushed forward or by fluctuation of subperiosteal abscess. Clinically, patient has acute otalgia and/or fever which has recurred or persisted after short course of antibiotics of acute otitis media attack. Hearing loss is usually conductive, with or without ear discharge.

Note: In infants and young children, recurrence of diarrhea or vomiting may also be presenting feature. In contrast, in masked mastoiditis, pain, fever, swelling and discharge are usually absent.

Tenderness in acute mastoid can be elicited in mastoid tip, zygomatic root, retroauricular groove (in acute otitis media—tenderness only over antrum and McEwen's triangle).

Postaural swelling: Initially, when cortex is intact and periosteum starts thickening with edema, there is blurring of bony character of mastoid (velvety feel). With increase in edema, retroauricular sulcus fills up and gets obstructed and pinna is pushed forward **(Figs. 5A to C)**. Later on, pus enters cortex and presents as subperiosteal abscess.

Postaural/subperiosteal abscess: Perichondrium is intact but bone gets eroded. It is the most common extratemporal complication of COM **(Fig. 6)**.

The various abscesses include **(Fig. 7)**:
- *Bezold abscess*: Abscess on internal/medial aspect of mastoid tip, deep to sternocleidomastoid muscle, pushing the muscle outwards and presents as a swelling in the upper part of neck. It can follow the posterior belly of digastric muscle and may present as swelling between angle of jaw and mastoid and can sometimes reach the parapharyngeal space. It is sudden in onset and patient may present with pain, fever and torticollis (spasm of SCM). History of purulent otorrhea should be taken.
- *Zygomatic abscess:* Infection of zygomatic air cells which are present at the posterior root of zygoma can lead to this type of abscess. It presents as a swelling in front of and above the pinna. Edema of the upper eyelids can be seen.
- *Meatal abscess (Luc's abscess):* Skin intact but pus is present in posterior-inferior wall of external auditory canal (EAC). Swelling is seen in deep part of bony canal and abscess can sometimes burst into the canal.

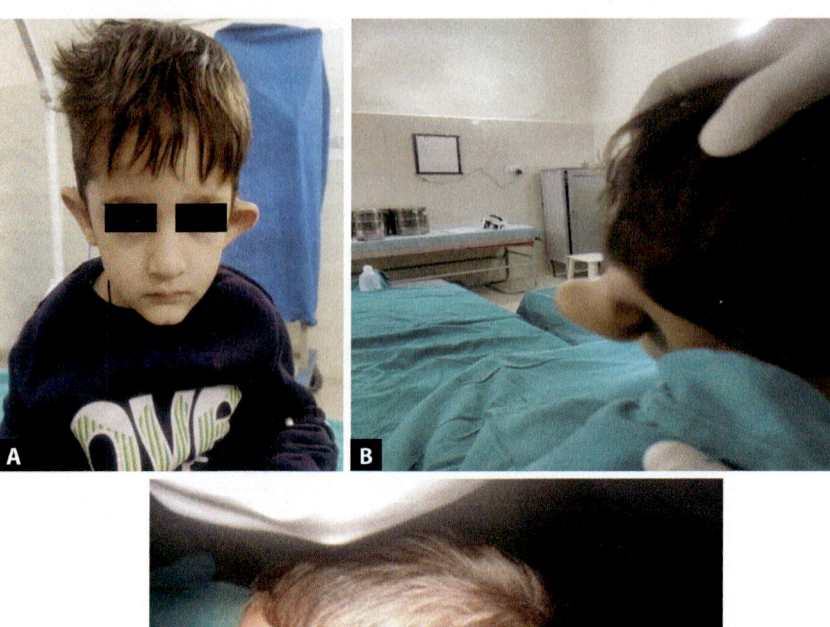

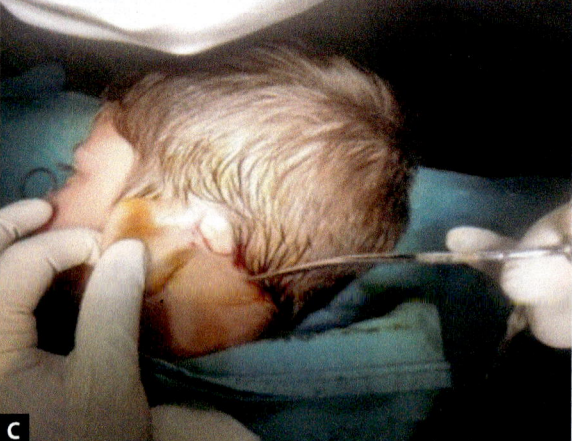

Figs. 5A to C: Postaural subperiosteal abscess pushing the pinna forward.

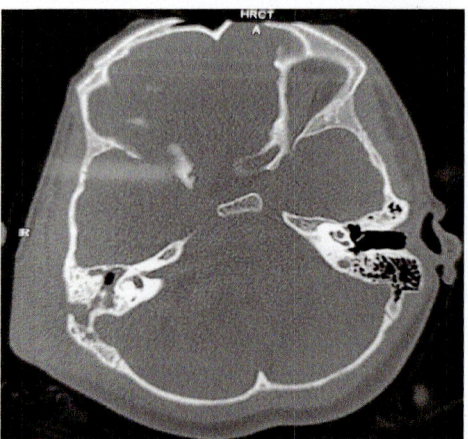

Fig. 6: High-resolution computed tomography (HRCT) temporal bone showing right-sided postaural mastoid abscess.

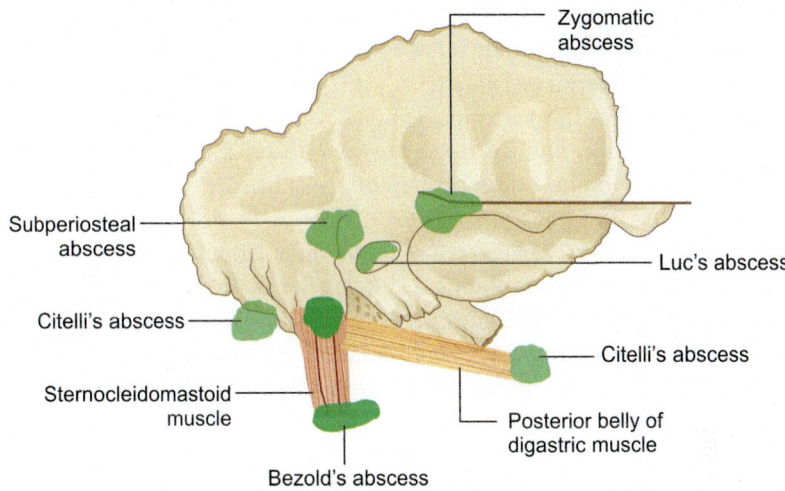

Fig. 7: Abscesses in relation to mastoid.

- *Citelli's abscess:* Abscess is formed posterior to mastoid more toward the occipital bone. Some authors are of the consideration that this abscess is formed anterior to mastoid along the posterior belly of digastric muscle.

General Condition

Patient is not well; there is feeling of listlessness, lack of concentration and nagging awkward feeling in ear. Children may have tendency to fall asleep for short period at odd times and there is decreased appetite/refusal for food. Temperature and pulse rate are raised, tongue furrowed, face is apprehensive.

Management: Acute mastoiditis is a surgical emergency.

Incision and drainage of subperiosteal abscess with cortical mastoidectomy under intravenous antibiotic coverage.

In masked mastoiditis, surgical treatment in the form of cortical mastoidectomy is performed. In chronic mastoiditis, modified radical mastoidectomy/radical mastoidectomy is performed.

Intracranial Complications

Intracranial spread is most dangerous in terms of morbidity and mortality.

Symptoms: They are generally of those due to compression of brain tissue, e.g., headache, malaise, fever, and drowsiness.

Principle of Treatment

Three stages are as follows:
1. Systemic broad-spectrum antibiotics
2. Neurological consultation and intervention
3. Treatment of primary otological pathology.

Antibiotics: Every treating ENT unit should make its generalized antibiotic guidelines/protocol depending upon availability of drugs, pattern of infecting organisms and bacterial resistance.

Large dose of antibiotics by intravenous route is advisable.

Treating surgeon should not wait for culture and sensitivity report. Antibiotics are given based on probability of causative microorganism and clinical response.

- *In acute infection:* Drugs effective against *Haemophilus influenzae*, ampicillin, and chloramphenicol (100 mg/kg/day).
- *In chronic infection:* Antibiotics effective against gram-negative infection especially *Pseudomonas aeruginosa*. Also, metronidazole (400–600 mg/8 hourly) for gram-negative anaerobes such as *Bacteroides fragilis* (chloramphenicol, penicillin, and metronidazole penetrate abscess capsule).

Treatment of primary ear disease: Acute otitis media—this is cured by antibiotics. Myringotomy may be required in some cases. In some patients cortical mastoidectomy is required. Some advocate routine exposure of sigmoid sinus and middle cranial dura

- *In chronic otitis media*-modified/radical mastoidectomy is done.
  Generally, these surgical otological interventions are contemplated once neurosurgical intervention has taken care of intracranial complication except in cases of lateral sinus thrombosis and extradural abscess where primary mastoid surgery is indicated.
- **Investigation:** Investigation and treatment should run concurrently. Delay in initiation of treatment while waiting for investigations increases morbidity.
- *High resolution CT scan temporal bone:* It is the gold standard especially for intracranial complications. Before the advent of CT scan, X-ray mastoid was the investigation of choice.
- Electroencephalogram (EEG)
- *Arteriography:* This shows distortion of vascular pattern especially in supratentorial mass.
- *Air encephalography and ventriculography:* These are not done these days.
- *Magnetic resonance imaging (MRI):* Few centers prefer this investigation because of absence of bone artifacts and ability to detect early infections.
- Lumbar puncture especially in meningitis.
  - **General points to remember:**
    - CSOM associated with otalgia is suggestive of impending intracranial lesion.
      - Presence of headache suggests intracranial complication has occurred.
  - Projectile vomiting and nausea indicate increased intracranial tension

- Drowsiness indicates that brain tissue is involved (compression)
- *Temperature and pulse rate changes:*
  - Raised temperature and pulse rate is suggestive of infection
    - Subnormal temperature and decreased pulse rate are suggestive of brain abscess.
      - If infection predominates [e.g., lateral sinus thrombosis (LST)]—swinging temperature with increase in temperature peak and pulse rate.
    - Presence of rigors suggests LST.
- *Differential diagnosis* (bedside evaluation of brain abscess, meningitis and LST)
  - *Brain abscess:* Patient is ill, drowsy, and listless and never feels well (Decrease appetite and body weight; patient is emaciated).
  - *Meningitis:* Patient is ill with severe headache and photophobia, projectile vomiting.
  - *LST:* In between rigor attacks, patient is active and cheerful.

■ EXTRADURAL ABSCESS

Most common of all intracranial complication arising from the infection of middle ear cleft. The pus collects between bone and otherwise tough duramater it is often associated with granulation tissue on the surface of dura.

In middle cranial fossa, dura may be stripped extensively resulting in significant intracranial mass resulting in raised intracranial pressure (ICP). The patient may present with focal neurological signs and papilledema. Mostly these abscesses are lateral and limited by arcuate eminence.

Rarely, it may arise medial to arcuate eminence and involve petrous apex causing irritative symptomatology of Gasserian ganglion of Vth and VIth cranial nerve (Gradenigo syndrome).

Posterior fossa extradural abscess: Spread of pus is limited by dural attachment laterally to sigmoid sinus canal, medially to internal auditory meatus and it generally produces sigmoid sinus—perisinus abscess.
- *Clinical features:* If there is ipsilateral headache especially deep-seated along with malaise, suspect extradural abscess. Classically, symptoms regress if there is free communication of abscess with middle ear and spontaneous aural discharge.
  - *Diagnosis:* HRCT temporal bone is diagnostic, and to look for concomitant/associated other intracranial complications.
  - *Treatment:* Exploration and drainage of pus.

Bone removal from area of healthy dura granulation tissue on dura left behind. Some authors advocate cauterization of granulation tissue using bipolar cautery.

SUBDURAL ABSCESS

Dura is very resistant to destruction. But sometimes infection causes necrosis of the dura leading to infection of subdural space commencing with collection of seropurulent effusion and ultimately to frank pus. Abscess may be small near to the site of dural penetration or may enlarge enough to cause signs and symptoms of space occupying lesion. Adjacent cortical veins involvement may occur leading to formation of multiple small abscess. Subdural abscess usually collects near falx cerebri. Usual findings are numerous multiloculated abscesses over convex surface of cerebral hemisphere and between hemispheres along the falx. Nonhemolytic streptococcus is most common infecting organism.

Clinical Features

Severe headache and drowsiness are usually the presenting features.
- Focal neurological symptoms—irritative (fits)
- Paralytic
- Drowsiness may progress rapidly to coma.
- Paralysis of one upper or lower limb with rapid progression to hemiplegia
- Hemianopia and hemianesthesia
- If dominant side involved—aphasia
- Epileptic fits of Jacksonian type starting locally and spread to involve full body, followed by weakness.
- Site of fits and pattern of weakness determines clinically the diagnosis of position of abscess.

Management

In subdural abscess, progression of disease and symptoms is fast.
Note: if there is no response to medical treatment in suspect cases of meningitis or if motor seizures occur—suspect subdural abscess.

Diagnosis

- HRCT temporal bone
- Cerebrospinal fluid (CSF) (lumbar puncture)
  - CSF pressure increased
  - Sugar normal
  - Culture sterile.

Treatment

- High dose of intravenous antibiotics (penicillin, chloramphenicol, and aminoglycosides)
- In patients with AOM—myringotomy and/or cortical mastoidectomy is done

- In patients with CSOM—MRM/radical mastoidectomy is done.
  Neurosurgical management: One or multiple burr holes are made for drainage of subdural fluid
- Antiepileptics are given to suppress convulsions.

LATERAL (SIGMOID) SINUS THROMBOPHLEBITIS

Lateral sinus thrombophlebitis is initiated with extradural perisinus abscess followed by suppurative blood clot in the lumen of the sinus. Partial breakdown of the infected clot leads to bacteremia, septicemia, and septic embolization.

Upward Extension of Thrombus

Thrombus extends from torcular Herophili upward to the superior sagittal sinus or invasion of superior and inferior petrosal sinus leads to involvement of the cavernous sinus. The spread of venous thrombophlebitis into the brain substance leads to brain abscess.

Downward extension of thrombus-thrombus may extend into internal jugular vein and involve subclavian vein.

In preantibiotic era, LST was mostly seen as a complication of ASOM. Nowadays, it is mainly seen as CSOM complication.

Most commonly organisms involved are beta hemolytic streptococci, but majority has mixed flora involving *Proteus mirabilis, Staphylococcus, Streptococcus pneumonia,* and *Bacteroides.*

Clinical Presentation

- *In preantibiotic era*:
  - Patients presented with high spiking fever (picket fence pattern, i.e., diurnal temperature spikes that exceed 103°F/39.4°C) associated with rigors with profuse sweating. Shivering during rigors may be so violent to shake the bed. There is headache and neck pain (pain in neck is due to inflammation of sternomastoid muscle). There may be emaciation with progressive anemia. With the extension of infected clot downward to internal jugular vein (IJV), there occurs perivenous inflammation and tenderness in upper neck and suppuration of jugular lymph nodes. Perivenous inflammation involving Jugular foramen leads to IXth, Xth, and XIth cranial nerve palsy. Raised intracranial pressure causes papilledema and vision loss.
  - Superior sagittal sinus involvement can lead to hydrocephalus. Cavernous sinus involvement causes chemosis and proptosis.
    - Thromboembolic phenomenon of infected clot may lead to lung involvement, subcutaneous tissue, large joints, pleuroperitoneal cavity, usually seen in masked lateral sinus thrombophlebitis (by masking effect of antibiotics as the primary ear pathology)

- *Nowadays:* Persistent fever with ill feeling, earache and neck pain, mastoid tenderness, and stiffness along sternomastoid muscle is consistent to lateral sinus thrombophlebitis. About 50% of patients have other associated intracranial complications especially meningitis and brain abscess. Papilledema is seen in 50% patients while some patients have altered sensorium as clinical finding. Downward extension of clot to IJV causes tenderness and localized edema over thrombosing IJV. Subclavian vein involvement causes engorged collateral vein over the shoulder and extensive intravascular clotting leading to thrombocytopenia. Pitting edema over mastoid and adjacent region due to thrombosis of mastoid emissary vein, known as *Griesinger's sign* may be seen.

  Patient with lateral sinus thrombophlebitis, who has swinging temperatures is an absolute emergency as the emboli from thrombus at lateral sinus is the cause of this clinical presentation and needs surgery as soon as possible.

Investigation

- Hemogram—anemia with increased total leucocyte count (TLC) and ESR or thrombocytopenia.
- Blood culture during "temperature peak" was initially the most important diagnostic test
- *Queckenstedt or Tobey-Ayer test:* It is done whenever lumbar puncture is indicated. The test involves measurement of CSF pressure and observing its changes on compression of one or both IJV. Normally, compression of one IJV causes rapid increase in CSF pressure by 50-100 mm Hg above the normal with equal rapid fall on release of pressure. In Lateral sinus thrombophlebitis, pressure over the vein on involved side causes no rise or very low rise in CSF pressure <20 mm Hg while pressure on normal side causes a rapid pressure rise to 2-3 times the normal value.
- *Lillie-Crowe test:* If one lateral sinus is occluded, digital compression of opposite IJV causes dilatation of retinal veins on retinoscopy.
- *High resolution CT scan:*
  Increased density of fresh clot:
  - Filling defect within the sinus (on contrast-enhanced CT scan)
  - Failure of opacification
  - *Septic thrombosis:* Intense inflammatory enhancement within sinus wall and adjacent dura
  - Tentorial enhancement from collateral venous flow
  - Helps to rule out complications such as brain abscess and subdural abscess
- Digital subtraction venography
- Radioisotope scanning (gallium) reveals hot spots of sepsis.

Management

Intravenous antibiotics are—penicillin, chloramphenicol and an aminoglycoside.
- Anticoagulants are now rarely used and are administered only if spreading thrombus reaching cavernous sinus.
- Temperature, pulse rate and respiration (TPR) and chest monitoring every 4 hours
- Neurological signs/symptoms charting every 12 hours
- If there is no improvement or there is deterioration—mastoid exploration is done within 48 hours.
- In cases of acute and coalescent mastoiditis—cortical mastoidectomy is done
- In cases of CSOM—radical mastoidectomy is done via postaural route
- Always expose the sinus plate; in case necrotic plate of bone is present—remove with probe and curette.
- If there is no bony necrosis, uncover the sinus with diamond burr and blunt dissection.

Expose the sinus upward up to sinodural angle and lower down to jugular bulb:
- If sinus is rough and bluish and compressible—insert small needle through the wall to seek the free flow of venous blood. In case of incorrect diagnosis of lateral sinus thrombophlebitis—seal the puncture site by keeping a piece of free muscle tissue.
- If sinus feels firm, white and opaque—suggests that the lumen is occluded with clot or fibrous tissue. Open the sinus with sharp instrument. Absence of blood or necrotic debris is known as "silent LST."
- If sinus wall is covered with granulation or if it is necrotic—open the sinus and remove the pus and necrotic tissue. Explore the sinus in both directions, till jugular and confluence of sinus superiorly.
- Previously it was the teaching that the clot removal should be extended in each direction until free flow of blood was established. Nowadays, it is necessary to remove organized thrombus and no longer explore the clot centrally until free flow is established.

Note: In coalescent mastoiditis if cortical mastoidectomy is performed, always expose sigmoid sinus even in absence of suspicious intracranial complication.

Ligation of Internal Jugular Vein is Indicated in:
- Refractory septicemia not responding to antibiotics and surgery
- Children showing embolization.

■ MENINGITIS

Meningitis is the most common intracranial complications secondary to middle ear infection with significant morbidity and mortality. In children,

AOM is most common cause and in adults, CSOM is mainly responsible for spread of infection from middle ear cleft to meninges due to spread through necrosing bone.

Causative Organisms

In AOM—*Haemophilus influenzae* type B and *Streptococcus pneumoniae* are most common.

Gram-negative enteric organisms such as *Proteus* and *Pseudomonas* and anaerobes like *Bacteroides* are common pathogen in CSOM.

Initially infection leads to exudative response in subarachnoid space resulting in raised CSF pressure. Later on, frank purulence accumulates in the basal cisterns. The free flow of CSF in ventricular foramina gets obstructed due to exudates leading to noncommunicating type hydrocephalus. While obstruction to CSF flow in the subarachnoid space produces communicating hydrocephalus. Spread of infection through Virchow Robin spaces leads to the formation of brain abscess. Also, pus collection in exit foramina of cranial nerves leads to cranial nerve palsies.

Clinical Features

Neck stiffness due to irritation of upper cervical nerve roots.
- Headache initially localized to ipsilateral side and becomes generalized and bursting later on.
- Malaise and high-grade fever (without spikes)
- Children generally have restlessness and frightfulness due to initial mental hyperactivity.
- Adults—anxiety with in between periods of drowsiness
- Photophobia
- Projectile vomiting
- Positive Kernig's sign, later on opisthotonos

Deterioration is clinically seen as:
- Altered delirium and stupor finally into coma
- Tendon reflex disappear, cranial nerve palsies, Cheyne-Stokes respiration and fixed dilated pupil, coma, and death

Diagnosis

Lumbar puncture—rise in CSF pressure (100-150 mm Hg) is initial finding. Later on, white cells appear in CSF followed by clouding/turbid CSF.

Microscopically
- Polymorphs (not usually seen in CSF) with number $0.1-10 \times 10^9$/L ($100-10,000/mm^3$)

- Protein content is raised from normal 150–400 mg/L to 2–3 g/L
- Chloride content lowered from 120 mmol/L (normal) to 80 mmol/L
- Glucose levels are lowered from normal 1.7–3.0 mmol/L to zero (diagnostic) Gram-staining and culture sensitivity.

CT scan—to rule out brain abscess/subdural abscess.

Note: Even if brain abscess leaks into CSF, or presence of subdural abscess, white blood cell (WBC) count rises significantly with raised CSF pressure. But blood sugar level is reduced in none of the two conditions.

Treatment

- Medical treatment of meningitis is foremost important.
  Lumbar puncture (LP) for diagnosis; also repeated LP is done to reduce intracranial pressure (second within in 24 hours, then daily till improvement).
- *Intravenous antibiotics:* Penicillin group and chloramphenicol
  Rifampicin for *Haemophilus influenzae* in chloramphenicol resistant infection.
  In presence of CSOM—antibiotic agent such as azlocillin, ticarcillin, and ceftazidime.
  In presence of anaerobic—metronidazole 400 mg intravenous TDS.

Surgical Treatment

- In AOM—myringotomy ± Grommet insertion (for repeated drainage).
- Coalescent mastoiditis—cortical mastoidectomy
- CSOM—radical mastoidectomy

Failure of medical treatment: Resistant infective organism:
- Persistent leakage from middle ear infection into CSF
- Leakage from Brain abscess
- Presence of unidentified concomitant complication.

■ BRAIN ABSCESS

Otogenic cause is one of the most important causes of brain abscess accounting for approximately 25% in pediatric age and 50% in adults. Temporal lobe involvement is twice as common as compared to cerebellum. Route of spread is mostly by direct extension from middle ear cleft infection.
- Temporal lobe abscess occurs mainly above tegmen plate.
- In cerebellar abscess, lateral lobe is involved mainly which may be adherent to the lateral sinus or to a patch of dura underneath Trautmann's triangle.

Bacteriology

The bacterial flora is mainly mixture of aerobes and obligate anaerobes. Anaerobic streptococci are the most common organisms. Pyogenic staphylococci are also common especially in children; *Streptococcus pneumoniae* and *Streptococcus haemolyticus* are also found. Gram-negative bacilli are *Proteus mirabilis*, *Escherichia coli* and *Pseudomonas aeruginosa*, and *Bacteroides fragilis*.

Clinical Features

Four stages are seen clinically:
1. *Encephalitis*: Formation of abscess starts with an area of cerebral edema and encephalitis and causes headache, fever, malaise, and vomiting followed by drowsiness.
   Note: If there is persistent headache in CSOM, always think of intracranial complications; and in presence of drowsiness think of sinister complications.
   Localized encephalitis can spread readily as generalized encephalitis, leading to stupor, coma, and then death.
2. *Latent period:* Transition from localized encephalitis to pus formation contained within a developing fibrous capsule. The stage lasts for 2–3 weeks and is mainly asymptomatic.
3. *Frank abscess:* This causes features of space occupying lesion along with focal neurological sign and raised CSF pressure. Malaise, anorexia, weakness, and lethargy are additional clinical findings. With raised intracranial pressure, pulse rate slows, and temperature falls to subnormal level. Drowsiness may alternate with periods of irritability.
   - Papilledema is seen earlier in cerebellar abscess than in temporal lobe abscess. If intracranial pressure keeps on raising, the patient goes into coma, the ipsilateral pupil dilates and finally each pupil gets fixed and dilated.
4. *Terminal stage/death:* Death occurs due to effect of raised intracranial pressure. Symptoms occur due to rupture of abscess into the ventricular system or subarachnoid space leading to fulminating meningitis and death.

Localizing features specific to the area involved are as below:

Temporal Lobe Abscess

- A cerebral abscess in the dominant hemisphere causes nominal aphasia.
- Visual field defects arise from involvement of the optic radiations.
- There is quadrantic homonymous hemianopia, affecting the upper part of temporal visual fields.
- Visual fields are lost on contralateral side of lesions because of damage to the fibers arising in both retinae of same side.
- This can be assessed by performing bedside conformation test for visual field.

- *Motor paralysis*:
  Two patterns are seen, they are as follows:
  1. Upward abscess spread affects facial movement on opposite side and then upper and lower limbs gets involved.
  2. Inward expansion firstly affects lower limb followed by upper limb and face.

Cerebellar Abscess

It causes weakness, ataxia, and past-pointing.
- Finger-nose test reveals intention tremors and past pointing.
- Dysdiadochokinesia is difficulty in rapid alteration of supination and pronation of forearm.
- Difficulty in rapidly touching each finger to the thumb tip.
- Spontaneous nystagmus may be present, which is coarse, irregular, and beating toward the side of lesion.
- Above mentioned clinical signs get easily obscured by rapidly progressive intracranial pressure.

Investigations

Computed tomography scan with or without intravenous Conray contrast is the most diagnostic for brain abscess and any other associated complications such as subdural abscess and lateral sinus thrombophlebitis.

Plain Computed Tomography

Low density area surrounded by finger like area of edema.

Contrast-enhanced Computed Tomography

Capsule enhancement—dense rim. If no ring enhancement—area of cerebritis not reached to stage of true abscess formation.

Other Investigations

- *Carotid angiography:* There is upward and medial displacement of middle cerebral artery in temporal lobe abscess.
- Plain X-ray may show displaced calcified pineal gland.
- *Electroencephalography (EEG):* It shows abnormal delta wave activity.

Lumbar Puncture

CSF shows increase in CSF pressure, raised protein, raised white cells, while blood glucose remains normal.

Treatment

Initially, in the absence of neurosurgeon, intracranial pus was drained at the same sitting of mastoidectomy, by opening the dura and needling the brain along the tract established by infection. Nowadays, standard guidelines are, giving high dose of intravenous systemic antibiotics; neurosurgical management of abscess and after a gap of 10–14 days, radical mastoidectomy is performed. In case of acute otitis media, myringotomy, or cortical mastoidectomy is be indicated. Urgent neurosurgical consultation should be done at the earliest. If raised intracranial pressure causes coma or rapid deterioration, intravenous dexamethasone (4 mg IV every 7 hourly) or IV mannitol (0.5 g/kg) should be given.

- Intravenous antibiotics are given at high dose, antibiotics which crosses blood-brain barrier; includes—penicillin, chloramphenicol, aminoglycosides (where *Pseudomonas* or *Proteus* is present), and metronidazole for *Bacteroides*.
- Neurosurgical intervention is performed, by either draining the abscess repeatedly through burr holes, or to excise it completely with its capsule. Repeated needle aspiration is indicated in very ill patients and can be safely done under local anesthesia. Primary excision of abscess is favored by many with the advantage of immediate decompression of brain. Drawbacks are extensive damage to cerebral tissue resulting in high chance of neurological deficit.
- Open operation is performed by incising the abscess and removing pus from abscess cavity under direct inspection. Anticonvulsants are given following surgical treatment of brain abscess especially temporal lobe abscess, to prevent epileptic seizures.

■ OTITIC HYDROCEPHALUS (PSEUDOTUMOR CEREBRI)

Otitic hydrocephalus also termed as benign intracranial hypertension or pseudotumor cerebri, is a syndrome of increased intracranial pressure with a normal ventricular system and cerebrospinal fluid of normal composition. It is the least common complication that is mainly seen in children and adolescents. It occurs due to obstruction of the lateral sinus affecting the cerebral sinus outflow or extension of thrombus to the superior sagittal sinus, blocking CSF resorption by Pacchionian bodies, thus increasing the CSF pressure.

Clinical Features

The clinical signs and symptoms seen are mainly due to raised intracranial tension. Headache, drowsiness, blurred vision, nausea and vomiting, and diplopia are the presenting complaints. Focal neurological signs are absent. Clinical examination reveals papilledema, lateral rectal palsy due to VIth CN stretching on one or both sides with history of recent AOM or COM.

Diagnosis

Lumbar puncture should be done with cautious lest herniation of cerebellar tonsil occurs.

Cerebrospinal fluid findings shows, raised pressure. Cerebrospinal fluid is sterile and biochemical tests are normal. Computed tomography scan shows normal ventricles.

Treatment

- Treat the persistent middle ear infection. Reduce ICP to prevent visual impairment by use of steroids/diuretics and hyperosmolar dehydrating agents and the coperitoneal shunting.
- Optic nerve sheath fenestration.

■ FURTHER READING

1. Dubey SP, Larawin V. Complications of chronic suppurative otitis media and their management. Laryngoscope. 2007;117(2):264-7.
2. Mawron SR, Ludman HS. Mawson's Diseases of the Ear, 5th edition. London: Hodder Arnold;1988.
3. Mustafa A, Heta A, Dreshaj Sh. Complications of chronic otitis media with cholesteatoma during a 10-year period in Kosovo. Eur Arch Otorhinolaryngol. 2008;265(12):1477-82.
4. Rupa V, Raman R. Chronic Suppurative Chronic suppurative otitis media: complicated versus uncomplicated disease. Acta Otolaryngol. 1991;111(3):530-5.

CHAPTER 14

Complicated Rhinosinusitis

Venkata Surya Phani Bhushan Durvasula,
Vikas Gupta, Parmod Kalsotra

■ INTRODUCTION

Complications of rhinosinusitis occur due to progression of sinusitis beyond paranasal sinuses (PNS). Complications are more common in children than in adults. Sixty to eighty five percent of orbital infections are the result of complication of sinusitis. In modern antibiotic era, the complications of sinusitis have dramatically fallen. But sinus infection is still one of the most common causes of ocular and orbital complications. Before discussing the complications of sinusitis, few important anatomical factors need to be reemphasized.

- Bony orbit is a quadrilateral pyramidal cavity, formed by seven separate bones. Roof of orbit is formed by the floor of frontal sinus, floor by roof of maxillary sinus. Medial wall by frontal process of maxilla, lacrimal bone, lamina papyracea of the ethmoid and body of sphenoid (just anterior to optic foramen). Lateral wall is the thickest and strongest of all the walls. It is formed by greater wing of the sphenoid bone posteriorly and frontal process of the zygomatic bone anteriorly **(Fig. 1)**.
- In frontoethmoidal fissure, are the anterior and posterior ethmoid foramen where in vascular and neural structures pass.
- *Congenital dehiscence:* Usually seen behind the trochlear fossa or supraorbital notch
    • At the junction of middle and outer thirds of the roof of orbit

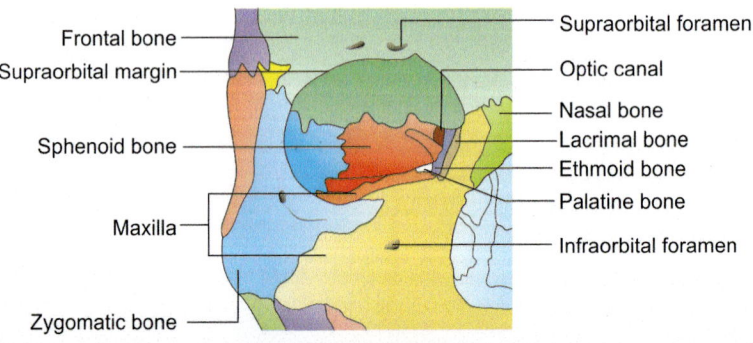

Bones of the orbit and some of the major landmarks
Fig. 1: Anatomy of orbit.

- At the junction of anterior and middle thirds of os planum
- Over the posterior ethmoidal cell
- Ophthalmic vein is completely valveless, resulting in a two-way communication between face, nasal cavity, sinus, and pterygoid plexus.
- Periosteum of the orbit (periorbita)—passes through suture lines to fuse with periosteum of other side. Periorbita becomes continuous with the tarsal plate which in turn prevents orbital effusion and infection in the orbit to spread through the lids.
- Orbital septum (palpebral ligament) forms a barrier between intraorbital and periorbital tissue.

MODE OF SPREAD OF SINUS INFECTION

- Through bony wall of sinus:
  - Congenital dehiscence
  - Fracture lines (after trauma)
  - Osteomyelitis in compact bone
  - Porous lamina papyracea
- Venous spread
  - Via valveless diploic veins of Breschet of the frontal, ethmoid and sphenoid bones which communicate with dural venous plexus.
  - Septic vein thrombosis
  - In patients with septicemia and pyemia

  Lymphatic spread (orbit is devoid of lymph nodes/lymphatics) unlikely to play a role in disease progression.
- Direct spread
  - Through inferior orbital fissure
  - Spread via perineural spaces—olfactory nerves to subarachnoid spaces
  - Spread via ethmoidal artery foramen.

CLASSIFICATION OF COMPLICATIONS

- Orbital
- Extraorbital
  - Intracranial
  - Bony

Orbital, intracranial and osseous complications are seen typically due to acute sinus, infection can also occur in chronic rhinosinusitis especially secondary to superimposed acute infection.

Orbital Complications (60–75%)

Orbital complications occur most frequently when ethmoid sinuses are involved followed by frontal and maxillary sinuses. Multiple complications can occur in the same patient.

Chandler classification (I to V) according to the progression of the infection **(Fig. 2 and Table 1)**.

I. *Preseptal cellulitis (Inflammatory edema) (50%):* Bacterial infection of eyelid and periorbital soft tissue, leading to local erythema and induration. Patient presents with fever, pain, conjunctival injection, epiphora and blurring of vision.

Infection of ethmoidal sinus will cause edema initially over the frontal process of maxilla above the internal palpebral ligament and later on, it will extend laterally.

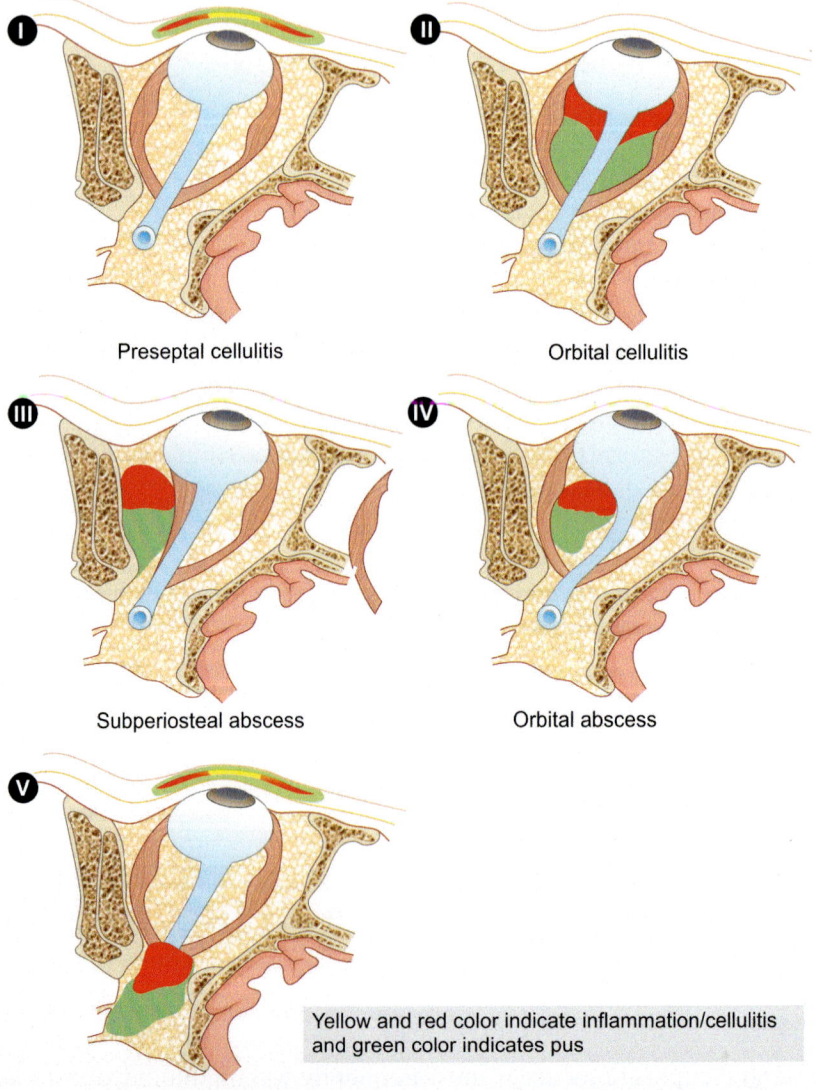

Preseptal cellulitis

Orbital cellulitis

Subperiosteal abscess

Orbital abscess

Yellow and red color indicate inflammation/cellulitis and green color indicates pus

Cavernous sinus thrombosis

Fig. 2: Chandler's classification (I to V).

TABLE 1: Orbital complications of rhinosinusitis Chandler's classification (1970).

• Type I: – Preseptal cellulitis	• Does not threaten the orbit • Inflammatory edema anterior to orbital septum	• Can be treated on OPD basis • Eyelid swelling (impeded venous drainage) • Chemosis is absent • Extraocular muscle mobility normal • Vision is normal • Mild proptosis
– *Postseptal (Type II to V):* Signs indicating postseptal are proptosis, gaze restriction, decreased vision, color vision defect, afferent pupillary defect. Urgent hospitalization and aggressive treatment are indicated		
• Type II Orbital cellulitis (Diffuse cellulitis)	Edema and inflammation of orbital contents. No frank pus	• Epiphora-blurry vision • Proptosis + • Chemosis + • Eyeball movement decreased
• Type III (Subperiosteal abscess)	Extraconal abscess	• Proptosis + • Chemosis + • Eye movement normal in early stages (Impaired extraocular muscle movement in advanced stage)
• Type IV (Orbital abscess)	Intraconal frank pus	• Proptosis ++ • Complete ophthalmoplegia • Vision loss
• Type V (Cavernous sinus thrombosis)	In addition, fever, headache, photophobia, proptosis, ophthalmoplegia, cranial nerve palsy III, IV, VI, V1, V2	Bilateral ocular signs and loss of vision

Eyelids are swollen and edematous but not tender. Eyelid edema occurs due to impedance in the drainage of blood flow of superior ophthalmic veins into the ethmoidal veins.

Extraocular movements are unrestricted with normal visual acuity. Mild proptosis may be seen due to concomitant edema of orbital contents.

II. *Orbital cellulitis (35%):* There is infection of soft tissue, periosteum, and orbital septum with a risk of permanent blindness. It is the most common complication in pediatric population and is mostly due to ethmoid sinusitis. There is diffuse edema of orbital contents and actual infiltration of extraocular orbital adipose tissue with inflammatory cells. Clinical features include erythema, induration of eyelids, proptosis, gaze impairment, eye pain, conjunctival chemosis and fever.

Ophthalmoplegia may be seen due to impaired extraocular muscle movement. There is no impairment of visual acuity.

III. *Subperiosteal abscess (15%):* There is pus collection between the periorbita and bony wall of orbit causing a space occupying lesion formation and displacing the globe in lateral and downward direction depending upon the location of subperiosteal abscess. Most commonly located at:
- Medial wall of the orbit with superomedial or inferomedial extensions from ethmoid sinusitis.
- Inferior wall of the orbit from maxillary sinusitis
- Superior wall of the orbit from frontal sinusitis.

Abscess may rupture through the orbital septum and present in the eyelid. Clinically, patient has chemosis and proptosis with globe pushed laterally or downward. Initially eyeball movements are normal but later on these may get impaired. CT scan is mandatory at this stage.

IV. *Orbital abscess (<1%):* It may be due to rupture of subperiosteal abscess or progression of orbital cellulitis leading to pus formation and collection in orbital tissue. Pus may find its exit pathway anteriorly through the lid. Clinically, exophthalmos and significant chemosis with severe proptosis and pain, complete ophthalmoplegia and visual impairment. There is risk of irreversible blindness.

V. *Cavernous sinus thrombosis (CST):* There is serious orbital and intracranial complication of rhinosinusltis with a high mortality rate even with rapid recognition and treatment.

It may be due to sphenoid, ethmoid or frontal sinusitis and/or orbital cellulitis through the valveless superior and inferior ophthalmic veins connecting the cavernous sinus. Extension of infection to intercavernous sinuses, to the contralateral cavernous sinus occurs within 24–48 hours of the initial presentation and results in appearance of symptoms in the opposite eye, which is the hallmark feature of CST. Clinical features of cavernous sinus thrombosis:
- Fever, toxemia
- Severe bilateral orbital pain, ptosis, periorbital edema
- Severe chemosis
- Severe proptosis, headache, trigeminal paresthesia
- Papilledema due to obstruction of venous drainage from the retina
- Progressive ophthalmoplegia and paralysis of extraocular muscles due to involvement of cranial nerves—III, IV, VI.
- Fixed dilated pupils
- Visual acuity impairment
- Additionally, marked edema over the mastoid emissary vein, marked meningismus, prostration. Frank meningitis may be seen in few patients.

Note: In patients with rapid progression of clinical signs, altered sensorium or ophthalmoplegia, one should suspect cavernous sinus thrombosis which has to be confirmed on contrast-enhanced computed tomography (CECT)/ magnetic resonance imaging (MRI) (shows filling defect).

Clinical Picture of Orbital Complications
- Clinical features of orbital involvement in a patient with a recent history of upper respiratory tract infection
- Erythema of eyelids
- Induration of eyelids
- Proptosis
- Diffuse orbital cellulitis and abscess–direct outward protrusion
- Subperiosteal abscess–lateral displacement of globe
- Gaze impairment, diplopia
- Ophthalmoplegia
- Pain in eyes (usually aggravated by eye movements)
- Conjunctival chemosis
- Fever (fever may be absent in immunocompromised patients)
- Restricted eyeball movements

Visual impairment may occur because of:
- Corneal ulceration (due to proptosis)
- Ischemic optic neuropathy
- Inflammatory optic neuropathy
- Central retinal artery occlusion

(*Note:* In children, orbital complications may sometimes be painless).

Intranasal: Intense engorgement of nasal mucosa and middle meatus blockage. Pus is usually thin and scanty.

Intracranial Complications (15–20%)
Intracranial infection due to sinusitis occurs either due to direct extension of infection or through hematogenous spread.

Thrombophlebitis originating in the mucosal veins can progressively involve the emissary veins of the skull, the dural venous sinuses, the subdural veins, and finally the cerebral veins. By this mode, the subdural space may be infected selectively without evidence of extradural infection or osteomyelitis.

Intracranial complications occur most commonly due to posterior spread of infection from frontal sinus.

Signs and symptoms of intracranial complications are:
- Soft tissue edema (superior eyelid or over frontal bone)

- High grade fever, severe headache, meningeal irritation, nausea, vomiting, diplopia, photophobia, altered sensorium, papilledema, focal neurological deficits.

Types of Intracranial Complications

- *Meningitis:* Headache, neck stiffness, high grade fever, it is mostly seen in children. Kernig's and Brudzinski's sign (neck rigidity) are positive. Lumbar puncture is diagnostic.
- *Epidural abscess:* It is the most common intracranial complication in children. Symptoms are somewhat similar to subdural empyema but are less severe. Fever, headache, local tenderness, altered sensorium are seen.
- *Subdural abscess/empyema:* It is the most common intracranial complication, secondary to acute or subacute frontal sinusitis in otherwise healthy adults. Headache, fever, meningismus, lethargy, altered sensorium, orbital cellulitis are common symptoms seen. Rapid progression can lead to increased intracranial pressure-leading to neurological dysfunction, coma, and death. It is a neurosurgical emergency.
- *Intracerebral abscess:* Epidural and subdural empyema can involve brain parenchyma and lead to formation of brain abscess. Headache is most common symptom while fever and altered sensorium is less common. Other symptoms are vomiting, lethargy, focal neurological deficit. Frontal lobe involvement mainly shows mood and behavioral changes with increase in intracranial pressure. Seizure may occur.
- *Brain infarction:* It is a rare vascular complication which occurs due to dural venous thrombosis, secondary to adjacent empyema.

Osseous Complications (5–10%)

Frontal sinus is the most common sinus involved with osteomyelitis.

Osteomyelitis: It may develop by spread of infection via marrow spaces or thrombosis in diploic veins-subperiosteal abscess and subsequently formation of bone sequestrum.

Frontal osteomyelitis is mainly seen in young adults while maxillary osteomyelitis is seen in infants.

Clinically skin is edematous or a mass is seen over the forehead or frontal bone (Pott's puffy tumor).

Pott's puffy tumor is subperiosteal abscess and osteomyelitis of anterior table of frontal bone presenting with headache, frontal swelling, fever. It may be associated with other intracranial complications such as epidural abscess and subdural empyema and intracranial abscess, if not managed adequately. Frontocutaneous fistula is a late complication. CT scan will reveal bony erosions. Diagnosis can be confirmed with Technetium-99m pertechnetate and Gallium-67 citrate bone scan.

Complications in chronic rhinosinusitis with or without nasal polyposis are less dramatic and rare but are more difficult to manage. There is bone erosion and expansion due to mucocele or polyp, osteitis, metaplastic bone formation and optic neuropathy.

Most common bacterial species seen in complicated sinusitis are *Haemophilus influenzae, Moraxella catarrhalis, Streptococcus pneumonia*. While *Staphylococcus aureus*, Diphtheroid and anaerobes are seen in odontogenic origin complication.

Diagnosis

Look for Red Flag Signs/Symptoms

Periorbital edema, erythema, displaced globe, double vision, ophthalmoplegia, severe unilateral or bilateral headache, reduced visual acuity, frontal swelling, sign of meningitis.

Admit patient suspected of intraorbital/intracranial complication. Visual acuity, pupillary reactivity and ocular motility assessment at regular intervals is indicated for post septal complications (especially by ophthalmologist team).

Investigations

- Blood counts, C-reactive protein
- CSF β-protein in patients who underwent FESS and presenting with meningitis
- Pus culture: Intranasal swab (direct or nasal endoscopy).

Nasal Endoscopy (Flexible/Rigid)

Intranasal: Intense engorgement of nasal mucosa and middle meatus blockage. Pus is usually thin and scanty.

Imaging

- *Plain X-ray* (Water's view) may reveal fluid accumulation, maxillary opacification
- *High Resolution CT scan* (Coronal/axial and sagittal—all three axis): This is diagnostic and extent of disease and localization of preseptal/postseptal complication is seen. HRCT with contrast is effective in assessment of sinus disease and sinogenic brain abscess and subdural empyema.
- *MRI* is done in case of coexisting orbital and intracranial complications (Diagnostic). Damaged tissue with edema is easily picked in T2i weighted images. Diffusion-weighted (DWI) are very useful in intracranial infections and orbital abscess.

Orbital Complications:
1. *Preseptal cellulitis* **(Fig. 3)**: Nonspecific findings including:
    a. Eye soft tissue swelling
    b. Thickening of preseptal tissue
2. *Postseptal cellulitis:* In addition to above, there is induration of extra conal, intraconal and retrobulbar fat without abscess formation.
3. *Subperiosteal abscess:* Lenticular rim enhancing collection is present in relation to lamina papyracea. Fat plane is intact between it and medial rectus. Globe displacement may be lateral in case of ethmoid sinusitis and anteroinferior in case of frontal sinusitis.
4. *Orbital abscess:* Multiple rim enhancing abscess with surrounding cellulitis and proptosis is seen in CT scan with contrast.
5. *Cavernous sinus thrombosis:* CT may be normal. MR venography is preferred that shows irregular filling defect due to absence of venous flow. In addition, thickening and increased signal intensity is seen in extraocular muscle in T2 weighted MRI.

Intracranial Complications:
1. *Meningitis:* Normal CT brain. Gadolinium enhanced MRI brain shows dural enhancement.
2. *Epidural abscess:* Hypodense or isodense crescent shaped collection in epidural space on plain CT head.
3. *Subdural abscess:* CT scan reveals hypodense collection along the cerebral hemisphere or along the falx. Radiologically, subdural empyema stays on one side of falx while epidural empyema can cross the midline, anterior to falx. MRI shows low signal on T1 and high signal of T2 with peripheral enhancement.

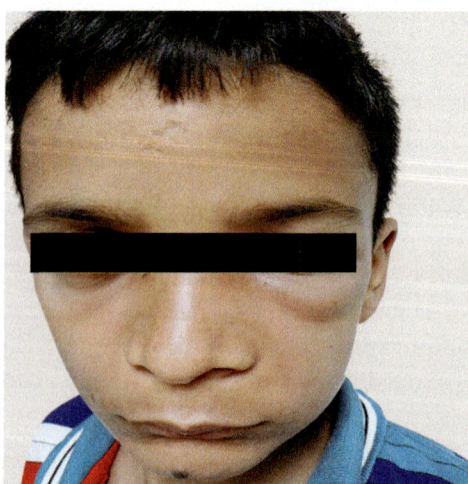

Fig. 3: Young child with typical clinical presentation of preseptal cellulitis with acute rhinosinusitis.

4. *Brain abscess:* CT scanning shows low-density lesion with peripheral enhancement. MRI study reveals cystic lesion with extending capsules on T2 images.

Radiological Findings of Osteomyelitis

Computed tomography scanning will reveal bony erosions of the involved sinus.

In Pott's Puffy Tumor, CT demonstrates an opacified frontal sinus with stranding and swelling of the overlying scalp. It will also show a defect in the anterior wall of the sinus **(Fig. 4)**.

Management (Flowchart 1)

Treatment of Orbital Complications

Medical:
- *Nasal decongestants:* Xylometazoline/oxymetazoline locally (intranasally)
- Antiallergic orally
- Intravenous antibiotics (broad spectrum)
- Antiviral and antimycotic in immunocompromised patients
- Steroid rarely indicated (only if patients get benefit from reducing intracranial and intraorbital edema).

Monitor temperature pulse respiration chart: Failure of temperature to drop steadily and rapidly to normal or reversal of downward direction of temperature curve within 24 hours, surgical intervention is required.
- *Stage I (preseptal)* can be managed on OPD basis with bed rest, cold compression, antibiotics (wide spectrum—oral/parenteral) and nasal decongestion.

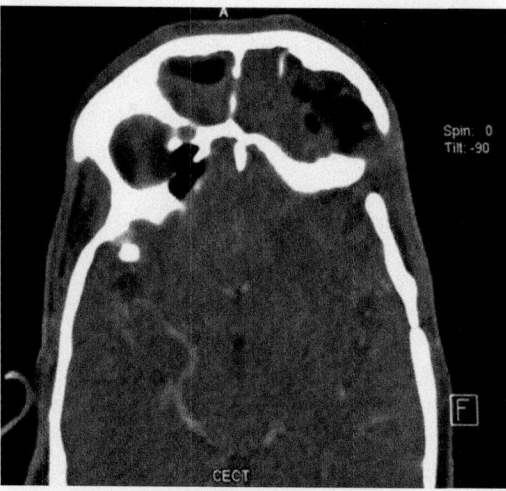

Fig. 4: Postcraniotomy persistent frontal sinusitis with frontal osteomyelitis.

Flowchart 1: Management algorithm of complicated acute rhinosinusitis.

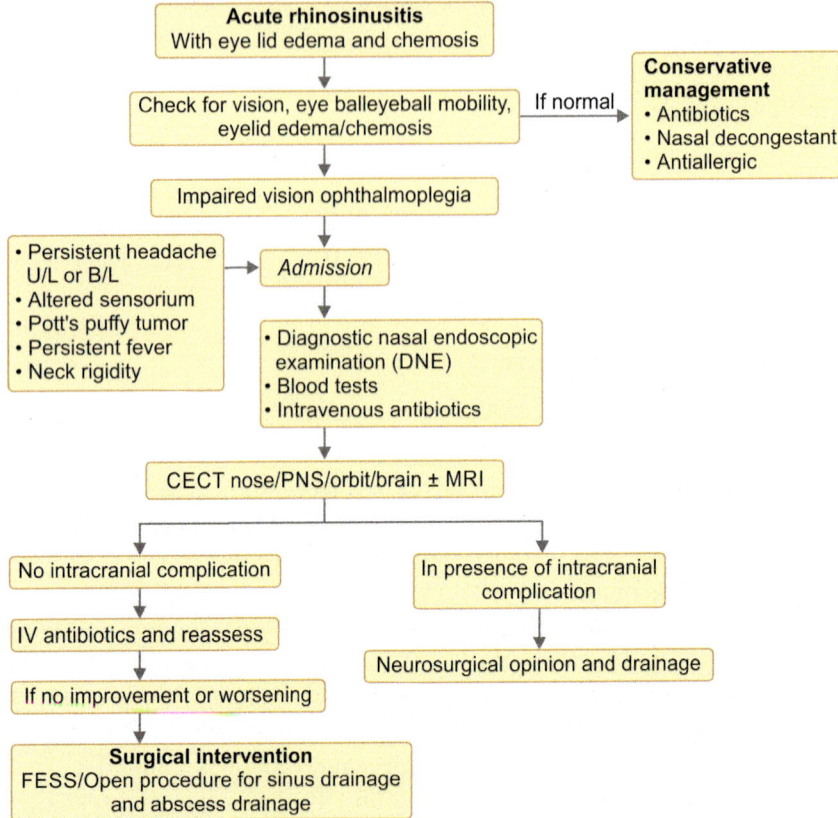

- *Stage II to V (postseptal):* Intravenous antibiotics (aerobic and anaerobic cover): Third generation cephalosporins, metronidazole and cloxacillin till culture and sensitivity is done.
- CT scan of nose and PNS especially in patient presenting with orbital/periorbital swelling or signs and symptoms of complicated sinusitis.
- Ophthalmologist opinion for documentation of proptosis, vision, ophthalmoplegia.
- Neurosurgical opinion in case of suspected intracranial complication.

Indications for surgery:
- Appearance of impaired visual acuity <20/60 or worse (early sign: loss of red color differentiation)
- Presence of intracranial complication
- Presence of subperiosteal or orbital abscess (radiologically)
- Decreased color vision
- Afferent pupillary reflex impaired

- Orbital signs not improving or worsening after 24 hours of intravenous antibiotics (diplopia, ophthalmoplegia, proptosis, chemosis).
- Most cardinal indication for Surgery
  - Decreased red color vision and visual acuity
  - Impaired ocular mobility

Surgical Procedure

Treatment for subperiosteal abscess:
- Done under general anesthesia
- *Can be open procedure/endoscopic:* Basic aim is to drain the primary sinus and establish the ventilation of sinus. Presence of acute inflammation induced hyperemia leads to more bleeding and makes classical FESS very difficult. However, in the presence of subperiosteal abscess, an endoscopic approach should aim at exposing the lamina papyracea above the maxillary antrostomy and then with a Freer's elevator the lamina should be carefully broken in a controlled manner to release the pus. In experienced hands it can be very gratifying procedure avoiding scar of external ethmoidectomy.
- *FESS:* To drain underlying sinus infection and to manage complication especially frontal sinus. Sometimes inability to obtain the access to the frontal sinus intranasally may necessitate a frontal trephination, to drain the frontal abscess.
- Endoscopic skull base surgery (transnasal intracranial surgery)

Open procedures include:
- External ethmoidectomy approach (Lynch–Howarth approach) and subperiosteal abscess is drained into the nasal cavity.
- In case of frontal sinus empyema, front ethmoidectomy or trephination through floor of frontal sinus should be performed.
- In maxillary antral disease, diagnostic and therapeutic maxillary antral lavage is sufficient in acute maxillary sinus while in complicated chronic maxillary sinusitis, Caldwell-Luc or *Horgan's approach* is indicated.

Since maximum complications are seen in acute sinusitis without preexisting chronic disease, a complete and meticulous ethmoidectomy is not indicated. In case of orbital abscess, after external ethmoidectomy, periorbita is widely exposed and linear incision made into it for drainage of orbital abscess.

After surgery, nonadherent dressing impregnated with antibiotic ointment, loosely packed and brought out through nostril. Antibiotics are given for 10–14 days or until temperature is normal for at least 1 week.

Treatment of orbital abscess:
- *Open approach:* External ethmoidectomy, incision and orbitotomy
- Transnasal endoscopic
- Combined open and endoscopic.
  This ideally includes active participation of ophthalmologic colleagues.

Treatment of cavernous sinus thrombosis (CST): On clinical examination of opposite eye, if there is appearance of chemosis/edema/proptosis and ophthalmoplegia: suspect cavernous sinus thrombosis.

Prolonged high dose broad spectrum antibiotics for at least 2 weeks beyond clinical resolution is advisable. Follow-up of at least 6 weeks is advised. Surgery is only indicated to drain primary nondraining sinus or abscess collection.

The role of anticoagulants in CST has remained controversial. Those in favor of anticoagulants suggest prevention of thrombus propagation and anti-inflammatory role whereas those against the anticoagulants are of opinion of increased risk of intracranial bleed. Generally, rapidly reversible anticoagulants are used such as unfractionated heparin with an aim to keep INR levels between 1.5 and 2.

Treatment of Intracranial Complications: Medical management begins with high dose of IV antibiotics that cross blood-brain barrier (third generation cephalosporin plus metronidazole). Anticonvulsant medication may also be started as incidence of seizure in intracranial complications is high. Neurological/intracranial complication is managed jointly by neurologist/neurosurgery team. If possible combined primary sinus drainage surgery in same sitting with neurosurgical intervention should be done. Primary HRCT of sinus is always indicated. Frontal sinus is most commonly underlying etiology of intracranial complication and in acute setting it is preferable to do frontal sinus trephine procedure with placement of external drain (some authors have advised endoscopic balloon sinuplasty). Definite frontal sinus surgery can be done in second sitting when patient is fully recovered from complication.

Neurological procedure:
- Epidural abscess with or without intracranial abscess and communication between paranasal sinus and intracranial compartment, combined ENT and neurosurgery approach is indicated. In the presence of uncomplicated epidural abscess—sinus trephination and drainage are done.
- In subdural empyema with or without intracranial abscess, draining of abscess along with drainage of subdural empyema is done. Craniotomy with burr holes is performed.
- Brain abscess resection via craniotomy is very rarely done. Nonsurgical management has been proposed if abscess is <2 cm or if patient is a poor surgical candidate. In case of solitary abscess or even multiple abscess

(provided no mass effect) with no communication between sinus and intracranial compartment: stereotactic aspiration is performed. Pus for culture/sensitivity is taken. Evacuation with craniotomy is indicated in recurrent abscess or a periventricular abscess for fear of its rupture into ventricular compartment refractory to repeated puncture/drainage and antibiotics.

Note: It is advisable to perform concurrent drainage of primary sinus disease and associated intracranial complication.

Treatment of Bony Complications:
- In presence of osteomyelitis, wide excision of necrotic bone till freely bleeding bone margins are seen
- Prolonged culture directed antibiotic therapy is given for 6 weeks
- Excessive osteomyelitis of anterior table can be removed using Riedel's procedure.

WARNING SIGNS/SYMPTOMS OF ORBITAL/INTRACRANIAL COMPLICATIONS

The warning signs and symptoms of orbital and intracranial complications are described in **Table 2**.

MUCORMYCOSIS

Rhinocerebral mucormycosis (black fungus) is a rapidly progressive angioinvasive fatal opportunistic fungal infection predominantly affecting people with immunocompromised state. It came to limelight during COVID-19 pandemic. In rhinocerebral mucormycosis, the disease

TABLE 2: Signs and symptoms of orbital and intracranial complications

Orbital	• Periorbital edema and/or erythema • Proptosis • Gaze impairment • Restricted ocular mobility • Blurred vision/double vision • Eye pain • Chemosis • Pupillary defects
Intracranial	• Fever • Unilateral/bilateral headache • Altered sensorium/lethargy* • Neurologic deficit* • Seizure* • Tender, swollen forehead

*Lethargy, seizure and neurologic deficit are more ominous signs of long-term morbidity, mortality, and prolonged hospitalization.

takes a rapidly progressive course by extending to neighboring tissues including the orbit and central nervous system, resulting in blindness and even death.

Risk Factors
- Patients with uncontrolled diabetes
- Patients receiving high doses of steroids for long time
- Previously immunocompromised patients, for example cancer patients, organ transplant patients, renal failure patients.

Red Flag Signs
- One sided facial pain and swelling/numbness of face
- Fresh onset of headache
- Nasal crusting and blood-stained nasal discharge
- Pain in eye, redness in conjunctiva (red eye), eyelid swelling, proptosis, double vision, ptosis, blurred vision, pain in eyes, vision loss
- Cough, dyspnea, hemoptysis, fever-suggestive of *pulmonary mucor*
- Palatal discoloration, loosening of tooth, discomfort in chewing
- Black spots on perioral area, perinasal area, and nasal bridge
- Unilateral otalgia
- Altered sensorium-points toward intracranial spread.

Diagnosis (Table 3)
- KOH wet mount-DEEP NASAL smear (in sterile saline) shows Broad, nonseptate hyphae fungal forms (branching at obtuse angle).
- Biopsy of lesion (Formalin for histopathological examination/special stain-PAS): Shows large fungal balls and single scattered thick nonseptate hyphae.
- Diagnostic nasal endoscopy (DNE) showing blackening of turbinate, nasal septum, and floor of nose **(Fig. 5).**
- *Eye examination:* Congestion/chemosis/pupillary reaction/eyeball movements in all quadrants (for extraocular muscles)/visual testing/fundus examination (central retinal artery occlusion)
- Check for color differentiation (inability to distinguish red color-first sign of impending visual loss)
- *Gadolinium-enhanced MRI nose, PNS and orbit (Diagnostic):* T1 (isointense), T2 (variable: fungal elements tend to show low signal).
- *CECT nose and PNS:* Retroantral soft tissue edema/infiltration, premaxillary edema, mucosal thickening of sinuses, osseous erosion.

Histopathology: Hallmark of disease in mucormycosis is tissue necrosis which results from angioinvasion and thrombosis of blood vessels.

TABLE 3: Clinical staging of rhino-orbito-cerebral mucormycosis.

Staging	Symptoms	Signs
Stage 1: Involvement of nasal mucosa	• Nasal stuffiness • Foul smelling nasal discharge • Epistaxis	• Foul-smelling mucoid or black tinged or hemorrhagic nasal discharge • Nasal mucosal inflammation, erythema • Violaceous or blue discoloration • Pale ulcer • Anesthesia • Ischemia • Eschar
Stage 2: Involvement of PNS	Symptoms in Stage 1 + Facial pain • Facial edema • Dental pain • Systemic symptoms (malaise, fever)	Signs in Stage 1 + • U/L or B/L localized or diffuse facial edema • Edema localized over the sinuses • Localized tenderness
Stage 3: Involvement of orbit	Symptoms in stage 1 and stage 2 + • Pain in eye • Proptosis • Ptosis • Diplopia • Loss of vision • Infraorbital and facial, V1 and V2 nerve anesthesia	Signs in stage 1 and stage 2 with conjunctival chemosis • Isolated ocular mobility restriction • Ptosis • Proptosis • Infra orbital nerve anesthesia • Supraophthalmic vein thrombosis • V1 and V2 nerve anesthesia and features of cranial nerves III, IV and VI palsy, indicating orbital apex syndrome/superior orbital fissure syndrome
Stage 4: Involvement of the CNS	Symptoms in stage 1 to stage 3 + • Bilateral proptosis • Paralysis • Altered consciousness • Focal seizures	Signs in Stage 1–3 + • Bilateral orbital edema indicates cavernous sinus thrombosis • Hemiparesis • Altered consciousness and focal seizures indicate brain invasion and infarction

Source: Honavar SG. Code Mucor: Guidelines for the Diagnosis, Staging and Management of Rhino-Orbito-Cerebral Mucormycosis in the setting of COVID-19. Indian J Ophthalmol. 2021;69:1361-5.

Treatment

1. Antifungal Therapy

I. *Amphotericin B*
    • It is the drug of choice (first-line)

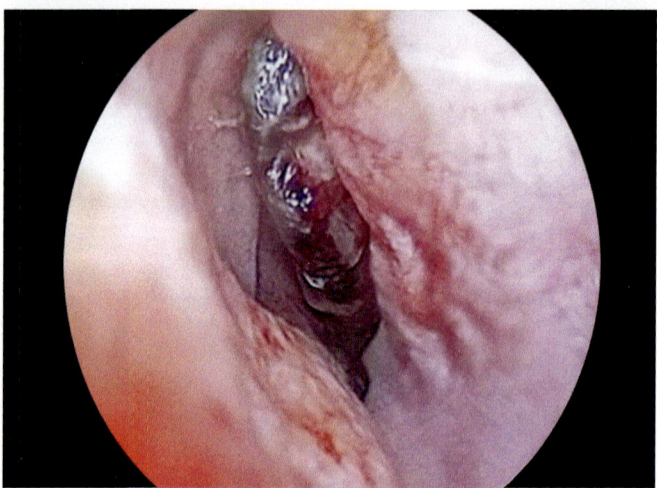

Fig. 5: Diagnostic nasal endoscopy (DNE) showing typical findings of mucormycosis.

- ABCD (Amphotericin B including colloidal dispersion): 0.5–1.5 mg/kg/day
- ABLC (Amphotericin B lipid complex): 5 mg/kg per day upto 2–3 g for 3–6 weeks
- L-AmB (Liposomal Amphotericin B): 5 mg/kg/day (Nose and PNS)
- 10 mg/kg/day (CNS)
- If liposomal is not available, Amphotericin B deoxycholate (1–1.5 mg/kg/day for 3–6 weeks).
- Start calculated dose of Amphotericin B from first day, avoid dose escalation

II. Posaconazole
- Used for salvage therapy but not primary therapy in the form of tablets/oral suspension/injection. Oral—300 mg BD on first day followed by 300 mg daily for 3–6 month or minimum of 6 weeks following clinical/radiological regression.
- Oral absorption is suboptimal if the patients have mucositis, diarrhea, on acid suppression therapy or poor oral intake.

2. Surgical Management

Extensive surgical debridement of all devitalized tissue is the core of mucormycosis therapy.
- Decreases the overall fungal load.
- Increases the penetrability of antifungal drug.
- Slows down the disease progression.
- Establishes histopathology.

Surgical approaches:
1. *Endoscopic approach:* Lesions limited to nasal cavity and paranasal sinuses.
2. Open approach
    I. *External ethmoidectomy and pansinusectomy:* It is done for lesions limited to nasal cavity and PNS without intracranial and orbital extensions. It involves exenteration of ethmoidal air cells and removal of necrotic turbinates and nasal septum.
    II. *Total maxillectomy:* It involves removal of entire maxilla with pterygoid plates. It is done for lesions with extensive involvement of maxilla along with **(Figs. 6A and B)**
        a. Extensive bone destruction
        b. Blackish discoloration and necrosis of skin
        c. Palatal destruction
        d. Soft tissue infiltration into pterygopalatine fossa, infratemporal fossa and into pterygoid plates.
        e. Rapidly spreading mucormycosis
    III. *Maxillectomy with orbital exenteration:* Extensive involvement of maxilla with extension into orbit.

Postsurgical management: After surgery for mucormycosis, the surgical cavity should be inspected regularly using nasal endoscopes. Repeated debridement needs to be done along with irrigation of the cavity with Amphotericin B. The cavity can also be packed with Amphotericin B gel or Amphotericin B nasal spray can be used. The surgery is supplemented with antifungal therapy either monotherapy or in combination.

The duration of antifungal therapy depends on following factors:
- Symptomatic improvement clinically
- Healthy looking cavity on nasal endoscopy
- Normal radiographic images
- Negative biopsy specimen and cultures from the affected site.

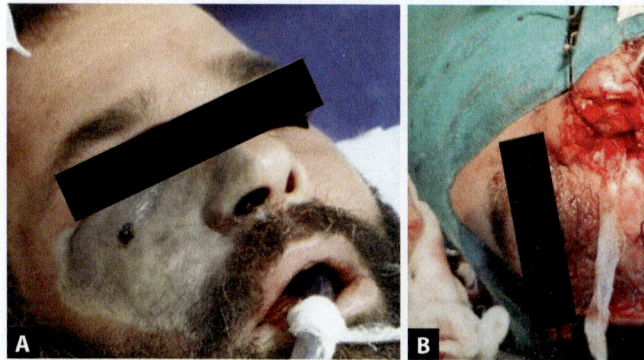

Figs. 6A and B: Preoperative and intraoperative clinical pictures of total maxillectomy.

3. Elimination or control of predisposing factors.
4. Antibiotics to control super added infections.

Prognosis

Surgery is the most important variable determining the outcome/prognosis of mucormycosis. Other factors which usually are associated with poor prognosis are:
- Intracranial involvement
- Absolute neutrophil count <1,000
- Facial and lid gangrene
- Hemiplegia
- Diabetic ketoacidosis
- Cavernous sinus thrombosis
- Orbital apex syndrome
- Altered sensorium at presentation.

■ FURTHER READING

1. Blitzer A, Lawson W. Fungal infections of the nose and paranasal sinuses. Part I. Otolaryngol Clin North Am. 1993;26(6):1007-35.
2. Chandler JR, Langenbrunner DJ, Stevens ER. The pathogenesis of orbital complications in acute sinusitis. Laryngoscope 1970:1414-28.
3. Diouf MS, Adama T, Ndiaye C, Amadou T, Deguenonvo R, Malick N. Complications of sinusitis: an 80-case series from the ENT and neurosurgery departments of the Fann university hospital center of Dakar, Senegal. Eur Ann Otorhinolaryngol Head Neck Dis. 2020;137(6):473-6.
4. Ferguson BJ. Mucormycosis of the nose and paranasal sinuses. Otolaryngol Clin North Am. 2000;33(2):349-65.
5. Giannoni CM, Stewart MG, Alfred IL. Intracranial complications of sinusitis. Laryngoscope. 1997;107:863-7.
6. Goldberg AN, Oroszlan G. Anderson TD. Complication of frontal sinusitis and their management. Otolaryngol Clin North Am. 2001;34:211-25.
7. Heinemen HS. Bacterial brain abscess. In: Braude AI (Ed). Infectious Diseases and Medical Microbiology, 2nd edition. Philadelphia: PA Saunders; 1985.
8. Honavar SG. Code Mucor: Guidelines for the Diagnosis, Staging and Management of Rhino-Orbito-Cerebral Mucormycosis in the setting of COVID-19. Indian J Ophthalmol. 2021;69:1361-5.
9. Jones NS, Walker JL, Barri S, Jones T, Punt J. The intracranial complication of sinusitis: can they be prevented? Laryngoscope. 2002;112:59-63.

Index

Page numbers followed by *b* refer to box, *f* refer to figure, *fc* refer to flowchart, and *t* refer to table.

A

Abrasion 100
Abscess 211*f*
  communication of 213
  drainage of 169
  epidural 230, 232
  extradural 213
  internal 230
  intracranial 236
  mastoid 210*f*
  meatal 209
  orbital 227, 228, 232
  parapharyngeal 156*t*
  perisinus 213
  peritonsillar 163*f*
  postaural 209, 210*f*
  posterior fossa extradural 213
  retropharyngeal 87, 154, 156*f*, 156*t*, 180, 185
  subdural 214, 230, 232
  submandibular space 158*f*
  subperiosteal 209, 211, 227, 228, 232
  tonsillar 162
  zygomatic 209
Accessory respiratory muscles 86
Acid 192, 194
  burns 198
  neutralization of 198
  sodium bicarbonate for 194
Acquired immunodeficiency syndrome 160
Actinomyces israelii 167
Actinomycosis 167
Acute epiglottitis 178, 181*f*
  clinical features of 179
Acute rhinosinusitis 232*f*
  management of 234*fc*
Acute vertigo 11, 26, 29, 30, 35, 40, 43, 45
  attack 11, 30, 44*fc*
  management of 108
  treatment of 46
Acyclovir 47, 55, 190
Adrenaline 1
Aerodigestive tract 192

Air
  embolism 96
  hunger 78, 86
Airway 88, 99
  bronchoscopy 177
  compromise 163
  distress 142, 174
  foreign body 81, 180, 185
  laryngeal 97
  management
    basics of 1
    immediate 135
  obstruction 84, 140
  oral 89, 185
  types of 97*t*, 98
Alcohol 19
  abuse 16
Alexander law 19
Alkaline
  agents 192
  burns 192
Alkalosis 23, 50
Almoor's approach 203
Alprazolam 33
Aminoglycoside 217
  ototoxicity 188
Amitriptyline 35
Ammonia 192
Amnesia, spontaneous 42
Amphotericin B 239
  deoxycholate 240
  lipid complex 240
Ampicillin 151, 181, 197, 212
  component 181
Analgesia 1
Anemia, progressive 215
Anesthesia 177
  general 78, 79, 93, 100
  local 93, 100
Animal bites 2, 3
Anisocoria 39
Antagonists 108
Anterior inferior cerebellar artery syndrome 14, 33
  typical of 40

Antibiotic 46, 87, 188, 209, 212
  intravenous 30, 219, 222, 233
  prophylaxis 121
  steroid cream 54
  systemic 7
  therapy 147
  topical 7
Anticogulants 64
Antidepressants, tricyclic 42
Antifungal therapy 239
Antihistamines 50
Antirabies
  management 8
  treatment 8
Antiseptics 6
Antitetanus
  management 8
  prevention 8
  serum 8
Antivertiginous drugs 42
Antiviral 47, 55, 190
  therapy 55
Apnea 96
Argon 72
Arnold-Chiari malformation 37
Arterial back pressure 146
Arterial blood gas 193
Aryepiglottoplasty 184
Arytenoids 133
  cartilage 139
  prominent 183
Asch forceps 105
Aspirin 64
Asthma, atypical 82
Ataxia 35, 42, 46
  cerebellar 40
Audiological tests 18
Audiometry 26
Aural fullness 15
Auscultation 174
Autoimmune 47, 49
Avitene 72
Avulsion 107

B

Bacillus
  licheniformis 7
  polymyxa 7
  subtilis 7
Bacitracin zinc 7
Bacteremia 215
Bacteriology 219
Bacteroides 215, 218, 222
  fragilis 212, 220
  melaninogenicus 165

Ball-valve obstruction 83
Barium-swallow 135
Barky cough 182
Bartonella henselae 168
Battle's sign 51
Bell's palsy 48, 55, 56
  causes of 48
  treatment of 55
Bell's phenomenon 50
Benzodiazepines 33, 35
Beta-blockers 35
Betahistine 31, 33
Bezold's abscess 158, 209
Binaural loudness balance, alternate 26
Binocular vision 13
Bismuth iodine-paraffin-paste 117
Bleach ingestion 195
Bleeding
  disorders 190
  sites, posterior 68
  transoral 145
Blind
  folded test 25
  nasal intubation 89
Blink reflex 53, 53*f*
Blood
  clot, inhalation of 100
  glucose 221
  loss 99
  pressure 61
Bloody purulent discharge 77
Body balance system 11, 24
Bone
  fragments of 103
  graft 120, 128
  plate osteosynthesis 113
  temporal 110, 128, 204, 210*f*
  zygomatic 110, 224
Bony
  complications, treatment of 237
  defects, nonanatomical 200
Boyce-Jackson position 79
Brain
  abscess 213, 215, 219, 233, 236
  infarction 230
Brainstem 28
  compression 34
  lesion 17
  stroke 39
  symptoms 39, 42
  tumor of 37, 53
Brandt Daroff exercises 35
Breath sounds, reduced 82
Breathy voice 86
Broad-spectrum antibiotic 54, 87

Bronchial obstruction 82
   types of 83
Bronchitis, laryngotracheal 180
Bronchoscopy 85*f*, 87, 148, 178
   procedure of 84
Bronchotomy 84
Brudzinski's sign 230
Bruit 141
Buccal mucosa 48
Budesonide 182
Bull's lamp 74
Burns
   degree of esophageal 196*t*
   oropharyngeal 193
   second degree 197

C

Calcium
   antagonists 31
   supplementation 73
Caldwell-Luc maxillary antrostomy 70
Caloric test 188
Canal occlusion, posterior 32
Canal wall tympanoplasty 207
Carbamazepine 35
Carbogen inhalation 190
Carbolic acid 74
Carbon dioxide 72
Cardiac arrest 96
Cardiac failure 190
Cardiovascular diseases 64
Carotid
   angiography 221
   arteriography 135
   artery 145
      external 69
      injury 143
      internal 69
      proximal 140
   blow-out 144
      management of 145
      morbidity of 146
      mortality of 146
   coverage 146
   sheath 154, 157
Cartilage fragments 139
Cat scratch disease 168
Caustic ingestion 192
   types of 194*fc*
Caustic lesion, grading system for 197*b*
Cavernous sinus thrombosis 227, 228, 232
   treatment of 236
Cavities, pleural 169

Cefoxitin 160
Cefuroxime 151
Cellulitis 160
   diffuse 227
   orbital 227
   postseptal 232
   preseptal 226, 232, 232*f*
Central nervous system 15, 36, 55
Central vestibular
   dysfunction 42
   pathway 19
Cephalosporins 197
Cerebellar function 17
Cerebellum 13, 37, 219
   lesions of 24
Cerebral tissue 222
Cerebrospinal fluid 104, 223
   leak 128
   otorrhea 128
   rhinorrhea 129
Cerebrovascular
   accident 39, 64
   disease 35
   disorders 37
Cervical
   infections 165
   injuries 142
   lymph nodes, ipsilateral 162
   mediastinotomy 169
   muscle spasm 42
   rotation 16
   spine 142
      injury 88-90, 100, 134, 142
   vertebrae 142
Cervicofacial actinomycosis 167
Chandler's classification 226, 226*f*
Chemoreceptor trigger zone 31
Chemosis 235, 236
   conjunctival 227
   severe 228
Chest
   injuries 92
   X-ray of 87, 135
Chevallet fracture 103
Chloramphenicol 160, 212, 217
Chlorhexidine 6
Choanal atresia 184, 185
   bilateral 184
Cholesteatoma 16, 56
Cholesteatosis, black 209
Chorda
   tympani functions 52
   tympanic nerve 52
Chorea 14

Chromic acid 65
Chronic obstructive airway diseases 92
Cinnarizine 31, 33, 42, 108
Cisapride 197
Citelli's abscess 211
Clindamycin 151, 160, 197
Clonazepam 33, 35
Clostridium perfringens 166
Clothesline 131
Cochlear function 205
Cochleosaccular dysfunction 49
Coils, use of 146
Cold air caloric test 206
Colloidal silver solution 7
Coloboma 185
Combitube 90
Compression plates 123
Computed tomography 44
    contrast-enhanced 152
Condyle 126
    neck fractures 126
Conjunctival injection 226
Consciousness, loss of 15
Conservative therapy 152
Continuous positive pressure ventilation 92
Contusion 100
    simple 133
Convergence movements 13
Cooksey Cawthorne exercises 35
Corneal irritation, signs of 51
Corticosteroids 50, 182
Cough 61, 82, 86, 173
Cranial dura, middle 212
Cranial nerve 49
    examination 17
Craniocorpography 27
Craniotomy 236
Crepitus 81, 141
Cribriform plate fracture 104
Cricoarytenoid joint movements 178
Cricoid cartilage 133
    fracture 139
Cricopharyngeal sphincter 78
Cricothyroid 91
Cricothyroidotomy 97, 136, 141, 177
Cricothyrotomy 88, 90, 94
    steps for 91
Cricotracheal anastomosis 139
Cricotracheal membrane 134
Croup 87, 182
Crusts 98
Cuneiform cartilage 184
Cup-shaped biopsy forceps 84
Cyanotic attacks 184

Cysts 7
Cytomegalovirus 187

D

Debridement 3
Deep cervical fascia 148
    middle layer of 148
    superficial layer of 148
Deep neck space 147*f*
    abscess, complications of 163
    infection 147, 152*fc*, 162*f*
        incisions for 153*f*
Dermis 4
Dermoplasty 72
Desaturation 184
Dexamethasone 31, 32, 130, 189
    transtympanic 189
Dextrose 190
Diabetes mellitus 26, 49, 51, 160, 188
Diagnostic nasal endoscopy 65, 240*f*
Diazepam 19, 32, 33, 35, 42, 46
Digastric muscle 127
Digestive tract injuries 143
Dimenhydrinate 31, 33, 108
Diphenhydramine 31, 33, 46
Diplopia 29, 235
Direction-fixed nystagmus 40
Disequilibrium 39
Disseminated intravascular coagulation 63
Distal carotid arteries 140
Distress, respiratory 182
Dix-Hallpike
    maneuver 43
    test 22
Dizziness 13, 23, 34, 42
    acute 32, 45
    central 14
    episodic 41
    physiologic 13
Doll's eye test 21
Domperidone 33, 42, 109
Dorello's canal 202
Double tube tracheostomy tube 96
Drainage
    surgical 160
    transoral 154
Droperidol 30
Drug therapy 30
Dysarthria 29, 39
Dysequilibrium 37
Dysesthesia 29
Dysgeusia 48, 52
Dysmetria 17

Dysphagia 29, 39, 81, 97, 151, 155, 163, 166, 192
   mild to moderate 143
Dysphonia 29, 166
Dyspnea 78, 141, 142, 155
   severe 155, 163

E

Eagleton's approach 204
Ear 2, 77
   anomalies 185
   canal, part of 77
   discharge 15
   disease, treatment of primary 212
   examination 43
   surgery of 56
   trauma 106, 109
Earache 15
Edema 50, 143, 173, 236
   inflammatory 226
   laryngeal 85
   periorbital 228
Egg shells 81
Electrocardiogram 44
Electrodes, placement of 53*f*
Electroencephalogram 27, 44
Electrolyte disturbances 55
Electromyography 54
Electroneuronography 58
Electronystagmography 27, 188
Electrophysiological test 52
Emetics, induction of 194
Emphysema 87, 96
   obstructive 82
   subcutaneous 85, 134
   surgical 96
Empyema 230
   subdural 236
Encephabol 35
Encephalitis 220
Endocrine systems 131
Endolymphatic sac decompression 32
Endoscopic appearance 196, 196*t*
Endoscopic nasal surgery 72
Endoscopy 87, 143
   esophageal 196
   role of 195
   triple 135
Endotracheal intubation 89
Endotracheal tube 89, 176, 176*t*
Epidermis 3
Epiglottis 184
Epiglottitis 178, 181*f*

Epilepsy 14, 35
Epiphora 226
Epistaxis 61, 73
   anterior 61, 63
   causes of 62*t*
   digitorum 63
   idiopathic 61
   management of 64, 71*fc*
   severe 69
Epley's maneuver 35
Epsilon aminocaproic acid 73
Erythema 166, 227
Erythrocyte sedimentation rate 189
Escherichia coli 165, 220
Esophageal
   airway 89
   perforation 81, 175, 193
   strictures 199
Esophagography 143
Esophagoscopy 148, 196
   complications of 81
   procedure 79
Esophagus 78, 131, 143, 169, 192, 195, 196
   lower end of 80
   weakness of 195
Ethmoid crest 70
Ethmoidal artery
   anterior 69
   posterior 69, 70
Ethmoidal sinus 226
Ethmoidectomy, external 235, 241
Ewald's laws 23
Explosions 2
External skeletal fixation 113
   methods of 113
   types of 113
Eye
   conjugate deviation of 17
   examination 17, 238
   pain 227
   protection 10
Eyelids 101
   erythema of 229
   induration of 227, 229

F

Face 225
   paralysis of 48
Facial
   appearance, asymmetrical 48
   artery, branch of 63
   bones 99, 112
   function, recovery of 52

hemianesthesia, ipsilateral 40
injury
　healing of 101
　treatment of 100
motion, impaired 48
nerve 59
　injury 101, 108
　motor fibers of 53
　neuroma 51
　palsy 50, 51
　surgery of 56
　testing 52
palsy 16, 40
　acute 48, 49*t*, 55, 58*fc*, 60
　bilateral 49*t*
paralysis 50, 204
sensation 39
trauma 71
Facio-masseteric nerve anastomosis 57
Famciclovir 190
Farrior's subcochlear hypotympanic approach 203
Fasciculus, medial longitudinal 13
Fastigial nuclei control 13
Fever 166, 226, 227
　high-grade 230
Fiber-optic endotracheal intubation 90
Fibrinolysis, systemic inhibitors of 73
Fibrous tissue 137
Fistula 207
　sign 16
　test 43, 206
　　false negative 207
　　false positive 207
　tracheocutaneous 98
　tracheoesophageal 98
　tracheoinnominate 98
Fits, epileptic 214
Fixation, internal 123
Flexible fiberoptic airway endoscopy 174
Fluid
　intravenous 46
　shifts 55
Foley's catheter 67
Forceps, types of 85
Fracture 105, 126
　displaced 120
　floating 110
　geriatric 127
　high-level 111
　horizontal 110
　lateral middle third 114
　line of 127
　longitudinal 107
　middle third 109, 113
　midface 109
　nondisplaced 119
　oblique 108
　orbital blow-out 118
　panfacial 128
　pyramidal 111
　subzygomatic 110, 111
　suprazygomatic 111
　transverse 111, 128
　treatment of 122
　types of 114
　unilateral 121
　unstable 117
Frank abscess 220
Free muscle tissue 217
Freer's elevator 235
Frenckner's approach 203
Frontal sinus fractures 119
Frontomaxillary suture 109
Frontozygomatic suture 109
Fukuda's stepping test 24
Fungi 7
Furstenberg' incision 161
Fusidic acid 7

G

Gait 11, 24, 25, 33, 40, 42
Ganciclovir 190
Gangliosides 31
Gas exchange, inadequate 175
Gastric
　lavage, induction of 194
　perforation 193
　　signs of 198
Gastrografin 135
　swallow 135
Gastrointestinal system 164
Gaze impairment 227
Geniculate ganglion 59
Genital hypoplasia 185
Gillies method 116
Ginkgo biloba extract 31
Glasgow Coma Scale 135
Glass fragments 81
Glottis 85
Gold standard test 135
Gradenigo syndrome 213
Granulation tissue 82
Granulomatous cheilitis 50
Griesinger's sign 216
Grisel syndrome 163
Growth retardation 185

Index

Guerin's fracture 110
Guillain-Barré syndrome 53
Gunn pupillary sign 129
Gunshot injuries 100

H

Haemophilus influenzae 7, 178, 182, 200, 212, 218, 231
Hair relaxers 192
Halmagyi's sign 21
Halmagyi's test 21
Halo sign 129
Head
    impulse test 21, 33, 45
    injuries 92
    maneuver 88
Headache 16, 228
    severe 214, 230
Hearing assessment, bedside 33
Hearing loss 15, 36, 40, 50, 188
    asymmetric sensorineural 190
    conductive 51, 107
    degree of 188
    idiopathic sensorineural 188
    risk of 208
    sensorineural 33, 49, 187, 208
    severity of 188
    sudden sensorineural 29, 187, 189*t*
Heart
    anomalies 185
    disease, ischemic 26, 64
Heimlich maneuver 88
Heliox 87
Helium-oxygen mixture 87
Hemangioma, subglottic 184
Hematemesis 143
Hematology 164
Hematoma 96, 100, 106, 134, 141, 143
    intraneural 58
Hemogram, complete 26, 51
Hemolytic streptococcal gangrene 165
Hemoptysis 141, 143
Hemorrhage 34, 76, 96
    cerebellar 41
    intracranial 34
    pontine 40*f*
    sentinel 145
    subarachnoid 15
    subglottic 173
Hemosinus 116*f*
Hemostasis 101
Hemostatic agents, topical 73
Hennebert's sign 23, 41, 207

Hepatic system 164
Herpes
    simplex virus 48
    zoster 55
        antiviral for 47
        oticus 48, 55
Herpetic vesicles 54
Hiatus-lumen appears 80
High-pressure oxygen 90
High-velocity blunt trauma 131
Hitzelberger sign 17
Hoarse voice 86, 174
Horizontal mattress suture 4, 4*f*
Hormonal influences 50
Horner's syndrome 39, 40, 164
House-Brackmann facial nerve grading system 60, 60*t*
Humidified air 182
Hydrochloric acid 198
Hydrogen peroxide 6
Hyoid bone fracture 133, 138
Hyperacusis 48
Hypertension 26, 64
    benign intracranial 222
Hyperventilation 23
Hypopharynx 77, 140
Hypotension 141
    orthostatic 16
Hypotympanum 202
Hypoventilation 68
Hypoxia 68

I

Iatrogenic trauma 148
Imipenem 160
Immobilization 125
    methods of 125
Incudostapedial joint separation 107
Infection 68, 97, 157
    acute 212
    bacterial 183, 200
    chronic 212
    extradural 229
    head and neck 147
    odontogenic 148
    pharyngeal 148
    prevention of 101
    spread of 200
    springs 155
Inflammatory reaction, severe 75
Inflatable cuff, care of 96
Injury
    esophageal 192

full thickness 2
glottic 139
laryngotracheal 121, 133
mandibular 90
mucosal 119
penetrating 59, 141
retrobulbar 99
special 138
supraglottic 139
tracheal 141
Inner ear
injury 107
membrane rupture 187
Innominate artery compression 174
Inoculum, bacterial 121
Intensive care unit 94
Intermaxillary fixation 123, 125
Internal jugular vein 143, 146
ligation of 217
Internal maxillary artery 69
embolization 71
ligation 70
transoral ligation of 70
Internal skeletal
fixation 113
suspension 113
Internal wire suspension, types of 114t
Intracranial complications 201, 211, 216, 229, 232
signs of 229, 237t
symptoms of 229, 237t
treatment of 236
types of 230
Intracranial pus 221
Intratemporal complications 201
Intrinsic brainstem lesion 35
Intubation 88, 89
Ionized calcium 23

J

Jarjavay fracture 103
Jaw thrust maneuver 88
Jugular foramen 215
Jugular vein 140
anterior 93
internal 143, 146

K

Kernig's sign 230
Kiesselbach's plexus 61
Kirschner wire 113, 114, 125
Kopfschuttel test 22

L

Labyrinthine
fistula 37, 206
peripheral 28
segment 59
Labyrinthitis 21, 28, 37, 46, 205
diffuse purulent 38
serous 38, 205
suppurative 206
Lacerations 81, 106
mucosal 137
Lacrimal apparatus 114
Lag screws 124
Lamina papyracea 69
Lansoprazole 184
Laryngeal membrane injuries 133
Laryngeal nerve, recurrent 96
Laryngofissure 137
Laryngogram 135
Laryngomalacia 173, 174, 183
Laryngopharynx 177
Laryngoscope 89, 95, 178
Laryngoscopy 84, 87
Laryngotracheal
anatomy 92
separation 131, 134, 136, 139
trauma, acute 133
Laryngotracheobronchitis 86, 182, 183f
Laryngotracheobronchoscopy 177
Larynx 48, 131, 176
Laser 72
debridement 3
laryngeal surgery 178
Latency 23
Lateral medullary
infarction 39
syndrome 40f
Lateral neck, X-ray of 156f, 159f
Leech, removal of 77
Lemierre's syndrome 164f, 165, 167
Lesions, peripheral 50
Light-headedness 16
Lillie-Crowe test 216
Liposomal amphotericin B 240
Lips 2, 6
border of 101
Little's area 61, 65
Lorazepam 33, 35
Low velocity trauma 131
Luc's abscess 209
Ludwig's angina 157, 159f
Lumbar puncture 218, 221, 230
Lumpy jaw 167
Lung, infection of 82

Lyme's disease 49
Lymph node, jugular 215
Lymphatic spread 225
Lynch incision 69

M

Mackintosh laryngoscope 178
Macroglossia 174
Magnetic resonance imaging 44, 152
Major vessels, injury of 142
Mandible
　ascending ramus of 126
　fracture of 120, 121*f*, 122*f*, 126
　special areas of 126
　X-ray of 151
Mandibular
　condyle, dislocation of 128
　injuries, severe 89
　right parasymphyseal fracture,
　　preoperative orthopantomogram
　　of 122*f*
Masseteric space 158, 161
Masticator space 161, 161*f*, 162*f*
Mastoid
　emissary vein 216
　reservoir 208
　tenderness 16
Mastoidectomy, cortical 56, 222
Mastoiditis 158, 208, 209
　acute 208, 208*f*, 209, 211
　chronic 208
　coalescent 217
　types of 208
Maxilla
　displacement of 100
　fracture 110
　margin 102
Maxillary artery, internal 69
Maxillary sinus 118
　antrostomy 117
　wall fracture, bilateral 116*f*
Maxillary sinusitis 228
Maxillectomy 241
　total 241, 241*f*
Maximal stimulation test 52
McEwen's triangle 209
McNaught keel 139
Meclizine 32, 33, 46, 108
Mediastinitis 163, 193
　descending necrotizing 168
Mediastinotomy, anterior 169
Mediastinum, superior 141
Medical therapy 152
Meleney's gangrene 165

Melkersson-Rosenthal syndrome 50
Meniere's disease 14, 22, 23, 29, 32, 39,
　　45, 207
　diuretic for 47
　mimicking 41
Meningitis 54, 213, 217, 230, 232
　treatment of 219
Mental status examination 173
Merocel
　pack 66
　removal of 72
Metallic foreign body 76, 78, 83*f*
Metallic tracheostomy tube 96
Metoclopramide 33
Metronidazole 160
　penetrate abscess capsule 212
Microfibrillar collagen 72
Micrognathia 174
Microlaryngeal surgery 177
Microlaryngoscopy, therapeutic 178
Middle cerebellar peduncle, part of 39
Middle ear 202*f*, 213
　trauma 107
Middle meatus 63
Middle meningeal artery 70
Middle turbinate basal lamella 70
Migraine 16
　vertebrobasilar 35
　vestibular 42
Molars, lower 165
Monocortical miniplates 124
Moraxella catarrhalis 231
Morbidity, causes of 1
Mortality, causes of 1
Motion sickness 42, 46
Motor
　coordination test 28
　output system 28
　paralysis 221
　weakness 15
Mouth 10
Mucormycosis 237, 240*f*
　therapy 240
Mucosa 75, 197
　laryngeal 81
　subglottic 176
Mucosal flap 70
Mucosal inflammation 61
Mucous membranes 164
Mumps 187
Murmur 141
Muscle
　buccinator 154
　constrictor 148
　paravertebral 157

Musculofacial flaps 141
Musculoskeletal system 164
Mycoplasma pneumoniae 182
Myonecrosis 166
Myringotomy 56, 212, 222

N

Narrow neck 131
Nasal
   airway 89
   balloon 68
   bone
      comminution of 103
      deviation of 102
      fracture 104, 105*f*
   cavity 68, 225
   decongestants 233
   endoscopy 231
   fractures 102
   packing, anterior 66, 66*f*, 68*f*, 105
   septum 61
      anterior 61
      deviated 67
   tampons 66
   tumors 71
Nasolabial artery 63
Naso-nasopharyngeal plexus 63
Naso-orbito-ethmoid 103*f*, 104*f*
   fracture 103
Nasopharyngeal portion 68
Nasopharynx 68
   carcinoma of 63
Nausea 14, 30, 31, 34, 42
Near syncope 16
Neck 131
   fascial planes of 149*f*
   plain radiographs of 134
   rigidity 230
   spaces of 148
   trauma 131
      different types of 132*fc*
Necrosis, tracheal 98
Necrotizing fasciitis 165, 165*f*, 166
Neodymium-doped yttrium-aluminum
        garnet 72
Neomycin 7, 74
Nephritis 160
Nerve
   anastomosis 57
   conduction velocity 54
   decompression 56
   excitability test 52
   grafting 57
   skip lesion of 52

Nervous system 164
Neural surgery 56
Neuritis 99
   vestibular 28, 29
   viral 47
Neurological
   deficit 141, 222
   diseases 92
   disorder 49, 50
   procedure 236
   signs 41
Neuroma, acoustic 41
Neuronitis, vestibular 39
Neuropathy
   alcoholic 51
   peripheral 24
Neuropraxia 204
Nitric acid 198
Noisy
   breathing 78
   respiration 86
Noncompression plates 124
Nose 10, 75
   blowing 61
   external 6
   picking 61
Nuclei, vestibular 41
Nylén-Bárány test 22
Nystagmus 30, 33, 36, 37, 38*t*, 41, 46
   downbeat spontaneous 19
   end-point 19
   gaze evoked 29
   head shaking 22
   jerk 18
   periodic alternating 20
   positional 22
   slow phase of 19
   spontaneous 12, 18, 19, 38, 43
   torsional 20
   upbeat spontaneous 20
   vertical 34

O

Obstruction, respiratory 68, 91
Obstructive oral cavity lesion 90
Ocular dizziness 14
Ocular palatal myoclonus 20
Oculomotor system 20
Odynophagia 77, 81, 143, 151, 158, 182
Ondansetron 33
Open-book fracture 102
Ophthalmic
   artery 70
   vein 225

Ophthalmoplegia 41, 228, 235, 236
Ophthalmoscopy 17
Optic
   nerve decompression 130
   neuropathy, traumatic 129
Optokinetic reflex 12, 13
Orbit, anatomy of 224*f*
Orbital abscess 227, 228, 232
   treatment of 236
Orbital complications 225, 232
   clinical picture of 229
   signs of 237*t*
   symptoms of 237*t*
   treatment of 233
Orbital exenteration 241
Orbital floor
   fracture 118
   status of 117
Orbital fracture, types of 118
Orbital periosteum 69
Oropharyngeal mass lesion 171
Oropharynx 77
   trauma 149
Orthopantomogram 121*f*
   postoperative 122*f*
Oscillopsia test 22
Osler-Weber-Rendu syndrome 72
Ossiculoplasty 59
Osteomyelitis 163, 229, 230, 233
   frontal 230, 233*f*
Osteosynthesis 125
   Champy's line of 124*f*
   load-bearing 125
   load-sharing 125
   types of 125
Otic capsule 59
Otitic hydrocephalus 222
Otitis
   externa 77
   infections 49
   media 37, 46
     acute 51, 58, 203, 205, 212, 222
     chronic 51, 54, 56, 58, 201*f*, 205, 207, 212
     complicated 200
Otolaryngological examination 16
Otolith
   bilateral loss of 12
   organ saccules 28
   unilateral loss of 12
Otologic surgery 56
Ototoxicity 22, 188
Overshoot saccades 24
Oxcarbazepine 35

Oxidized cellulose 72
Oxycel pledgets 65
Oxygen
   administration 87
   cylinder 95
   inhalation 87

P

Pacchionian bodies 222
Pain 155, 226
   abdominal 193
   control 101
   retroauricular 48
Palatine artery 63
Pallor 46
Palpable laryngeal fractures 137
Palpitation 15
Pansinusectomy 241
Papilledema 220
Papilloma, juvenile 173
Papillomatosis
   laryngeal 178, 185
   respiratory 185
Para labyrinthitis 205
Parainfluenza virus 182, 183
Paralabyrinthitis 205
Paralysis 48
   respiratory 92
Paranasal sinus 63, 99, 224
Parapharyngeal abscess 156*t*
   management of 160
Parapharyngeal space 158
Paraplegia 142
Parasymphysis 121, 126
Paresis, unilateral 48
Paresthesia 15
   trigeminal 228
Parotid duct 102
   laceration of 102
Parotid space 161, 162*f*
Paroxysmia, vestibular 46
Partial thromboplastin time 64
Past-pointing test 25
Pectus excavatum 184
Pediatric stridor 171
   causes of 178, 186*fc*
   management of 186*fc*
Pediatric tracheostomy 93
   tube 176*t*
Pendular tracking test 24
Penetrating neck trauma 132, 139
   management of 141
Penicillin 212, 217
   plus 160

Pentoxifylline 35
Pericardial cavities 169
Pericarditis 167
Perilabyrinthitis 205
Perilymph fistula 23, 41, 44, 46
Peritonsillar space 161
Peritonsillitis 156*t*
Personal protective equipment 10
Petrositis 201, 202, 203
    acute 202, 203
    chronic 202, 203
Petrous apex 204*f*
    syndrome, principle of 203
Pharyngoesophageal sphincter 131
Pharynx 143
Phenytoin 19
Phonophobia 42
Photophobia 42
Physiotherapy 57
Pin fixation, external 128
Pinna 6
Platysma 80
Pneumatized mastoid 208
Pneumomediastinum 85
Pneumonia, migratory 82
Pneumonitis 167
Pneumothorax 82, 85, 97
Polymyxin B sulfate 7
Polyneuritis 49
Polysomnography, overnight 87
Polyvinyl alcohol 72
Pontine syndrome 39
Posaconazole 240
Postauricular incision 59
Postcraniotomy 233*f*
Posterior inferior cerebellar artery 14
    syndrome, typical of 41
Posterior nasal
    artery branch 63
    bleed 61
    packing 68*f*
Posterior wall fractures, treatment of 119
Poststapedectomy 205
Post-traumatic nerve deafness, management of 109
Potassium 190
    hydroxide 192
    titanyl phosphate 72
Pott's puffy tumor 230
Pott's spine 151
Povidone iodine 6
Pregabalin 54
Pregnancy 60, 61
Pressure testing 23

Pretracheal fascia 148
Prochlorperazine 33, 46
Promethazine 31
Proptosis 227, 235, 236
    mild 227
    severe 228
Proteus mirabilis 215, 220
Protozoa 7
Pseudomonas aeruginosa 7, 212, 220
Pseudotumor cerebri 15, 222
Psychotic reaction 55
Pterygoid plexus 225
Pterygomaxillary dysjunction 111
Ptosis 39, 228
Pulmonary function tests 92
Pulsatile oscillopsia 41
Pulse 152
    loss of 134
    oximetry 182
Pure tone audiometry 51
Purpura, signs of 64
Pyrexia 81
    of unknown origin 79
Pyriform margin 102
Pyritinol 35

Q

Quadriplegia 142

R

Radical mastoidectomy 207
    modified 58
Radiopaque
    foreign body 79, 82
    rhinolith 76*f*
Rail-road technique 96
Ramadier-Lempert approach 203
Ramsay Hunt syndrome 48, 204
Reconstruction plate 124
Rectus muscle, external 202
Red flag signs 238
Reflex
    cough 82
    laryngopharyngeal 184
Refractory epistaxis 64
Rehabilitative therapy 35
Renal failure, acute 163
Renal system 164
Respiration 152
    mouth-to-mouth 88
Respiratory cycle 174
Respiratory distress, severe 182
Respiratory failure 175

Respiratory insufficiency 92
Retinal slip 12
Retroauricular sulcus fills 209
Retrocochlear pathology 191
Retropharyngeal space 154, 155
Retrotracheal space 155
Rheomacrodex 190
Rhinocerebral mucormycosis 237
Rhinolith 75
Rhino-orbito-cerebral mucormycosis 239*t*
Rhinoscopy, anterior 104
Rhinosinusitis
    acute 232*f*
    Chandler's classification, orbital
        complications of 227*t*
    chronic 231
    complications of 224
    secondary 76
Rigid fixation 123
Ring sign 129
Rinne's test 18
Road traffic accidents 131
Romberg's test 24, 43
Rotational chair testing 28
Rotational vertigo, episodes of 35
Rubella 187
Ryle's tube 197

S

Saccade movements 13
Saccadic
    eye movements 24
    pursuit 23
    system 13
Saline 190
Saliva
    dribbling of 50
    drooling of 155, 179, 182
Salivary gland infection 148
Scabs 98
Scalp 100
Scar 98
    formation 2
Schirmer's test 52
Schwannoma 190
Sclerosis, multiple 28, 37, 41, 53
Scopolamine transdermal patch 42
Screaming tinnitus 40
Sea-saw nystagmus 20
Seiffert's operation 70
Seizures 15
Sensation, characteristics of 14
Sensorium 15
Sepsis, signs of 81

Septal fragments, telescoping of 102
Septal perforation 65
Septic thrombosis 216
Septicemia 215
    signs of 159
    symptoms of 159
Septoplasty 67
Shock 193
    hypovolemic 68
    septic 167
Shoulder roll 94
Siegel's examination 16
Siegel's speculum 23
Sigmoid sinus 213
Silver
    compound 7
    nitrate 74
    sulfadiazine 7
Sinister symptoms 193
Sinonasal surgery 64
Sinus 63, 225
    drainage surgery, primary 236
    infection 224
        mode of spread of 225
        recurrent attacks of 64
    thrombophlebitis 216, 217
        lateral 215
Sinusitis, complications of 224
Skeletal
    Fixation
        external 113
        internal 113
    suspension, internal 113
    system 131
Skew deviation 20, 21, 33
Skin 94
    graft, use of 72
    stapling 5
Skull fracture 100
Sleep study 87
Smooth pursuit
    eye movements 23
    system 12
Sneezing 61
Snellen's eye 22
Sniffing position 155
Sodium
    bicarbonate 194
    hydroxide 192
Soft palate 48
Soft tissue 101
    edema 229
        element of 87
    injuries 100

neck 152, 174
    X-ray of 86, 151, 181*f*
  wounds, types of 100
Sore throat 155
Spaces above hyoid bone, infection of 157
Spaces below hyoid bone, infection of 163
Sparing fracture 59
Sphenoid 110
Sphenopalatine 63, 69
  artery 63
Spinal board 142
Spinocerebellar ataxia 37
Spinothalamic tract 41
Squamous cell carcinoma 199
Stapedial reflex 52
Staphylococcus 106, 161, 215
  aureus 7, 155, 158, 164, 167, 178, 182, 231
  epidermidis 167
Static imbalance 18
Steeple sign 183*f*
Steinmann pins 113
Stellate ganglion block 190
Stenosis 78
  subglottic 171, 176, 178, 184
  tracheal 98
Stenson's duct 161
Sternomastoid muscle 169, 215
Sternothyroid muscle 169
Steroids 32, 55, 87, 189, 233
  intratympanic 189
  systemic 189
  therapy 55
Stop-valve obstruction 83
Streptococcus
  haemolyticus 220
  pneumonia 167, 215, 218, 220, 231
  pyogenes 167, 182
Stridor 78, 86, 141, 171, 172*b*, 174
  biphasic 79, 172, 182
  causes of 179*t*, 180*t*
  fluctuation of 173
  inspiratory 172, 179
  types of 171, 172*f*
Stroke 27, 39
  acute ischemic 32, 34
Stylomastoid foramen 51
Subclavian steal syndrome 16
Subglottis 87, 178
Submandibular gland 144
Submandibular space 157
  abscess 158*f*
Subperiosteal abscess 209, 211, 227, 228, 232
  treatment of 235
Sudden sensorineural hearing loss 29, 187, 189*t*
  causes of 187*t*
Sulbactam 151, 181
Sulfur granules 167
Sulfuric acid 198
Superior semicircular canal dehiscence 41
Supraglottis 177
Supraglottitis 178
Suprasternal notch 93
Surgical therapy 32
Surgical treatment 56
  principles 153
Swelling, postaural 209
Swollen joints 64
Sylvian gyrus 12
Symphysis 121, 126
Syncope 16
  vasovagal 15
Syphilis, congenital 207
Syringobulbia 20
Syringomyelia 20

T

Tachycardia 81
Tachypnea 81
Tandem gait test 43
Tear
  drop sign 118
  dural 104
  mucosal 81
Tegmen tympani 58
Temperature pulse respiration chart 233
Temporal bone 110, 128, 204, 210*f*
  fractures 57, 128
  trauma 57
Temporal lobe abscess 220
Temporary balloon occlusion test 146
Tenacious mucus 95
Tetanus
  spores, germination of 2
  toxoid 8
Thoracic counterpart 141
Thornvaldt's approach 204
Threatened carotid blow-out 145
Thrombocytopenia 62
  chemotherapy-induced 61
Thromboembolic phenomenon 215
Thrombophlebitis 167, 200
Thrombus, upward extension of 215
Thudicum speculum 66
Thumb 79, 94
  sign 181*f*

Index

Thyrohyoid membrane 133
Thyroid 144
   artery, inferior 169
   cartilage 134, 137
   gland 144
   pedicle 157
   vulnerability of 133
Thyroiditis, acute suppurative 166
Thyrotomy, midline 137
Tilley's forceps 76
Tinnitus 15, 36, 188, 189
Tissue
   subcutaneous 4, 80
   types of 2
Tobey-Ayer test 216
Tongue 48
Tonsillitis, bacterial 165
Tooth, removal of 127
Topographic testing 52
Torticollis 159, 209
Toxemia 228
Toxic shock syndrome 67, 164, 166
Trachea 94, 96, 178
Tracheal injury 141
   signs of 141
   symptoms of 141
Tracheitis, bacterial 180, 182
Tracheoarterial fistula 98
Tracheobronchial tree, mucosa of 82
Tracheostomy 88, 90, 91, 95, 97, 141, 176, 185
   change of 96
   complications of 96
   elective 92
   emergency 94
   indications for 91, 91*b*
   midline dissection 95*f*
   percutaneous dilatational 93
   tube 95
      care of 95
      size of 98, 98*t*
Tracheotomy 91
Tranexamic acid 73
Transantral approach 70
Transcervical drainage 154
Transcranial Doppler 41
Transfixation 114
Transient ischemic attack 27
Transnasal endoscopic sphenopalatine artery ligation 70
Transosseous wiring 113
Trauma 1, 49, 64
   care 1
   faciomaxillary 99
   mild frontal 102
   moderate frontal 102
   severe frontal 102
   site of 140*f*
Traumatic labyrinthine dysfunction 43
Trichloroacetic acid 65
Tripod fracture 115, 115*f*
Trismus 89, 90
Tubal patency 16
Tuberculosis 160
Tullio's phenomenon 37, 41
Tullio's sign 23
Tumor 37, 53, 78
Tuning fork test 18
Turbulent airflow, signs of 171
Tympanic membrane 204
Tympanomastoidectomy 56

U

Unreliable topographic test 52
Unterberger's test 24
Upper airway obstruction, acute 86
Upper cervical nerve roots 218
Upper gastrointestinal contrast 198
Upper respiratory tract infection 61
Upper tracheal impaction 82

V

Valacyclovir 55, 190
Vasovagal reflex 68
Ventilation, transtracheal 90
Verapamil 35
Vertebrobasilar insufficiency 39, 44
Vertical mattress suture 5, 5*f*
Vertigo 13, 34, 37, 38*t*, 41, 46, 59, 189, 207
   acute 11, 26, 29, 30, 35, 40, 43, 45
      central 32, 34, 36*t*
      peripheral 36*t*
      stages of 35
   attack of 34
   benign paroxysmal positional 14, 35, 38, 43, 44
   central 30*t*, 37
   complicated 27
   concussion 35
   intermittent 41
   maneuver-induced 22
   migraine associated 45
   momentary 41
   paroxysmal attacks of 41
   peripheral 15
   positioning 31

maneuvers 47
post-traumatic 42
psychogenic 47
refractive 31
subjective 14
true 42
Vestibular
  dynamic visual acuity test 22
  evoked myogenic potentials 28
  function test 27
  schwannoma 23, 41, 188
  suppressants drugs 33*t*
  syndrome, acute 11
  visual stimuli 42
Vestibule 205
Vestibulo-ocular reflex 11, 21
Vestibulospinal
  reflex 12
  tracts 12
Vincent's organism 157
Virucidal agents 8
Viruses 7
Visceral space, anterior 163
Vision, blurring of 226
Visual acuity 12
  impaired 234
Visual blurring 51
Visual component testing 23
Visual dysfunction 15, 39
Visual impairment 228, 229
Visual suppression 36
Visual system 12
Vitamin
  C 73
  K 73
Vocal cords 171
Vocal fold
  immobility 139
  palsy 174

Voluntary motor units, loss of 54
Vomiting 14, 30, 31, 46, 100, 202
  induction of 194
von Willebrand disease 61

W

Wallenberg's syndrome 21, 39, 40*f*
Walsham forceps 105
Weber's test 18, 188
Wheezing 82, 172
Wire osteosynthesis 123
Woodruff's plexus 63, 64
Wound 2, 8, 100
  assessment of 2
  cleaning of 101
  closure of 138
  edge of 3, 101
  etiology of 1
  incised 100
  lacerated 100
  management 1
  traumatic 138*f*

X

Xylocaine 1, 66, 90
  spray of 67, 77

Z

Zygoma 115, 117
  fracture of 114
Zygomatic complex fracture 115*f*, 116*f*
  classification of 117*t*
Zygomaticofrontal suture 109
Zygomaticomaxillary
  buttress 110
  complex fracture 114, 116
  sutures 115